Advance Praise for
The LGBT Casebook

"The title of *The LGBT Casebook* does not do full credit to this rich source of information and clinical support for all health care professionals, at every stage of learning and practice. Given the prevalence of LGBT individuals in society, and the stresses to which their sexual orientations subject them, most of us will see LGBT patients, and few of us, whatever our own orientations, are prepared to offer them the expertise they deserve. It's all in this Casebook, in well-organized and eminently readable form. Kudos to editors Levounis, Drescher, and Barber! Their book should be on the bookshelf of each of us."

Nada L. Stotland, M.D., M.P.H., Professor of Psychiatry, Rush Medical College; Past President, American Psychiatric Association

"A book that should be read by everyone! *The LGBT Casebook* brings homosexuality out of the psychiatric closet and into the 21st century. Based on solid evidence from the scientific literature, this book breaks common myths and stereotypes, helping the reader truly understand gays, lesbians, bisexuals, and transgendered women and men. It reaches deep into the mind of LGBT people to explore the psychological distress caused by homophobia and stigma; describes the 'legal standing' of LGBT family relationships; and shows the practicing mental health clinician how to manage the most common psychiatric conditions affecting individuals in today's LGBT communities."

Analice Gigliotti, M.D., Past President, Brazilian Association on Studies of Alcohol and Other Drugs (ABEAD)

"This brilliantly edited volume is an essential reference and a must read for all therapists who treat LGBT patients and their families. The unique issues LGBT patients bring to therapy are interwoven with the common clinical problems in everyday practice, as the case studies illustrate beautifully. A groundbreaking contribution to the field!"

Steven S. Sharfstein, M.D., President and CEO, Sheppard Pratt Health System, Baltimore, Maryland; Clinical Professor and Vice Chair, Department of Psychiatry, University of Maryland School of Medicine; Past President, American Psychiatric Association

"[For] difficulty in treating special populations, this book is a must. The case studies lend themselves to everyday problems, concerns, and solutions."

Steven S. Kipnis, M.D., FACP, FASAM, Medical Director, New York State Office of Alcoholism and Substance Abuse Services

"*The LGBT Casebook* is a must read for all therapists, including those in the field of addiction counseling. The authors have simplified the daunting task of educating the therapeutic community regarding proper understanding of the LGBT patient. The early chapters do an excellent job of reviewing how the basic life issues affect this special population. The full range of behaviors and psychological mechanisms used by these patients are fully discussed, including the many behavioral and psychological elements that the LGBT person uses to hide important aspects of the self. Also discussed is how to deal with the sexual identity question in the patient-therapist relationship in this special patient population.

Later chapters use case histories to illustrate how the various psychiatric diagnoses affect the LGBT patient. These chapters include many pearls of wisdom and contain a summary of key points, questions with correct answers, and a reference list. The chapters on parenting and those on substance abuse are of special importance.

This book more than accomplishes its goal to help clinicians better understand the mental health needs of lesbian, gay, bisexual, and transgender people. It brings a better understanding of the common problems that these special patients face every day, such as what it means to be 'in the closet' and what it means to 'come out' to oneself and others. I congratulate the authors for providing the mental health professional with an excellent guide towards proper understanding of the LGBT patient with a psychiatric diagnosis."

Nicholas A. Pace, M.D., FASAM, Clinical Associate Professor of Medicine, New York University Langone Medical Center

The **LGBT** Casebook

The **LGBT** Casebook

Edited by

Petros Levounis, M.D., M.A.

Jack Drescher, M.D.

Mary E. Barber, M.D.

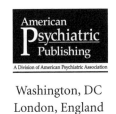

American **Psychiatric** Publishing

A Division of American Psychiatric Association

Washington, DC
London, England

If you would like to buy between 25 and 99 copies of this or any other American Psychiatric Publishing title, you are eligible for a 20% discount; please contact Customer Service at appi@psych.org or 800–368–5777. If you wish to buy 100 or more copies of the same title, please e-mail us at bulksales@psych.org for a price quote.

Manufactured in the United States of America on acid-free paper
16   15   14   13   12   5   4   3   2   1
First Edition

Typeset in Adobe's Minion and Trade Gothic

American Psychiatric Publishing
A Division of American Psychiatric Association
1000 Wilson Boulevard
Arlington, VA 22209-3901
www.appi.org

Library of Congress Cataloging-in-Publication Data
The LGBT casebook / edited by Petros Levounis, Jack Drescher, Mary E. Barber. — 1st. ed.
    p. ; cm.
  Includes bibliographical references and index.
  ISBN 978-1-58562-421-8 (pbk. : alk. paper)
  I. Levounis, Petros. II. Drescher, Jack, 1951- III. Barber, Mary E., 1967-
  [DNLM: 1. Homosexuality—psychology—Case Reports. 2. Bisexuality—psychology —Case Reports. 3. Gender Identity—Case Reports. 4. Mental Disorders—complications —Case Reports. 5. Mental Disorders—therapy—Case Reports. 6. Transsexualism—psychology—Case Reports. WM 611]
  616.85'83—dc23
                                                                2012010020

British Library Cataloguing in Publication Data
A CIP record is available from the British Library.

Contents

PART I. Basic Principles

PART II. Case Studies

Contributors

Andrew J. Anson, M.D.
Chief Resident in Psychiatry, St. Luke's and Roosevelt Hospitals, New York, New York

Kenneth Ashley, M.D.
Director of Mental Health Services, Peter Krueger Clinic, Beth Israel Medical Center, New York, New York; and Assistant Professor of Psychiatry and Behavioral Sciences, Albert Einstein College of Medicine, Bronx, New York

Mary E. Barber, M.D.
Clinical Director, Rockland Psychiatric Center, Orangeburg, New York; and Assistant Clinical Professor, Columbia College of Physicians and Surgeons, New York, New York

Philip A. Bialer, M.D.
Attending Psychiatrist, Memorial Sloan-Kettering Cancer Center; and Associate Professor of Clinical Psychiatry, Weill Cornell Medical School, New York, New York

John K. Burton, M.D.
Assistant Professor of Clinical Psychiatry, Division of Child and Adolescent Psychiatry; and Center for Psychoanalytic Training and Research, Department of Psychiatry, Columbia University, New York, New York

Stephan Carlson, M.D.
Medical Director of Addiction Psychiatry Services, Department of Psychiatry and Behavioral Sciences, Staten Island University Hospital, Staten Island, New York

Kenneth M. Cohen, Ph.D.
Clinical Psychologist, Counseling and Psychological Services, Gannett Health Services, Cornell University; and Lecturer, Human Development, Cornell University, Ithaca, New York

Jack Drescher, M.D.

Clinical Associate Professor of Psychiatry and Behavioral Science, New York Medical College; and Training and Supervising Analyst, William A. White Institute, New York, New York

Laura Erickson-Schroth, M.D., M.A.

Resident, Department of Psychiatry, New York University, New York, New York

Nanette Gartrell, M.D.

Williams Institute Visiting Scholar, UCLA School of Law; Guest appointment, University of Amsterdam, The Netherlands

Ronald E. Hellman, M.D.

Director, LGBT Affirmative Program, South Beach Psychiatric Center, Brooklyn, New York

Karine J. Igartua, M.D., C.M., F.R.C.P.C.(C)

Codirector, McGill University Sexual Identity Centre; Service Chief, Psychiatric Emergency Services, McGill University Health Centre; Vice-President, Quebec Psychiatrists' Association; and Assistant Professor, Faculty of Medicine, McGill University, Montreal, Quebec, Canada

Dickson Jean, M.D.

Assistant Professor of Psychiatry and Behavioral Sciences, Albert Einstein College of Medicine, Bronx, New York; and Psychiatrist, Peter Krueger Clinic, Beth Israel Medical Center, New York, New York

Helene Kendler, L.C.S.W.

Supervising Psychotherapist, South Beach Psychiatric Center, Brooklyn, New York

Robert M. Kertzner, M.D.

Associate Clinical Professor of Psychiatry, UCSF, San Francisco, California; and Adjunct Associate Research Scientist, Columbia University, New York, New York

Steven Joseph Lee, M.D.

New York, New York

Ubaldo Leli, M.D.
Lecturer in Psychiatry, Department of Psychiatry, College of Physicians and Surgeons, Columbia University; and Faculty Member, Columbia Center for Psychoanalytic Training and Research, New York, New York

Petros Levounis, M.D., M.A.
Director, The Addiction Institute of New York; Associate Chair for Clinical Services, Department of Psychiatry and Behavioral Health; Chief, Division of Addiction Psychiatry, St. Luke's and Roosevelt Hospitals; and Associate Clinical Professor of Psychiatry, Columbia University College of Physicians and Surgeons, New York, New York

Vittorio Lingiardi, M.D.
Psychiatrist and Psychotherapist; Professor, Faculty of Medicine and Psychology; and Director, Clinical Psychology Specialization Program, Department of Psychodynamic and Clinical Psychology, Sapienza University of Rome, Rome, Italy

Lorraine Lothwell, M.D.
Clinical Instructor, New York University Child Study Center and Bellevue Hospital Center, New York, New York

Anthony Lujack, M.D., J.D., M.S.
Psychiatry Resident, Beth Israel Medical Center, New York, New York

Scot G. McAfee, M.D.
Vice Chairman for Education and Residency Training Director in Psychiatry, Maimonides Medical Center, Brooklyn, New York; and Assistant Professor of Clinical Psychiatry, New York Medical College, Valhalla, New York

Christopher A. McIntosh, M.D.
Staff Psychiatrist, Centre for Addiction and Mental Health, Toronto, Ontario, Canada

Nicola Nardelli, Psy.D.
Doctor of Psychology, Department of Dynamic and Clinical Psychology, Faculty of Medicine and Psychology, Sapienza University of Rome, Rome, Italy

Aaron Patterson, M.D., M.B.A., M.A.
Psychiatry Resident, Beth Israel Medical Center, New York, New York

Jennifer C. Pizer, Esq.
Legal Director and Arnold D. Kassoy Senior Scholar of Law, The Williams Institute on Sexual Orientation and Gender Identity Law and Public Policy, UCLA School of Law, Los Angeles, California

Daniel Safin, M.D.
Assistant Professor of Psychiatry and Behavioral Sciences, Albert Einstein College of Medicine, Bronx, New York; and Psychiatrist, Division of Psychosomatic Medicine, Beth Israel Medical Center, New York, New York

Ritch C. Savin-Williams, Ph.D.
Professor, Human Development, and Director, Sex and Gender Lab, Cornell University, Ithaca, New York

David K. Schwing, L.C.S.W.
Private Practice of Psychotherapy, Licensed Systems–Centered Practitioner, New York, New York

Shane S. Spicer, M.D.
Assistant Clinical Professor of Psychiatry, Department of Psychiatry, Columbia University College of Physicians and Surgeons; and Medical Director, Center Recovery, The Lesbian, Gay, Bisexual and Transgender Community Center, New York, New York

Serena Yuan Volpp, M.D., M.P.H.
Unit Chief, Residency Training Unit, Bellevue Hospital Department of Psychiatry; and Clinical Associate Professor of Psychiatry, New York University School of Medicine, New York, New York

Khakasa Wapenyi, M.D.
Director of Mental Health and Behavioral Sciences, Mount Sinai Comprehensive Health Program–Downtown, Mount Sinai Medical Center; and Assistant Professor, Department of Psychiatry, Mount Sinai School of Medicine, New York, New York

Eric Yarbrough, M.D.
Attending Psychiatrist, Department of Psychiatry and Behavioral Health, St. Luke's and Roosevelt Hospitals, New York, New York

Disclosure of Interests

The following contributors to this book have indicated that they had no competing financial interest in or other affiliation with a commercial supporter, a manufacturer of a commercial product, a provider of a commercial service, a nongovernmental organization, and/or a government agency, during the year preceding manuscript submission:

Andrew J. Anson, M.D.
Kenneth Ashley, M.D.
Mary E. Barber, M.D.
Philip A. Bialer, M.D.
John K. Burton, M.D.
Kenneth M. Cohen, Ph.D.
Jack Drescher, M.D.
Laura Erickson-Schroth, M.D., M.A.
Nanette Gartrell, M.D.
Ronald E. Hellman, M.D.
Karine J. Igartua, M.D., C.M., F.R.C.P.C.(C)
Dickson Jean, M.D.
Helene Kendler, L.C.S.W.
Robert M. Kertzner, M.D.
Steven J. Lee, M.D.
Ubaldo Leli, M.D.
Petros Levounis, M.D., M.A.
Vittorio Lingiardi, M.D.
Lorraine Lothwell, M.D.
Anthony Lujack, M.D., J.D., M.S.
Scot G. McAfee, M.D.
Christopher A. McIntosh, M.D.
Nicola Nardelli, Psy.D.
Aaron Patterson, M.D., M.B.A., M.A.
Jennifer C. Pizer, Esq.
Daniel Safin, M.D.
Ritch C. Savin-Williams, Ph.D.
David K. Schwing, L.C.S.W.
Shane S. Spicer, M.D.
Serena Yuan Volpp, M.D., M.P.H.
Khakasa Wapenyi, M.D.
Eric Yarbrough, M.D.

Foreword

PEOPLE IN THE LGBT COMMUNITY are just like everyone else. We have the same aspirations to be safe, to find a fulfilling purpose, to love and be loved, and to be valued for who we are and what we accomplish. Like others, some of us have problems with substance abuse and mental illness because we are human and a proportion of all people experience addiction and/or mental illness.

Being lesbian, gay, bisexual, or transgender often means experiencing social challenges such as bullying or family rejection. It can mean ambivalence about self-worth due to societal messages about identity and acceptance. It can mean facing barriers to success such as discrimination in employment or housing as well as assault and harassment just because of who or how you are in the world.

As a result, certain behavioral health issues may be unique to the LGBT experience. The LGBT population has higher rates of suicide, substance abuse (including tobacco), depression, and anxiety, as well as rates of schizophrenia and bipolar disorder similar to those in the general population. Some subsets of the LGBT community also face higher rates of serious physical conditions such as obesity, HIV/AIDS, and breast cancer.

Nationwide, LGBT consumers face serious limitations in the availability of specialized, culturally appropriate behavioral health services. For example, the SAMHSA study Substance Abuse Treatment Programs for Gays and Lesbians showed that only 6% of substance abuse treatment facilities surveyed across the nation offered special programs for LGBT clients. Mental health service providers are similarly limited.

Services should be designed specifically to meet the needs of LGBT communities. Behavioral health providers can work with LGBT experts and stakeholders as well as utilize SAMHSA's training and resources to expand awareness of the LGBT experience.

The LGBT Casebook includes numerous case studies illuminating conflicts and discussions prominent in the LGBT community. It is a critical resource for those interested in meeting the needs of this population that is, on the one hand, just like everyone else and, on the other hand, unique. I applaud the authors and editors for offering this critical resource to the LGBT community and those who serve them.

Pamela S. Hyde, J.D.

Nominated in 2009 by President Barack Obama and confirmed by the U.S. Senate, Pamela S. Hyde, J.D., is the Administrator of the Substance Abuse and Mental Health Services Administration (SAMHSA), a public health agency within the U.S. Department of Health and Human Services.

Preface

HOW CAN I BEST TREAT THIS PATIENT? Psychiatrists and other mental health professionals ask this question as they assess any new patient. For the clinician less familiar with the issues common to lesbian, gay, bisexual, and transgender (LGBT) people, a presenting patient may induce particular anxiety.

This manual's main goal is to help clinicians better address the mental health needs of LGBT people in the context of illustrating problems they face in their everyday lives. Some problems are common to most or all LGBT people, such as being in the closet and coming out. Some problems affect only a segment of the population, as in the case of chemical dependence or dealing with a serious mental illness such as schizophrenia.

This book's first five chapters introduce clinicians to some basic principles of the life issues affecting LGBT populations. These are followed by twenty case studies with discussion by the case authors. Each case study presents an LGBT patient with a DSM-IV-TR (American Psychiatric Association 2000) diagnosis (Axis I, Axis II, V codes, or some combination thereof), and the clinical presentation illustrates a way of working with the patient. For practitioners with little experience in this area, the book's intent is to show the intersection of psychiatric diagnosis with the context of LGBT lives. Those already familiar with working with LGBT people are certain to find new pearls of wisdom and new insights.

The reader can choose to dive into this book at the beginning and read it cover to cover, gaining insights into the full diversity of the LGBT population as well as the breadth of DSM diagnoses. Alternatively, a clinician could go directly to a chapter of interest, perhaps one dealing with the diagnosis of a patient currently in treatment, for specific suggestions. However you, the reader, approach this book, our hope in creating it is that you will find it of benefit to both your patients and yourself.

While we are proud of this groundbreaking volume, we also wish to acknowledge some of the pillars on which this book rests. These include the Association of Gay and Lesbian Psychiatrists Annual Symposia (www.aglp.org), the *American Psychiatric Press Textbook of Homosexuality and Mental Health*

(Cabaj and Stein 1996), the *Journal of Gay and Lesbian Mental Health*, and the Group for Advancement of Psychiatry (2011) LGBT Mental Health Syllabus. All of these, valuable references themselves, are important resources that helped provide the momentum and lay the foundational knowledge base for this work.

Petros Levounis, M.D., M.A.
Jack Drescher, M.D.
Mary E. Barber, M.D.

References

American Psychiatric Association: Diagnostic and Statistical Manual of Mental Disorders, 4th Edition, Text Revision. Washington, DC, American Psychiatric Association, 2000

Cabaj RP, Stein TS: The American Psychiatric Press Textbook of Homosexuality and Mental Health. Washington, DC, American Psychiatric Press, 1996

Group for Advancement of Psychiatry: LGBT mental health syllabus. Available at: http://www.aglp.org/gap. Accessed October 27, 2011.

PART I

BASIC PRINCIPLES

What's In Your Closet?

JACK DRESCHER, M.D.

BEING "IN THE CLOSET" is a colloquialism used to describe those who
are either hiding their homosexual feelings or hiding a lesbian, gay, or bisexual
(LGB) identity.[1] The term is closely linked to "coming out of the closet," which
refers to either revealing one's homosexual feelings and attractions or accepting
and declaring an LGB identity (see below and Chapter 2, "Coming Out to Self
and Others"). As one historian notes, this usage of "coming out" is relatively
recent:

> Nowhere does [the term *coming out of the closet*] appear before the 1960s in the
> records of the gay movement or in the novels, diaries, or letters of gay men and
> lesbians.... Like much of campy gay terminology, "coming out" was an arch play
> on the language of women's culture—in this case the expression used to refer to
> the ritual of a debutante's being formally introduced to, or "coming out" into,
> the society of her cultural peers.... Gay people in the prewar years, then, did not
> speak of *coming out of* what we call the "gay closet" but rather of *coming out into*
> what they called "homosexual society" or the "gay world." (Chauncey 1994,
> pp. 6–7; italics in original)

---

[1] There are some similarities between the developmental trajectories of lesbian, gay, and
bisexual (LGB) populations and those of transgender (T) populations. However, there
are also differences, some of which are discussed in greater detail in chapters 8, 15, 21,
24, and 25. This chapter mostly refers to "LGB" populations but refers to "LGBT" populations where the latter seems applicable.

Yet as Western societies increasingly became aware of issues surrounding homosexuality, the meaning of LGB culture's "coming out of the closet" expanded to describe revelations of other kinds of secrets, conjoined in part with another popular expression, "having a skeleton in one's closet." For purposes of this volume, however, *being in the closet* or *being closeted* refers to a range of behaviors and psychological mechanisms used to avoid knowledge of or discussions about either one's own homosexuality or that of others.

The Need to Hide

From a cross-cultural perspective, LGB people are often compared to members of other stigmatized minority groups. As with racism or anti-Semitism, for example, a stigmatized group member can reject the majority's perspective (move to a gay enclave), reach an accommodation (accept the role of token lesbian), or try to assimilate (hide one's bisexuality and try to pass as straight). Among racial or religious minorities, family and community offer their members role models of how to cope with the majority's prejudices. LGBT people, however, are often subject to stigmatizing attitudes from their own families and communities; as some have put it, "being born into the enemy camp" often creates an early need to hide.

As portrayed in literature, theater, films, or even by a patient in psychotherapy, one prevailing theme of the closet is that revealing one's sexual feelings or identity leads to problematic consequences. While the discovery of one's LGB identity may not necessarily be dangerous in one's current life circumstances, it may have been so in one's past. These difficulties often stem from normal socialization processes. Children learn to defensively hide feelings and thoughts that may be unacceptable to those around them, sometimes learning quickly and at other times through trial and error that some parts of themselves are unacceptable to others. Among children who grow up to be LGB, antihomosexual attitudes toward same-sex feelings of attraction or affection can lead to social difficulties. As a result, children may learn to conceal important aspects of their personalities.

Although *homophobia* has entered the language as an overarching term, most LGB people have been subject to several antihomosexual attitudes that include not only homophobia but also heterosexism, moral condemnations of homosexuality, and antigay violence.

Weinberg (1972) defined *external homophobia* as the irrational fear and hatred that heterosexual people feel toward LGB people and *internal homophobia* as the self-loathing LGB people felt for themselves. *Heterosexism* (Morin and Garfinkle 1978) is often confused with homophobia in popular usage. Heterosexism is a belief system that naturalizes and idealizes heterosexuality and either dismisses or ignores an LGB subjectivity. In its most benign form, it is a broad assumption that everyone is heterosexual, rendering LGB people invisible: commercials showing heterosexual couples kissing because they bought the advertiser's product; day care forms that only have spaces for "father" and "mother"; medical intake forms that do not take into account that patients can be married to someone of the same sex. In other words, in contrast to homophobia, heterosexism does not necessarily imply malice or ill will toward LGB individuals.

Yet heterosexist attitudes, sometimes implicitly and at other times explicitly, tend to equate the nonheterosexual with the immoral. Consequently, there are ideological examples of heterosexism. These include valuing heterosexual relationships above same-sex ones, opposing gay parenting regardless of a gay parent's actual qualities, or regarding LGB people as innately unsuited for certain jobs (teacher, scout leader, psychoanalyst). Here heterosexism verges on *moral condemnations of homosexuality* (Drescher 1998), which regard homosexuality as intrinsically harmful to the individual, to the individual's spirit, and to the social fabric. Those who morally condemn homosexuality frequently claim they do so out of love for some other cherished value such as literal interpretations of the Bible or "traditional marriage." Sometimes these moral condemnations are expressed in secular terms as well. For example, psychiatrists of the nineteenth century condemned "homosexuals" for engaging in sexual practices that were counter to "evolutionary design" because they (seemingly) interfered with heterosexual reproduction (Krafft-Ebing 1886/1965). A common religious example in today's world is the view espoused by those who claim to "hate the homosexual sin" while "loving the homosexual sinner."

Unfortunately, not everyone distinguishes "homosexuals" from their homosexuality. Just as many LGB people experience same-sex attractions as intrinsic to their identities, so do perpetrators of *antigay violence*. *Gay bashing* originally described actions by groups of young men who descended on LGBT meeting areas and, armed with bats, clubs, or other weapons, attacked anyone they believed to be lesbian, gay, bisexual, or transgender. Not all LGBT people have personally experienced antigay violence, but most have legitimate concerns about potential physical attacks. However, when public policy debates about the civil rights of LGB people become heated and strident, homophobic statements and moral condemnations of homosexuality are often experienced as *verbal gay bashing*. Verbal and political attacks have been shown to increase both minority stress and psychological distress in LGB populations (Rostosky et al. 2009).

One consequence of a developmental history involving exposure to antihomosexual attitudes is that many gay people have a difficult time acknowledging their homosexual feelings and attractions, either to themselves or to others. Most gay people are born into and raised in environments intolerant of open expressions of same-sex feelings or intimacy. Gender-atypical children, boys whose behavior is not conventionally masculine or girls who are not typically feminine, experience similar disapprobation—even if they do not grow up to be gay. Many LGBT people report having been bullied and traumatized either for coming out as

LGBT or for being perceived as such (Russell et al. 2011; Ryan et al. 2009). Such experiences, actual or anticipated, have caused many an LGB person to hide important aspects of the self. Some develop techniques for hiding that often persist into young adulthood and middle age, and sometimes even into senescence. There are both behavioral and psychological elements to this hiding.

Don't Ask, Don't Tell

As it is often assumed that one is heterosexual unless declared otherwise, it is not uncommon for many LGB people to adapt to heterosexist assumptions by hiding their homosexuality, both from themselves and from others. In rudimentary terms, and in popular understanding, a person "in the closet" is simply withholding information from others. However, closets are not always so simply constructed, and there are often complex variations and selective forms of "closetedness." For example: having an openly LGB personal life but telling no one at work; moving to another city where one lives as openly gay, but telling no one back home; or selectively telling (coming out to) some family and friends but not wanting everyone in one's social circle to know. Deciding whom to tell and where to come out are often daily activities that can have rational and irrational aspects. For example, it is rational for an openly married Canadian lesbian to choose not to reveal her homosexuality (or marital status) when traveling for work purposes to a Middle Eastern or African country where open expressions of homosexuality are considered a crime. It was also rational, before the 2011 repeal of the military's Don't Ask, Don't Tell policy, for U.S. gay military personnel to remain in the closet.

As a hiding mechanism, some LGBT people learn to speak without revealing the gender of the person being discussed or without providing any gendered details of their personal lives. Some may avoid references to gender altogether: "I went out last week with *someone* I've been dating for a few months. *We* went to a show in *their* part of town. *We* talked about the possibility of going out of town next weekend." A naïve listener hearing a man speaking these words might make the heterosexist assumption that he was discussing a relationship with a woman. For these and other reasons, clinicians should learn to ask direct and open questions about relationships—questions that do not presume all patients are heterosexual. When a clinician does not ask, a patient may not tell.

Orientation Versus Identity

Beyond the behavioral dimensions of telling or not telling, there are psychological mechanisms that operate in maintaining a closeted state of mind. Such operations are often described in LGB memoirs and autobiographies, and patients frequently describe them in clinical practice (Drescher 1998; Drescher and Byne 2009). Understanding these mechanisms requires defining some terms. (For more definitions of terms, please see the Glossary at the end of this book.)

A *sexual orientation* refers to a person's erotic response tendency or sexual attractions, be they directed toward individuals of the same sex *(homosexual)*, the other sex *(heterosexual)*, or both sexes *(bisexual)*. While engaging in sexual behavior is volitional, the direction of erotic responsiveness usually is not. Sexual orientation has at least three components—desire, behavior, and identity—which may or may not be congruent in an individual. Clinicians should not assume congruence among these three components solely on the basis of information about one or two of them.

Sexual identities, sometimes referred to as *sexual orientation identities,* are the subjective experiences of one's sexual desires or attractions. Further, the subjectivity of a sexual identity is shaped by culture and language, often with little or no regard to prevailing scientific categories of sexuality (Diamond 2008; Drescher 1998). Adopting a *lesbian, gay,* or *bisexual* identity involves some measure of self-acceptance of one's homosexual desires. A person who adopts such an identity might believe that one is "born gay," although the causes of homosexuality (and heterosexuality for that matter) are unknown (Drescher 2002). In some but not all cases, adopting a bisexual identity may serve as a transitional identity that precedes fully accepting a gay or lesbian identity. However, not everyone who experiences homoerotic desire or participates in homosexual behavior develops an LGB identity. For individuals who acknowledge their homosexual orientation without identifying as LGB, their homosexual identity may not be synonymous with their homosexual orientation (American Psychological Association 2009; Drescher and Byne 2009; Worthington et al. 2002). Figure 1–1 outlines four broad "homosexual identities" to illustrate ways in which patients manage their same-sex feelings.

Closeted individuals are unable to acknowledge to themselves or to others that they have homoerotic feelings and fantasies. This is a psychological state of mind reported retrospectively by individuals only after they have moved on to a later stage, commonly captured in the expression, "I didn't want to/couldn't admit those feelings to myself." For such individuals, feelings of same-sex attraction are unacceptable and unavailable to direct awareness and not integrated into the public persona. It is entirely possible for an individual to remain in this stage for a lifetime. Subjectively, a closeted person may tell herself she really does not have same-sex feelings or, if she is aware of the feelings, may attribute some other meaning to them besides homosexuality (e.g., "a passing phase"). Clinically, it is rarely therapeutic to tell a person in such a state of mind, "You are gay, but you just don't know it."

Hidden from the self as well as from others, a closeted individual may not act on same-sex feelings at all or may do so only in a dissociated state. Harry

Stack Sullivan's (1956) formulations of dissociative operations are extremely useful in understanding and therapeutically working with such individuals. In Sullivan's view, most people use a range of dissociative defenses in everyday life. In Sullivan's continuum of dissociative phenomena, *selective inattention* is a nonpathological process that makes life more manageable, analogous to tuning out the background noise on a busy street. Clinical presentations of being in the closet may lie somewhere in severity between selective inattention, most commonly seen in the case of a patient thinking about "the possibility" she might be gay, and severe dissociation, in which any hint of same-sex feelings resides totally out of conscious awareness.

Being able to reveal one's sexual identity in some settings while having to hide it in others can foster dissociative splits in everyday life—as in the case of gay military personnel before the repeal of Don't Ask, Don't Tell. Although this approach may be adaptive in certain circumstances, more severe dissociative activities that separate self-states can prevent a gay person from paying attention to the full consequences of hiding activities. Hiding activities can lead to errors in judgment, and this offers one possible explanation for how some heterosexually married, socially conservative politicians and religious figures have enmeshed themselves in embarrassing same-sex scandals.

Homosexually self-aware individuals are able to acknowledge, at least to themselves, that they have homoerotic or same-sex feelings and attractions. However, their subjectivities and behaviors may vary. A self-aware person may choose not to act on the feelings or may act on them secretly. Some behaviorally closeted individuals are homosexually self-aware and some are not. Some homosexually self-aware individuals consider the possibility of accepting and integrating these feelings in a public way. This subjectivity has been described as a normative phase in eventually coming out and affirmatively accepting an LGB identity (Cass 1979). However, not everyone accepts these feelings, as in the example of a homosexually self-aware individual seeking a religiously celibate lifestyle as a way to avoid the conflicts that would ensue from adopting a problematic LGB identity.

Non-gay-identified describes a fourth homosexual identity. Individuals in this category are aware of same-sex feelings, do not deny them, may be public about them with others, may act on the feelings (Pathela et al. 2006), and may even have earlier come out as LGB. However, these individuals consciously struggle against accepting same-sex attractions or relationships as part of their public identity. They may heterosexually marry. Because many people go through a phase of rejecting their homosexual feelings before accepting an LGB identity (Cass 1979), it is sometimes assumed that all individuals can, will, or should overcome this period of rejection. However, this is not always the case. Some may seek out ways to change their sexual orientation and, in an effort to disidentify with homoerotic feelings and activities, claim an identity as either

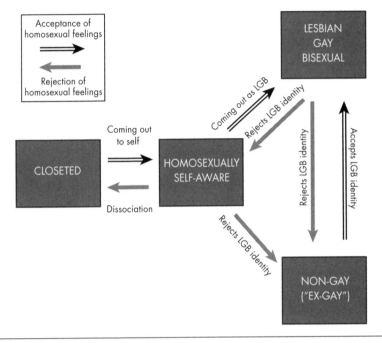

FIGURE 1–1. **Sexual identities (homosexual orientation constant).**

LGB=lesbian, gay, or bisexual.

Source. Adapted from Drescher and Byne 2009.

"ex-homosexual" or "ex-gay." A recent scholarly review of scientific research on whether such individuals have actually changed their sexual orientation is neither convincing nor compelling (American Psychological Association 2009). In recent years the issue has generated great cultural controversy (Drescher and Zucker 2006). However, while the non-gay identified may not be able to change their sexual orientation, they have tried to establish some control regarding their public identities.

For example, a man with a homosexual orientation may not accept his same-sex feelings. He might choose to marry a woman and to maintain an ostensibly heterosexual lifestyle. He may never lose his homosexual desires and, even if consciously aware of them, still not identify as gay. He may have a history of homosexual encounters and may even continue to engage in clandestine homosexual relationships while at the same time expressing disdain for the "gay lifestyle" and the gay community. He may seek religious or professional help and even his wife's complicity to shore up his nongay identity.

The four homosexual identities outlined above—closeted, homosexually self-aware, LGB, nongay—are not conceived as being on a developmental continuum. These subjectivities do not necessarily offer any diagnostic information about an

individual. In addition, they are not mutually exclusive; there can be overlap between them and differing motivations within them. For example, non-gay identified individuals may be motivated by religious beliefs, fear of estrangement from
family, a wish to live a conventional heterosexual lifestyle, or some combination of
these. Furthermore, sexual identities are not immutable. Although it may be difficult if not impossible to change one's sexual orientation (American Psychological Association 2009), it is possible to change attitudes about one's sexuality. Because the subjectivities outlined above are shaped by individual and cultural
factors, there is a wide range of psychosocially constructed attitudes and responses
that people may develop toward their own homosexuality.

Coming Out

Coming out is a commonly shared cultural experience defining a modern LGB
identity (see also Chapter 2). In everyday usage, as noted earlier, coming out, or
"coming out of the closet" means telling another person that one is gay. Anthro-
pologists and social scientists (Herdt and Boxer 1993) have described it as a ritual process of passage that requires an LGB person to 1) unlearn the principles
of natural or essentialist heterosexuality, 2) unlearn the stereotypes of homosexuality, and 3) learn the ways of the LGB culture they are entering. Coming
out means breaking with expectations that all sexual identities are heterosexual
ones.

Years spent in the closet can make the prospect of revealing one's LGB identity an emotionally charged experience (Gershman 1983; Magee and Miller
1994). When LGB people do choose to come out, it is usually because hiding
and separating aspects of the self is too problematic or painful (see Chapter 14,
"Posttraumatic Stress Disorder"). However, the process is not just about telling
others. There are intrapsychic and interpersonal aspects of the coming out process. In psychological terms, coming out can integrate dissociated aspects of the
self. Further, constant hiding may create difficulties in accurately assessing other
people's perceptions of oneself. Being in the closet may also have an impact on
self-esteem, making it difficult to feel one's actual accomplishments as reflec-
tions of one's own abilities. Consequently, coming out may involve integrating
not only one's sexual identity but also other aspects of one's affects and personality. Further, as LGB people in a heterosexual world repeatedly face moments in
which they have to decide whether or not to reveal themselves, coming out is a
process that potentially never ends. In that ongoing process, LGB people must
decide on a daily basis whether to reveal and to whom they will reveal—an experience that may have no exact parallel for those with heterosexual identities,
which are publicly enacted but usually not named or declared.

Although coming out can be integrative in the broadest sense, individual
personality differences as well as cultural and family dynamics can play out in

different ways if and when an LGB person decides to come out. A therapist needs to be aware of the different levels involved. For example, a patient can use coming out as a vehicle for maintaining compliant defenses in a particular social environment, for expressing anger at family members, or for other purposes. In other words, simply declaring oneself to be LGB does not necessarily lead to integration.

Each individual's experience of the coming out process can be unique. *Coming out to oneself* is a transition from a closeted subjectivity to a stage of homosexual self-awareness, often described retrospectively in LGB memoirs and autobiographies as a subjective experience of inner recognition. At times, coming out to oneself may precede an actual sexual experience. In some cases, people report a long-standing fear that they might be LGB, which had prevented them from acting on their feelings. Alternatively, the moment of coming out to oneself may occur in a sexual encounter, sometimes described as "a switch being turned on." When describing the moment of coming out to oneself, LGB people may use phrases like "coming home" or "discovering who I really am."

Such a pivotal moment is sometimes charged with excitement and trepidation. It is a realization that previously unacceptable or dissociated feelings and desires are part of one's self. Sometimes self-awareness can be a frightening prospect. It is also, in part, a verbal process in which one learns how to explain, in ways that are acceptable to the self, previously inarticulate feelings and ideas. It involves recapturing disavowed experiences through a continuing process of linguistic coding that gives previously unacceptable feelings new meanings—in effect, learning a new language of the self (Drescher 1998).

Coming out to oneself is often followed by *coming out to others*. This may involve making contact with other LGB people. At other times, it may mean telling a close heterosexual friend, family member, teacher, religious leader, or co-worker. The revelation to a trusted person is not always greeted with enthusiasm, particularly in settings where homosexuality is a subject that does not come up in "polite company." Some heterosexual individuals experience coming out as the breaking of a social taboo, hearing the announcement as a comment about the LGB person's sex life. They may feel, or even ask aloud, "Why do you have to talk about it?," unaware that when LGB people come out, they are not talking about their sex lives. As a public rite of passage, coming out says as much about an LGB person's sex life as wedding ceremonies say about the sex lives of heterosexual couples. In an effort to claim a normative identity, coming out is a way to explain to others that one's public life will unfold somewhat differently from those of heterosexual family and friends.

In this ongoing process, every situation in which an LGB person comes out may be associated with anxiety, a sense of relief, or both. The process can be complicated by fears of rejection. Such fears often play a significant role in an LGB person's decision about whom one should tell and whom one should not.

In some instances, reluctance to come out reflects an accurate assessment of potentially critical or rejecting reactions from friends and family members. In others, the assessment is inaccurate and opportunities for closeness are lost.

If one senses, accurately or inaccurately, that one cannot come out at home, moving to another city offers opportunities to come out among strangers. It is often an exhilarating experience to come out in a new, faraway place where one is not known to either family or friends. After making such a move, some people completely sever relations with their past lives. Others, after gaining comfort in their new lives, use the increased confidence that comes with psychological integration to come out to friends and family back home.

Coming Out Later in Life

The most common narratives of coming out involve doing so in adolescence or in one's twenties or thirties. However, there are some who come out as LGB in middle life or later. Some of these individuals have heterosexually married and raised families, and their coming out is precipitated by having an "empty nest" when the last child leaves home. Some may have been aware of their same-sex attractions for a long time, whereas others may have experienced them intensely only later in life.

Coming out late in life has its own special set of challenges (Olson 2011). Common points of entry into the LGB community, such as gay bars and dance clubs, are usually designed for the pleasure of younger people. LGB people who come out in later life are often in need of interpersonal skill-building and may not be welcome in venues catering mainly to younger people. As a result, a preexisting sensation of alienation from the straight community can sometimes turn into feelings of alienation from the more visible younger LGB community (which some mistakenly believe to be the *entire* gay community). However, as social acceptance of homosexuality has increased and more people have come out, there is a growing LGB infrastructure for older people. These include LGBT community centers and national organizations for older people, such as SAGE (Services and Advocacy for Gay, Lesbian, Bisexual and Transgender Elders). Those living in less populous areas without a supportive gay infrastructure often use the Internet to ease social isolation.

Coming Out as Double Minority

In a white-male-dominated society, being black, Hispanic, Asian, or Native American *and* LGBT is referred to as "double minority" status. Being a member of a double minority often entails interpersonal, familial, and cultural issues. Coming out as LGBT to one's ethnic or racial community of origin may be difficult if this community regards openly LGBT identities as an unwanted majority influence intruding on their culture of origin. Some clinical issues among double minority members include not feeling accepted by either one's ethnic or racial minority group or gay culture ("No group wants all of me"); having difficulty choosing a primary group identification ("Am I ethnic minority first or gay first?"); and dealing with overt and covert racism, homophobia, and sexism (within both the minority communities and the gay community). Often, members of double minorities are able to find support groups in LGBT community centers, where these exist, or through online support groups.

Conclusion

Given the social stigma attached to homosexuality, the ubiquity of antihomosexual attitudes in the culture, and the possibility of losing family and friends, why would an LGBT person come out at all? Despite the possible dangers of doing so, coming out is often experienced as an integrative process that serves to affirm one's sense of worth. As hiding from oneself depends upon dissociative defenses, coming out holds the possibility of psychological integration. Of course, the needs to find a balance between dissociation and integration will vary depending on an individual's specific life situation and personality. Nevertheless, comfort with one's own feelings plays an important role in social and psychological development. Coming out offers LGBT people the possibility of integrating a wider range of previously split-off feelings, not solely sexual feelings. Greater ease in expressing one's thoughts and feelings both to oneself and to others can lead to an enormous enrichment of one's life, work, and relationships.

What is the role of the clinician in the coming out process? A therapist might decide that it is preferable not to take a position on whether or not the patient comes out, perhaps even defining that stance as a "neutral" one. However, doing nothing is rarely an option. For example, a therapist can help a patient come out by offering direct feedback based on information the patient provides. If a patient's heterosexually married neighbor regales her with stories about his wife's gay friends and associates, a therapist might reasonably assume the neighbor might accept her if she comes out to him. On the other hand, coming out to others can sometimes be fraught with risks a therapist cannot predict. Thus, sometimes it may be unwise to advise a patient to come out to someone whose actual views the therapist does not personally know. Nor can a therapist fully predict the consequences of such a revelation on the relationship of those two people. As there are many closets, there are many different ways to come out. There is no single correct way to do so, a fact that may be overlooked by a therapist in a well-intentioned effort to affirm a patient's homosexuality and have the patient come out indiscriminately. Therapeutic interventions that involve coming out may require supervision or consultation with a more experienced colleague. Helping patients come out to others can be a challenging task and needs to be addressed with each patient in a way that recognizes individual differences. Recognition and respect for individual differences will allow a multiplicity of possibilities in the coming out process. In this way, patients may find their own way and define their own identities.

Key Points

- *Being in the closet* or *being closeted* refers to a range of behaviors and psychological mechanisms used to avoid knowledge of or discussions about one's own homosexuality or that of others.

- LGBT people are often subject to antihomosexual attitudes (homophobia, heterosexism, moral condemnations of homosexuality, antigay violence) that create an early need to hide.

- Although not all LGBT people have personally experienced antigay violence, most have legitimate concerns about potential physical attacks.

- *Sexual identities,* or *sexual orientation identities,* are not immutable, are not on a developmental continuum, do not offer diagnostic information, are not mutually exclusive, and can have differing motivations within them.

- Because being in the closet relies on dissociative defenses, coming out can lead to psychological integration and an enrichment of one's life, work, and relationships.

References

American Psychological Association: Report of the American Psychological Association Task Force on Appropriate Therapeutic Response to Sexual Orientation. Washington, DC, American Psychological Association, 2009

Cass VC: Homosexual identity formation: a theoretical model. J Homosex 4:219–235, 1979

Chauncey G: Gay New York: Gender, Urban Culture, and the Making of the Gay Male World, 1890–1940. New York, Basic Books, 1994

Diamond LM: Female bisexuality from adolescence to adulthood: results from a 10-year longitudinal study. Dev Psychol 44:5–14, 2008

Drescher J: Psychoanalytic Therapy and the Gay Man. Hillsdale, NJ, Analytic Press, 1998

Drescher J: Causes and becauses: on etiological theories of homosexuality. The Annual of Psychoanalysis 30:57–68, 2002

Drescher J, Byne W: Homosexuality, gay and lesbian identities, and homosexual behavior, in Kaplan and Sadock's Comprehensive Textbook of Psychiatry, 9th Edition. Edited by Sadock BJ, Sadock VA, Ruiz P. Baltimore, MD, Lippincott Williams & Wilkins, 2009, pp 2060–2090

Drescher J, Zucker KJ (eds): Ex-Gay Research: Analyzing the Spitzer Study and Its Relation to Science, Religion, Politics, and Culture. New York, Harrington Park Press, 2006

Gershman H: The stress of coming out. Am J Psychoanal 43:129–138, 1983

Herdt G, Boxer A: Children of Horizons: How Gay and Lesbian Teens are Leading a New Way Out of the Closet. Boston, MA, Beacon Press, 1993

Krafft-Ebing R: Psychopathia Sexualis (1886). Translated by Wedeck H. New York, Putnam, 1965

Magee M, Miller D: Psychoanalysis and women's experiences of "coming out": the necessity of being a bee-charmer. J Am Acad Psychoanal 22:481–504, 1994

Morin S, Garfinkle E: Male homophobia. J Soc Issues 34:29–47, 1978

Olson LA: Finally Out: Letting Go of Living Straight, A Psychiatrist's Own Story. Miami, FL, InGroup Press, 2011

Pathela P, Hajat A, Schillinger J, et al: Discordance between sexual behavior and self-reported sexual identity: a population-based survey of New York City men. Ann Intern Med 145:416–425, 2006

Rostosky SS, Riggle ED, Horne SG, et al: Marriage amendments and psychological distress in lesbian, gay, and bisexual (LGB) adults. J Couns Psychol 56:56–66, 2009

Russell ST, Ryan C, Toomey RB, et al: Lesbian, gay, bisexual and transgender adolescent school victimization: implications for young adult health and adjustment. J Sch Health 81:223–230, 2011

Ryan C, Huebner D, Diaz RM, et al: Family rejection as a predictor of negative health outcomes in white and Latino lesbian, gay, and bisexual young adults. Pediatrics 123:346–352, 2009

Sullivan HS: Clinical Studies in Psychiatry. New York, WW Norton, 1956

Weinberg G: Society and the Healthy Homosexual. New York, Anchor Books, 1972

Worthington RL, Savoy H, Dillon FR, et al: Heterosexual identity development: a multidimensional model of individual and group identity. Couns Psychol 30:496–531, 2002

Questions

1.1   Which of the following is *not* an antihomosexual attitude?

    A. Homophobia.

    B. Heterosexism.

    C. Moral condemnation of homosexuality.

    D. Antigay violence.

    E. Coming out.

The correct answer is E.

While *homophobia* is more generally used, most LGB people have been subject to other antihomosexual attitudes that include heterosexism, moral condemnations of homosexuality, and antigay violence as well. Early exposure to these attitudes leads children who grow up to be LGB to conceal important aspects of their personalities.

1.2 A psychological mechanism used to maintain a closeted identity is

    A. Integration.
    B. Dissociation.
    C. Gay-bashing.
    D. "Love the sinner."
    E. Gender-atypical behavior.

The correct answer is B.

Sullivan's formulations of dissociative operations include a nonpathological process that makes life more manageable, analogous to tuning out the background noise on a busy street. Being able to reveal one's sexual identity in some settings while having to hide it in others can foster dissociative splits in everyday life.

1.3 A non-gay-identified individual with same-sex attractions

    A. May be aware of same-sex feelings but not act on them.
    B. May have come out as gay earlier in life and then repudiated that identity.
    C. May heterosexually marry.
    D. May struggle against having those feelings.
    E. All of the above.

The correct answer is E.

Not all individuals with same-sex attractions accept an LGB identity. Some may try, without much success, to change their sexual orientation.

Coming Out to Self and Others

Developmental Milestones

Kenneth M. Cohen, Ph.D.
Ritch C. Savin-Williams, Ph.D.

THE PROCESS OF COMING OUT to self and others is frequently an evolving and lengthy one. It consists of multiple developmental milestones, the order and timing of which vary across individuals. Although few aspects of the self are as essential as sexual and romantic longings, individuals with same-sex attractions may struggle to recognize and embrace their underlying sexuality. They may be unaware or distrusting of their sexuality because of limited sexual experience, conservative attitudes, attenuated libido, or excessive self-monitoring of expressed behavior (Wiederman 1999). Some hesitate to adopt a socially stigmatized identity, and others loathe being narrowly defined by their sexuality.

In this chapter we delineate developmental milestones that, together, constitute the coming-out process. After considering the deceptively simple construct of who is gay, we review what is known about early feelings of being different from one's peers, the onset of same-sex attractions, sexual questioning, first sexual experiences, recognition and self-labeling, disclosure to others, and self-acceptance. Clinical recommendations are interspersed throughout and conclude the chapter.

Who Is Gay

Assuming patients are heterosexual unless proven otherwise can lead clinicians to make insensitive remarks and erroneous clinical assessments. Notwithstanding a verbal disclosure, the determination of sexual orientation is surprisingly complex and depends largely on the way in which "gay" is defined. Thus, it is necessary to distinguish among three related, but distinct, sexual domains: sexual orientation, sexual behavior, and sexual identity (see also the Glossary at the end of this book).

Domains of Sexual Orientation

Sexual orientation refers to the predominance of erotic thoughts, feelings, and fantasies one has for members of a particular sex (LeVay and Baldwin 2012). Likely present from birth or an early age, sexual orientation is usually considered immutable, stable, and resistant to conscious control. Sexual orientation should not be equated with sexual identity or sexual behavior, because most sexual-minority (i.e., nonheterosexual) individuals do not identify as gay or report engaging in same-sex behavior, especially during adolescence (Savin-Williams 2005). Although the relationship between sexual orientation and romantic attractions is unclear, the two certainly overlap.

Sexual behavior refers to the sexual activities in which an individual engages. Definitions of what constitutes "sex" vary across individuals and cohorts. We define *sex* as any manner of genital contact between two or more people. Influenced by cultural and individual factors, such as religion and race/ethnicity, one's choice of sexual partners may not always be consistent with one's underlying romantic and sexual-orientation desires. For example, domain incongruence is common among African American men who are on the "down low," participating in explicit sex with women and clandestine sex with men. Identifying as heterosexual, they may be unreceptive to safer-sex messages directed toward gay and bisexual men and consequently may be at increased risk for HIV and other sexually transmitted infections (Denizet-Lewis 2003).

Sexual orientation identity is a socially constructed label self-chosen to represent sexual feelings, sexual behavior, and romantic interests. Although options are usually limited to those available within a given culture and historic time, contemporary youths are increasingly rejecting sexual orientation identity labels (e.g., lesbian, gay, bisexual) in favor of less confining and simplistic descriptions that better represent their sexual and gender expressions, such as "mostly straight," "sexually fluid," and "boidyke."

It is essential that clinicians assess all sexual and romantic domains because these often are at variance with each other within the patient and thus are individually misleading. This is especially true among youths and those conflicted about their sexuality. Consider the case of a young woman who is sexually attracted to both sexes (bisexual sexual orientation), has sex only with males (heterosexual behavior), falls in love with women (homosexual romance), and identifies as lesbian for political and social reasons. Or the young man with homoerotic desires (homosexual sexual orientation), sexual experiences with males and females (bisexual behavior), romantic relationships with women (heterosexual romance), and a heterosexual identity. Depending on the questions asked, radically different conclusions about their sexuality will be reached.

Prevalence of Sexual Minorities

Data from four waves (12 years) of the National Longitudinal Survey of Adolescent Health confirm that estimating the number of nonheterosexual individuals depends on which of these sexual domains is assessed. Prevalence rates varied between 1% and 16% and were highest among females, among those who identified as "mostly heterosexual," and in measurements of same-sex attractions (Savin-Williams and Ream 2007; Savin-Williams et al. 2012). By age 28, 2% and 4% of men and women, respectively, identified their sexual orientation as gay, lesbian, or bisexual; however, more than 6% of men and nearly 20% of women claimed that they were not exclusively heterosexual. The implication is clear: Not all patients with same-sex sexuality necessarily identify as such, act on this, or disclose it to others, perhaps especially not to clinicians perceived to have narrowly defined values.

Developmental Milestones

"Coming out" is often characterized as an invariant, universal progression from initial unawareness and confusion to eventual identity pride and synthesis (e.g., Cass 1979). Despite the heuristic appeal and widespread popularity of stage-based coming-out models, such linear and idealized portrayals are not empirically substantiated (Savin-Williams 2005). For example, whereas identifying as gay or bisexual usually precedes same-sex dating or disclosure to others, some youths have a committed same-sex romantic relationship prior to self-labeling and have same-sex activities only after self-identification. Many contemporary youths do not experience sexual confusion, nor are they particularly "proud" to be gay—it is just who they are. As developmental milestones increasingly overlap, clinicians should be wary of assumptions about "normal" or "typical" developmental trajectories. The coming out process is best understood by an individual's achievement of developmental sexual milestones that increasingly occur without respect for tradition, timing, and order.

Feeling Different

Many sexual minorities recall growing up with an internal feeling of being sexually different or with behaviors and interests that are discrepant from those of their peers. This divergence from other children begins around age 7 or 8, but it can appear as early as first memories and is often the consequence of being called sissy or tomboy. In one study, by age 8 years, two-thirds of youths who later identified as gay or lesbian were considered gender atypical by others. More than half reported that their parents experienced them as gender inappropriate, and half of such parents attempted to change the youth's gender presentation (D'Augelli et al. 2008).

Same-sex-oriented patients frequently disclose ongoing feelings of differentness related to perceived gender inadequacy that may be characterized by deficient gender conformity (e.g., low masculinity in males), elevated gender nonconformity (e.g., high femininity in males), or both. Indeed, in one study, men reported that their initial feelings of being different were determined less by "inappropriate" sexual longings than by the shame generated by gender ineptitude (Troiden 1979). By adolescence, however, virtually all men with same-sex attractions recalled feeling *sexually* different because of their homoerotic interests, sexual interactions with males, and negligible erotic attraction for females. Most lesbians recalled similar feelings, with only half ascribing it to their sexuality (Schneider 2001).

Although the correlation between same-sex attractions and gender-atypical behavior is imperfect, many studies document a strong association (Cohen 2002). Perhaps not surprisingly, it is easier to conceal the behavioral expression of one's homoeroticism than to conceal gender nonconformity, possibly because the latter is less subject to conscious control. When atypical gender expression evokes peer bullying, the ridicule is frequently couched in antigay banter. An effeminate boy being called "gay" and a masculine girl "lesbian" by peers are seldom accusations about their erotic proclivities but statements about their gender nonconformity. Indeed, gender-transgressing heterosexuals also suffer harassment at the hands of intolerant peers. The inverse is true as well: sexual minorities who appear gender conforming are more likely to escape stigmatization and ridicule.

Same-Sex Attractions

The time frame for first same-sex attractions is broad, extending from first memories onward, though usually occurring years before the onset of puberty. Although it is not certain exactly when same-sex attractions first emerge, a sharp decline (of 4 years) has been observed during the past two decades in the recalled age of first attraction, especially among girls, not as a consequence of earlier pubertal onset but due to a growing cultural awareness of nontraditional sexualities. Contemporary youths now have a language, and thus a meaning, for experiences formerly considered unspeakable. Whereas previous cohorts of boys reported awareness earlier than girls, this is far less true today, likely a result of growing acceptance of female sexuality (Diamond and Savin-Williams 2009; Rosario et al. 1996).

Relative to males, female eroticism is more frequently experienced as romantic than physical. For example, girls were more likely to remember their first same-sex attraction as an emotional attachment or crush; boys, as a sexual thought, arousal, or behavior (Savin-Williams and Diamond 2000; Troiden 1979). It is unknown whether this reflects differences in biology, socialization, or both. The sexual attractions of females often are more dependent on interpersonal relationships and more influenced by cultural and social contexts, such as conversations and university courses (Diamond 2008). The implication is that women are more responsive to external circumstances and thus sexually more variable across their life course (Baumeister 2000; Diamond 2008; Peplau et al. 1999).

As a predictor of sexual orientation, the presence of same-sex attractions may not be the best developmental indicator. Recent research documents that many heterosexually identified individuals report some degree of same-sex attractions or behavior (Vrangalova and Savin-Williams 2012). In addition, as many as 80% of lesbians and 60% of gay men experience opposite-sex attractions and fantasies (Rosario et al. 1996). Developmentally, sexual and romantic attractions that are consistent with one's sexual orientation emerge earlier than those that are not, and early sexual attractions are unrelated to the timing of other developmental milestones, such as coming out to self and others, dating, and accepting one's sexuality.

Overall, most youths report that they were not disturbed by their early homoeroticism because it felt natural and enjoyable, simply a reflection of who they were (Savin-Williams 2005). When, however, these desires failed to dissipate with time, suspicion that one might be lesbian, gay, or bisexual could prompt a period of sexual uncertainty, questioning (and possibly a visit to a clinician to help with its resolution), or elaborate denial. Increasingly, however, contemporary youths do not question their sexuality because they know almost simultaneously that their same-sex attractions signify a sexual-minority status.

Questioning Assumed Heterosexuality

Same-sex attractions eventually take on sufficient meaning that individuals recognize they might not be totally heterosexual. Emerging clarity can elicit further sexual questioning, the resolution of which may not include the assumption of a sexual-minority identity label. Believing that it is a phase or experimentation, or that everyone is similarly homoerotic, allows individuals to minimize or discount their sexual desires. Others consider their sexual fantasies—but not themselves—to be gay, or if they are willing to assume more personal responsibility, they may concede that they are "slightly" gay (read: *bisexual*).

Mental health professionals can be especially effective in helping patients work through a challenging developmental milestone that is sometimes characterized by fear and sadness but more often manifests as sexual confusion. Sexual orientation clarification begins with educating patients about the distinctions among sexual orientation, behavior, and identity. Exploration of sexual behavior, emotional connectedness, attractions, and sexual fantasies before and during orgasm allows the clinician to inform patients about sexual domain inconsistencies and those elements that matter most (erotic attraction, crushes) and least (behavior, identity) in determining sexual orientation. This form of education is especially useful when treating gay men who report sexual orientation confusion, because they tend to place excessive weight on their emotional connections with females while minimizing their erotic attractions toward males. For many, this allows them to maintain hope for an eventual heterosexuality. This distinction, however, may be less clear among women, for whom emotional affiliation is more closely related to sexual orientation and often *precedes* sexual arousal. Whether these distinctive gender patterns hold for contemporary youth is not yet clear. For example, sexual fluidity, once thought to be the province of young women, is now reported among young men as well (Savin-Williams et al. 2012).

Inviting patients to recount their history of same-sex attractions facilitates understanding and organization of their past while illustrating its omnipresence. Clarity increases as memories previously considered innocuous assume greater meaning and support the "normality" and intractability of the patient's homoeroticism. As a revised narrative evolves, defenses and confusion often give way to recognition and understanding, if not yet acceptance and pride.

Same-Sex Behavior

Although the average age of the first same-sex encounter is 14 years, engaging in such behavior can precede, co-occur with, or follow other developmental milestones. In fact, 5%–10% of boys and 20% of girls embrace a same-sex identity *prior* to experiencing same-sex behavior (Savin-Williams 2005). Contrary to stereotypes, and surprisingly to many clinicians, relatively few gay- or lesbian-identified individuals participate exclusively in same-sex behavior across the life course. Although individuals from a variety of sexual orientations acknowledge same-sex encounters, those who are primarily homoerotic pursue such interactions with greater frequency and enthusiasm and obtain greater physical and emotional satisfaction.

In contrast to women, same-sex-attracted men report slightly earlier and more same-sex behavior with a greater number of partners, usually before heterosexual experiences. First homoerotic relations for women typically occur with a friend or someone they are dating, but for men they are far more likely to take place in the context of a purely sexual interaction, despite stated preferences for "relationship sex" (Savin-Williams 2005).

Lesbian and bisexual women are more likely than men to participate in heterosexual sex within a dating or friendship relationship, beginning at an earlier age and prior to same-sex contact. Although women's documented sexual fluidity may explain their greater participation and assumed interest in heterosexual encounters, they may also be exposed more than gay men to sexual invitations when dating. Nonetheless, both sexes typically experience first heterosexual sex within a dating relationship (Baumeister 2000; Diamond 2008; Diamond and Savin-Williams 2009).

Self-Identification

Coming out to oneself—the recognition that one's same-sex attractions, crushes, fantasies, or behaviors are meaningful and signify a nonheterosexual sexuality—is a milestone that can be both terrifying and relieving. Although this previously occurred well into one's twenties, contemporary cohorts are recognizing and naming their sexuality while still in high school or in some instances as young as age 10 (Savin-Williams 2005). Whereas young men may take months or years to progress from recognizing to naming their feelings, young women typically make the transition far more quickly. It is not uncommon for women to recognize, name, and disclose to others their homoeroticism all within a few days or months, or even shortly after entering a same-sex romantic relationship. Bisexual individuals may take longer to reach this developmental milestone, perhaps because their sexual identity is somewhat more fluid over time. Often, their preference for sexual and romantic involvement with one sex solidifies with age (Rust 2002).

Transcending historic notions of sexuality and related classifications, some young women and men are redefining sexual identity categories or rejecting them altogether. Rejecting narrow definitions of sexuality based on unidimensional, fixed precepts, a growing constituency of youth refuse labels, embrace notions of sexual fluidity, and characterize their sexuality as an interaction between their erotic preferences and their gender identity (e.g., a male-identified woman attracted to males who identifies as "gay male"). Self-definitions may be dynamic and unspecified (omnisexual, pansexual, heteroflexible), a conduit for amalgamating multiple identities (bi-lesbian, half-dyke, transboi), or rejection of sexual taxonomy altogether (unlabeled, undeclared, or simply "I love Rachael").

Others eschew sexual labels because they fear negative social and cultural repercussions or prefer to emphasize other aspects of self considered more important (e.g., religion, race, ethnicity). Still others reject traditional classifications because of the associated stereotypes that they find unacceptable. Consequently, individuals may acknowledge same-sex attraction and behavior but deny that they are gay, lesbian, or bisexual.

Studying female sexuality over a decade, Diamond's (2008) prospective longitudinal investigation found that many same-sex-attracted women considered their sexuality to be fluid and that most had experienced several changes in sexual identity since childhood. Common was the belief that sexual labels are limiting and that individual characteristics can trump gender in determining romantic interest. Although some women eventually embraced a heterosexual label, they insisted that their same-sex attractions persisted.

Stereotypes associated with terms such as *lesbian, bisexual,* and *gay* prevent some homoerotic individuals from recognizing and naming, in some form, their sexuality, and that can impede self-acceptance. Clinicians can encourage this process by gently posing the question, "What if you *are* gay/lesbian/bisexual?" and encouraging full articulation of implications and consequences before attempting to challenge and educate the patient. Permitting detailed expression of anticipated losses in relationships, identity, and expected heterosexual life, as well as shame-related personal beliefs (e.g., one is immoral, weak, mentally ill), facilitates the grieving that is often necessary for eventual acceptance.

Disclosure

Coming out to others is a lifelong process during which same-sex-attracted individuals repeatedly face the decision whether to reveal their sexuality to family, friends, coworkers, and new acquaintances. Despite minimal empirical support, mental health professionals generally believe that self-disclosure, when appropriately delivered, is a positive behavior that facilitates personal integrity, identity synthesis, and psychological health—especially over time as it replaces diminishing fears of ridicule and threats to physical safety (Cohen and Savin-Williams 2004).

For young men, disclosure to others usually first occurs several years after coming out to self. As noted previously, the gap between the two for young women is somewhat less. Increasingly, the recipient of first disclosure for both young men and women is a best female friend, though it is no longer rare to first reveal one's sexuality to a sibling, another same-sex-attracted peer, or a supportive heterosexual male friend. When objects of disclosure are carefully chosen, reactions are almost always positive, even celebratory. Indeed, today's generation of MTV-viewing, Internet-porn-consuming young adults consider sexual diversity to be normal and positive and thus are typically nonplussed when peers come out (Savin-Williams 2005). Thus, it is not uncommon for friends to progress quickly from mild surprise (or amused confirmation) to resolute determination that they will help find their same-sex-attracted friend a sexual or romantic partner.

Unique challenges may confront gender-nonconforming and ethnic and racial minority youth. The latter may face additional barriers to coming out to self and others as they reconcile an "atypical" sexuality that is unacceptable to their primary community (Greene 1994) (see also the subsection "Coming Out as Double Minority" in Chapter 1 of this book, "What's In Your Closet?"). Beleaguered by charges of betraying their ethnic/racial community by voluntarily adopting a "white man's disease," they may be left alone to navigate, or abandon altogether, the process of sexual development in mostly white gay subcultures in which racism can be unrecognized or unchallenged. However, some experience considerable support from their ethnic/racial community if it emphasizes family centeredness and protection of "one of our own." Gender-nonconforming individuals whose behavior and interests deviate significantly from those of their peers must also reconcile a lifetime of ridicule and harassment for a gender presentation that was likely linked by others to homosexuality long before they themselves realized the connection. Suffering verbal and physical abuse by peers may leave these patients with posttraumatic stress disorder symptoms (see Chapter 14, "Posttraumatic Stress Disorder") and resistance to accepting a homoerotic label that acknowledges the shameful truth of peer accusations.

Disclosing one's sexuality to others may be embraced as a means for obtained personal authenticity, social support, interpersonal closeness, freedom from the trepidation of discovery and anticipated rejection, dissuasion of a heterosexual suitor, and, when the other is similarly homoerotic, a potential romantic or sexual partner (Savin-Williams 2005). Reasons for withholding disclosure can include fear of the unknown, avoidance of disappointing others, belief that they will become irrevocably boxed in ("What if I later discover I'm not gay, or that I like a girl? What will people think!"), and dread of rejection because of their sexuality. It is noteworthy that youths are increasingly worried about being chastised or rebuked by insulted friends not because of their sexuality per se, but for failing to share it sooner.

Young people may delay disclosing to parents not because the parents are deemed unimportant, but precisely because they are considered to be so very important. Thus, they may first want to be certain about their sexuality before they make this final, most highly significant, disclosure. They may also delay coming out to parents because of the general discomfort youths of all sexual orientations often experience when discussing sexual matters with parents; the implied commitment to a sexuality not yet fully embraced; or fear of emotional devastation and financial ruin (e.g., lost academic financial support) should parents reject their child. Surprisingly, even gay-affirming parents with gay friends may be among the last to know about their child's sexuality because the youth may wish to avoid confronting anticipated parental enthusiasm and encouragement intended to nudge the youth toward self-disclosure and dating sooner than she or he would like.

Nevertheless, adolescents who come out to a parent (usually their mother) while living at home, despite stereotypes and highly publicized instances of abuse and condemnation, seldom receive an ongoing severely negative response. Parental reactions vary from celebration to rejection, but with time most eventually accept what they had long suspected (Savin-Williams 2001). Similar to their children, parents have been helped by normalizing media portrayals and the coming out of friends and coworkers. Indeed, a growing complaint by youths is of parents "outing" their children by directly inquiring about possible homosexuality. Except in extreme situations, such as when a youth's life or health is at risk, we recommend that clinicians advise parents that it is best to allow young people to decide on their own when to come out to parents and others.

Romantic Relationships

Desire for a committed romantic relationship is articulated by most sexual-minority individuals, but until recently, such a relationship was considered to be unobtainable until living away from home, safely isolated from the judgmental and punitive eyes of parents and peers. Thus, it is common to have a first same-sex date when one is a freshman in college or first entering the workforce. Although most youths continue to postpone dating until such times, growing cultural acceptance of sexual diversity and peer support (e.g., school-based Gay-Straight Alliance clubs) are motivating young people to come out while still in high school, where they can date or take a same-sex friend or partner to the prom.

This increasing acceptance was documented by Diamond and Lucas (2004), who found that sexual-minority youths did not differ from heterosexual youths in number of romantic relationships, especially among those who were most out and thus more able to identify and attract potential dating partners. Youths who had romantic relationships were less likely to report feeling depressed and anxious (cause and effect were not addressed). However, sexual-minority youths were more likely than heterosexual youths to fear not finding the type of relationship they wanted, and sexual-minority young men, in particular, faced obstacles to developing highly intimate same-sex relationships during their teen years (Diamond and Dubé 2002).

As with heterosexual dating, few of these early relationships are enduring, yet they afford important opportunities for psychosocial exploration, development and integration of emotional and sexual intimacy, and acquisition of a positive identity. Clinicians can reassure those who are pining for romance that they are not alone in desiring a romantic attachment, because many, if not most, sexual-minority individuals are seeking emotional intimacy. Locations and strategies for finding partners mirror those of heterosexual persons, although unique challenges should be acknowledged. For example, sexual-minority individuals must search within a smaller pool of potential homoerotic partners containing many who are closeted and perhaps unidentifiable. Consequently, they may convey interest toward heterosexual individuals whom they erroneously believe to be romantically or sexually available, creating possibly dangerous repercussions.

Self-Acceptance and Synthesis

Considered in many coming-out models to be among the final developmental stages, acceptance of one's sexuality and its synthesis with other aspects of personal identity can be achieved at any point in the life course. Bisexuals, lesbians, and gay men who attain sexual identity synthesis recognize the importance of their same-sex sexuality but no longer experience it as all-consuming or overarching; it is simply one of many aspects of self. Thus, a woman who earlier defined herself as a lesbian schoolteacher would now see herself as a schoolteacher who happens to be attracted to women.

Despite stereotypical representations of the tragic lives of gay youths, contemporary studies find that sexual-minority youths are as content with their lives as are heterosexual youths (reviewed in Savin-Williams 2005). For example, two-thirds of lesbian and gay adolescents reported feeling anywhere from indifferent to very good about their sexuality; less than one-tenth expressed a desire to "not be gay." If given the option, most would not take a "magic pill" to make them straight. Youths also can be content with their same-sex orientation without identifying as a sexual minority. For example, a now-dated study, the findings of which remain true, documented that whereas many youths feel good shortly after identifying as gay, others are positive about their sexuality prior to identifying (Sears 1991). Individuals might never identify as gay yet nonetheless accept and integrate their same-sex attractions with other domains of their life.

Those who remain ambivalent, conflicted, or rejecting of their sexuality often experience low self-esteem and attenuated life satisfaction. Clinicians can assist same-sex-attracted patients to accept, and even experience pride about, their sexuality. Whether they identify as a sexual minority is less important than acquiring the ability to integrate their sexuality with other essential elements of their lives, the results of which are authenticity, peace, and positive social interactions.

Notable and challenging exceptions to these outcomes are sexual minorities who, often for cultural reasons, are unable or unwilling to live a sexually open and integrated life. For example, foreign nationals temporarily residing in North America (e.g., for education, as a visiting scholar, on a work visa) or members of conservative racial/ethnic groups or religiously orthodox communities may have limited opportunities for sexual authenticity if they wish to avoid real or feared widespread social admonishment in their own country or culture. In such cases, help in clarifying their sexuality (especially by disentangling obligation from desire) is usually followed by exploration of viable options. For example, patients returning home to a country in which homosexuality is condemned may choose to address their lack of heterosexual interest by concealing their sexual orientation and maintaining a façade of perpetual bachelorhood (for males) or a defined role as family caregiver (for females); participation in underground sexual or gender communities, if any exist, may be the sole avenues for sexual expression. Alternatively, closeted sexual minorities may arrange to marry someone also on the "down low" and thus serve as each other's cover while publicly fulfilling societal mandates for heterosexual coupling and, perhaps, procreation. Or they may reveal their sexual orientation to a potential or current spouse and negotiate a financially stable relationship devoid of sexual intimacy (perhaps after one or more children are conceived) in which discreet sexual infidelity is permitted. Identifying nontraditional routes for integrating personal authenticity and sexual/romantic gratification while ensuring community acceptance is more than some sexual minorities believe possible. Such options may also be sufficient for reinstating hope for a fulfilling, albeit untraditional, life.

Clinical Implications

Same-sex-attracted patients present for mental health services with diverse needs, including those unrelated to their sexuality. Even supportive mental health providers are limited by patients' current understanding of and ability to communicate their same-sex sexuality, which will depend on the developmental milestones these individuals have experienced. Those with accepted and integrated sexualities often require little more than acceptance, respect, and appreciation of the unique developmental and social issues faced by sexual minorities as the clinician addresses the primary concerns that prompted treatment. Whereas some lesbians, gays, and bisexual individuals present with explicit sexual-minority concerns that they permit the clinician to freely explore, more often homoerotic awareness or concern arises indirectly and unexpectedly, such as following unrelenting peer harassment, the end of a relationship, or perceived job discrimination. Some youths may be unwillingly mandated by their parents to seek treatment for gender-atypical behavior and for suspected, or recently discovered, homoeroticism. Still others may repudiate their homosexuality while struggling to achieve or maintain sexual arousal during heterosexual encounters. They may request medical intervention for what they believe to be a physiological problem. Not uncommonly, these patients are prescribed medication to treat impotence or are referred to a urologist for this purpose without adequate assessment of underlying sexual attractions and fantasies, especially those experienced during masturbatory orgasms.

Support of same-sex-attracted individuals and their families requires planning and foresight, beginning with consideration of the first impressions they will receive of the clinician's workplace (office decorations, staff diversity, phrasing of intake forms and oral history). Additionally, medical personnel and staff benefit from sexual diversity training (continuing education, periodic staff training) and familiarity with gay-friendly community resources. Treatment is enhanced and follow-up improved when patients are referred to compassionate and conversant medical specialists. The following recommendations, previously suggested by Cohen and Savin-Williams (2004), should inspire comfort and trust among sexual-minority patients.

Physical Environment

The office environment can convey safety and reflect appreciation for diversity with information pamphlets (e.g., on coming out, same-sex relationships, safer-sex practices, sexually transmitted diseases, HIV/AIDS), lesbian- and gay-oriented magazines (e.g., *Curve, The Advocate*), and gay-affirming posters (same-sex couples, organizations) in the waiting room. Even discrete placement of a rainbow flag, pink triangle, or "safety zone" symbols can inspire comfort among sexual minorities (and their families and allies) who are aware of their meaning. Positioning affirmative gay-themed books (e.g., *Mom, Dad. I'm Gay* and *The New Gay Teenager*) at eye level in the clinician's office can further enhance patient confidence and trust. The Gay and Lesbian Medical Association (GLMA 2006) recommends prominently displaying a nondiscrimination policy statement, in which sexual orientation is included, and establishing unisex restrooms to lessen discomfort among transgender patients.

Intake Form

Intake forms are opportunities to convey recognition that not all patients are heterosexual, by using gender-neutral or bigendered language and assessing all domains of sexuality. Queries about current and past sexual behavior should include the options *males, females,* or *both.* Documentation of sexual identity should encourage truthful disclosure by allowing patients to choose between *heterosexual, lesbian, gay, bisexual, questioning, uncertain,* and *other* (space provided for elaboration). The GLMA (2006) suggests including standard questions about safer sex: "Do you need any information about safer sex techniques? If yes, with: men, women, both" and inquiries about sexual concerns: "Are you currently experiencing any sexual problems?"

Clinical Interview

Using nonoppressive, nondiscriminatory language when taking oral histories validates and supports same-sex-attracted individuals while alerting heterosexual patients to diverse sexualities and modeling respect for those who are not straight. Rather than inquiring about "significant others" or "partners," vague terms that are easily dismissed, it is preferable to ask, "Have you ever been sexually active with a boy/man or a girl/woman, or both?" or "Are you currently dating someone, perhaps a girl/woman or a boy/man, or both?" Questions about sexual behavior should be specific without presupposing heterosexuality. For example, penile-vaginal intercourse should be distinguished from vaginal-object and anal intercourse. It is especially important to use behavior-based language when treating patients who eschew sexual-minority labels but nonetheless engage in same-sex behavior. In such cases, risk assessment and promotion of safer-sex practices is achieved by discussing risky sexual behavior rather than by addressing disavowed sexual identity categories, such as "gay male," that clinicians often use to alert patients to risk.

Following the initial assessment, clinicians can further convey receptivity to diverse sexualities by conducting a detailed sexual history that incorporates timing of and reactions to sexual milestones, social support network, parental reactions, harassment/violence, and other sex- and gender-related psychosocial stressors.

Despite growing awareness and acceptance of nontraditional sexualities, especially in younger cohorts, cultural and religious renunciation of homosexuality prompts some homoerotic individuals to request help with changing their sexual orientation. Although they experience their sexuality as ego-dystonic, they should be informed that to date there is scant evidence that sexual orientation can be altered (American Psychological Association 2009). Whereas sexual identity and behavior are matters are choice, and thus changeable, scientific research has yet to demonstrate that therapy can alter sexual orientation. Rather, the clinician should facilitate self-acceptance and integration of personal identities (including sexual) by challenging stereotypes, educating, and reducing isolation and loneliness.

Key Points

- The process of coming out to self and others consists of multiple developmental milestones, the order, timing, and experience of which vary across individuals.

- The determination of sexual orientation is complex and depends largely on the way in which "gay" is defined. Thus, it is necessary to distinguish among three related domains: sexual orientation, sexual behavior, and sexual identity.

- Estimating the number of nonheterosexual persons depends on which of these sexual domains is assessed, with prevalence rates varying between 1% and 16% across studies.

- The coming out process is best understood by an individual's experience of developmental milestones, including feeling different from peers, being aware of same-sex attractions (with or without attractions to the opposite sex), questioning an assumed heterosexuality, desire for and expression of same-sex sexual behavior, self-identification as not exclusively straight, disclosure of that information to others, romantic relationships with those of the same sex, self-acceptance of one's same-sex sexuality, and synthesis of that understanding with other aspects of one's personal identity.

- Recommendations are offered to clinicians that should inspire comfort and trust among their nonheterosexual patients.

References

American Psychological Association: Report of the American Psychological Association Task Force on Appropriate Therapeutic Responses to Sexual Orientation. Washington, DC, American Psychological Association, 2009

Baumeister RF: Gender differences in erotic plasticity: the female sex drive as socially flexible and responsive. Psychol Bull 126:247–374, 2000

Cass VC: Homosexual identity formation: a theoretical model. J Homosex 4:219–235, 1979

Cohen KM: Relationships among childhood sex-atypical behavior, spatial ability, handedness, and sexual orientation in men. Arch Sex Behav 31:129–43, 2002

Cohen KM, Savin-Williams RC: Growing up with same-sex attractions. Curr Probl Pediatr Adolesc Health Care 34:361–369, 2004

D'Augelli TR, Grossman AH, Starks MT: Gender atypicality and sexual orientation development among lesbian, gay, and bisexual youth: prevalence, sex differences, and parental responses. Journal of Gay and Lesbian Mental Health 12:121–143, 2008

Denizet-Lewis B: Double lives on the down low. The New York Times Magazine, August 3, 2003, pp 28–33, 48, 52–53

Diamond LM: Sexual Fluidity: Understanding Women's Love and Desire. Cambridge, MA, Harvard University Press, 2008

Diamond LM, Dubé EM: Friendship and attachment among heterosexual and sexual-minority youths: does the gender of your friend matter? J Youth Adolesc 31:155–166, 2002

Diamond LM, Lucas S: Sexual-minority and heterosexual youths' peer relationships: experiences, expectations, and implications for well-being. J Res Adolesc 14:313–340, 2004

Diamond LM, Savin-Williams RC: Adolescent sexuality, in Handbook of Adolescent Psychology, 3rd Edition. Edited by Lerner RM, Steinberg L. New York, Wiley, 2009, pp 479–523

Gay and Lesbian Medical Association: Guidelines for care of gay, bisexual, and transgender patients. 2006. Available at: http://www.glma.org/_data/n_0001/resources/live/GLMA%20guidelines%202006%20FINAL.pdf. Accessed November 3, 2011.

Greene B: Ethnic-minority lesbians and gay men: mental health and treatment issues. J Consult Clin Psychol 62:243–251, 1994

LeVay S, Baldwin J: Human Sexuality, 4th Edition. Sunderland, MA, Sinauer Associates, 2012

Peplau LA, Spalding LR, Conley TD, et al: The development of sexual orientation in women. Annu Rev Sex Res 10:70–99, 1999

Rosario M, Meyer-Bahlburg HF, Hunter J, et al: The psychosexual development of urban lesbian, gay, and bisexual youths. J Sex Res 33:113–126, 1996

Rust PC: Bisexuality: the state of the union. Annu Rev Sex Res 13:180–240, 2002

Savin-Williams RC: Mom, Dad. I'm Gay. How Families Negotiate Coming Out. Washington, DC, American Psychological Association, 2001

Savin-Williams RC: The New Gay Teenager. Cambridge, MA, Harvard University Press, 2005

Savin-Williams RC, Diamond LM: Sexual identity trajectories among sexual-minority youth: gender comparisons. Arch Sex Behav 29:419–440, 2000

Savin-Williams RC, Ream GL: Prevalence and stability of sexual orientation components during adolescence and young adulthood. Arch Sex Behav 36:385–394, 2007

Savin-Williams RC, Joyner K, Rieger G: Prevalence and stability of self-reported sexual orientation identity during young adulthood. Arch Sex Behav 41, 2012

Schneider MS: Toward a reconceptualization of the coming-out process for adolescent females, in Lesbian, Gay, and Bisexual Identities and Youth: Psychological Perspectives. Edited by D'Augelli AR, Patterson CJ. New York, Oxford University Press, 2001, pp 71–96

Sears JT: Growing Up Gay in the South: Race, Gender, and Journeys of the Spirit. New York, Harrington Park Press, 1991

Troiden RR: Becoming homosexual: a model of gay identity acquisition. Psychiatry 42:362–373, 1979

Vrangalova Z, Savin-Williams RC: Mostly heterosexual and mostly gay/lesbian: evidence for new sexual orientation identities. Arch Sex Behav 41, 2012

Wiederman MW: Volunteer bias in sexuality research using college student participants. J Sex Res 36:59–66, 1999

Questions

2.1   Which of the following populations will likely show the largest prevalence rate?

        A. Males who engage in same-sex behavior.

        B. Females who identify as mostly heterosexual and report same-sex attraction.

        C. The combination of gay and bisexual males.

        D. Females who identify as bisexual.

The correct answer is B.

As stated in the text: "Prevalence rates varied between 1% and 16% and were highest among females, those who identified as "mostly heterosexual," and when same-sex attractions were measured."

2.2 Which of the following statements is *false*?

  A. Coming out is usually an invariant, universal progression from initial unawareness and confusion to eventual identity pride and synthesis.
  B. Many contemporary youths do not experience sexual confusion, nor are they particularly "proud" to be gay—it is just who they are.
  C. The coming out process is best understood by the achievement of developmental sexual milestones that increasingly occur without respect for tradition, timing, and order.
  D. Some youths have a committed romantic relationship prior to self-labeling and have same-sex activities only after self-identification.

The correct answer is A.

Despite the heuristic appeal and widespread popularity of stage-based coming-out models, linear and idealized portrayals of identity development are not empirically substantiated.

2.3 Parental reactions to their child coming out are best characterized as:

  A. Rejection, with most gay youths being thrown out of the home.
  B. Varying reactions across families, from celebration to rejection.
  C. Pride because of having a legally protected minority within the family.
  D. Stable reactions that seldom change across time, whether they involve celebration or rejection.

The correct answer is B.

Parental reactions vary, from celebration to rejection, but with time most eventually accept what they had long suspected.

From Outlaws to In-Laws

Legal Standing of LGBT Americans' Family Relationships

Jennifer C. Pizer, Esq.

WHAT IS THE "LEGAL STANDING" of lesbian, gay, bisexual, and transgender (LGBT) family relationships in the United States today? As this chapter is finalized in early 2012, six states and the District of Columbia issue marriage licenses equally to same-sex and to different-sex couples.[1] The laws of another five states allow same-sex couples to assume the same legal rights and responsibilities that different-sex couples may assume, but by entering a civil union rather than by marrying.[2] Four states permit same-sex couples to acquire a similarly complete set of state law rights and duties by registering a domestic partnership, which lacks a formal ceremony through which the new legal status is created.[3] Considering these 16 jurisdictions, more than one-third of the U.S. population now lives where state law offers same-sex couples full rights and duties through a state-conferred legal status. Recent studies indicate that 14% of same-sex couples in the United States are married (Badgett et al. 2011). In at

---

[1] The states are Connecticut, Iowa, Massachusetts, New Hampshire, New York, and Vermont.

[2] These states are Delaware, Hawaii, Illinois, New Jersey, and Rhode Island.

[3] These states are California, Nevada, Oregon, and Washington.

least five more states, same-sex couples may register for a more limited state-conferred status entailing decision-making authority in various contexts and sometimes other state law rights as well.[4] Many cities and counties also have registries in which same-sex couples may register their domestic partnership. But because family law rules operate at the state level, these local registries can provide only limited rights and recognition related to functions controlled at the local level.[5]

Two other areas of "family relationship recognition" make up the big picture—the private sector and the federal government. In the private sector, employee benefits (including health insurance for family members and the ability to take family medical leave) are valuable parts of compensation. Thanks to two decades of advocacy by employee groups and others, many of the largest companies voluntarily offer family benefits to employees with a same-sex life partner, and often also to those with an unmarried different-sex partner, as a matter of compensation equity.[6]

Lastly, because of the so-called Defense of Marriage Act (DOMA) enacted by Congress in 1996, federal law ignores the marital status of married lesbian and gay couples. This means the estimated 50,000 to 80,000 married same-sex couples in the United States are treated for federal law purposes as single, despite having full legal responsibilities and rights under state law.[7] Because of Obama administration policy changes, the picture has improved for federal employees, for whom workplace benefits now include recognition of same-sex partners and children for many benefits such as family medical leave, bereavement leave, and relocation benefits, but not spousal health insurance.[8] In addition, the Administration has been making changes in agency regulations to per-

---

[4] These states include Colorado, Hawaii, Maine, Maryland, and Wisconsin.

[5] These rights and recognitions can include health insurance and other family benefits for local government employees who have an unmarried life partner of the same or different sex, as well as family discounts at county museums and "family member" visitation privileges in local facilities such as hospitals and jails.

[6] According to survey data, 39% of Fortune 1000, 57% of Fortune 500, and 83% of Fortune 100 companies offer their employees benefits to cover a same-sex partner (Human Rights Campaign 2009). Note that these voluntary benefits are a term of employment and generally end when an employee leaves a job, and that an employer's choice to recognize its workers' family relationships does not entail recognition by government or other private parties, such as other businesses. In addition, despite the example set by these large companies, it is estimated that 70%–80% of private businesses, employing millions of workers, do not offer domestic partner benefits (Kaiser Family Foundation and Health Research and Educational Trust 2009). These conditions contribute to the reality that those in same-sex relationships tend to be uninsured and underinsured to a disproportionate extent (see Ponce et al. 2010).

[7] See Williams Institute S.598 testimony (Badgett et al. 2011).

mit some protections for same-sex partners in areas where private institutions receive federal funds, such as requiring fairness in hospital visitation, home mortgages and rental housing, and certain protections against partner impoverishment from the cost of long-term nursing home care.[9] At the same time, these improvements do not fully alleviate the financial, practical, and emotional harms that DOMA inflicts by requiring the vast body of federal law and regulations to treat married lesbian and gay people as *un*married.[10]

The U.S. constitutional system of state sovereignty with mandatory interstate cooperation makes things considerably more complicated. Although state family law and related rules sometimes vary greatly, individual states have evolved independently and voluntarily to the current status in which they usually respect the marriages and parent-child relationships that other states allow for their own residents, even if a particular state's own rules are different. Thus, when heterosexual couples and their families move to a new state, they sometimes find themselves subject to new, unexpected rules, but married couples can expect to remain married, and to remain legally bound to their children, whether their parental ties exist as a result of the adults' legal relationship or from an adoption decree or other court order. Further, when a married, heterosexual couple travels and faces a question of whether their home state's law or the different law of the place they are visiting controls, there generally is a settled approach for deciding which state has a stronger interest in enforcing its law. This system of interstate cooperation—often called "comity law"—exists against the backdrop of the U.S. Constitution's "Full Faith and Credit" and "Privileges and Immunities" clauses, which call upon states to respect one another's sovereignty while facilitating fair treatment of those who travel.

In the past roughly 15 years, however, about four-fifths of the states have created antigay exceptions to these rules, with three-fifths having done so by amending their constitutions. State family law rules have varied in the past, such as in their treatment of women and in criminalization or acceptance of interracial relationships. But the opposition to equal treatment of LGBT people—especially following law reform movements that largely have eliminated differential laws based on race, national origin, and sex—has been in dramatic con-

---

[8] The presidential memorandum providing some family benefits for federal workers with a same-sex partner, but not spousal health insurance, is posted at http://www.whitehouse.gov/the_press_office/Memorandum-for-the-Heads-of-Executive-Departments-and-Agencies-on-Federal-Benefits-and-Non-Discrimination-6-17-09.

[9] The presidential memorandum requiring hospitals that receive federal funding to respect patient wishes concerning visitation and surrogate decision making, if those wishes were put in writing, is available at http://www.whitehouse.gov/the-press-office/presidential-memorandum-hospital-visitation.

[10] See Williams Institute S.598 testimony (Badgett et al. 2011).

trast to the predictability and practicality achieved over the years for heterosexual couples and their families. These politics have forged an interstate legal landscape that is discriminatory and confusing in complex new ways. However, the consequences—unintended by many voters—are inspiring stronger calls for reform, including for interim steps to reduce the harms in the meantime.[11]

Indeed, laws and court rules are changing at an encouraging pace, although not nearly fast enough for the roughly 9 million people living in the United States today who identify as LGB or T (Gates 2011), of whom nearly 600,000 are in same-sex relationships (Gates and Cooke 2011), with roughly twenty percent of them raising 250,000 children (Badgett 2010).

In the United States, only 21 states and the District of Columbia explicitly protect workers against sexual orientation discrimination on the job, and only 7 explicitly protect against gender identity discrimination (National Gay and Lesbian Task Force 2011); federal law does not explicitly forbid either form of employment bias, though some protection exists under more general laws and the U.S. Constitution.[12] State and federal antibias protections are similarly inadequate regarding education, housing, health care services, financial services, and other commercial transactions. And even where civil rights laws are comprehensive and civic leaders trumpet a welcoming climate, antigay attitudes remain pervasive (Sears and Mallory 2011). Great numbers of LGBT Americans thus still live in fear of losing financial and personal security.

Why the Law Matters to Mental Health Professionals

Why discuss the state of the law in a book about mental health needs? There are several reasons. First, it is helpful for health professionals to grasp how the legal system's inclusion or exclusion of same-sex couples may be causing or exacerbating a patient's anxiety, depression, or other psychiatric conditions. In addition, from a practical perspective, mental health professionals may need to know who has decision-making authority and/or responsibility if a patient becomes incapacitated, and with whom a patient's information may be shared if a

---

[11] For example, in addition to the regulatory changes referenced above, President Obama also has endorsed the Respect for Marriage Act, which would repeal DOMA (http://www.whitehouse.gov/blog/2011/07/19/president-obama-supports-respect-marriage-act). It now has 32 sponsors in the Senate and 138 sponsors in the House of Representatives.

[12] Note that the federal and state constitutions apply only against government, and separate civil rights laws are required to constrain the conduct of private businesses and individuals.

patient cannot say. Absent a formal designation by the patient, state law usually allocates authority according to legally recognized family relationships. Absent a competent spouse, the law usually empowers adult children, siblings, or other relatives to speak for one who is incapacitated. Likewise, a parent may consent to or refuse medical care for a minor child as long as the parent has a legal tie to the child. Those with deeply meaningful but legally unrecognized relationships usually have no right to make decisions or even to receive information. The legal status of relationships also frequently determines whether a person is eligible for health insurance as a member of the primary insured's family, or for victim services or compensation when a loved one has been injured or killed.

It therefore can be necessary for mental health professionals to consider at the start of a treatment relationship, and to reconfirm over time, who plays an important role in a patient's life and whether those whom a patient would wish to be involved in his or her care have the necessary authorization.

Origins of Law Reform

Historically, American law has not treated LGBT people and their families fairly and with respect. Until recently, the law—like the health professions—did not recognize sexual orientation and gender identity as characteristics that exist along a spectrum for everyone. The tide was turning by 1996, when the U.S. Supreme Court was asked to consider the validity of a state constitutional amendment approved by Colorado's voters to negate antidiscrimination laws enacted by the municipalities of Aspen, Boulder, and Denver to protect lesbians, gay men, and bisexual persons. Colorado's Amendment Two required that protections for LGB people could be passed only at the state level. The U.S. Supreme Court concluded the amendment was invalid because, by closing the doors of local government and requiring that just this minority group take its requests for help to the state level, it violated the federal guarantee of equal protection.[13]

In 2003, the U.S. Supreme Court invalidated the remaining state sodomy laws as inconsistent with constitutional guarantees of individual liberty. Justice Kennedy's lead opinion expresses concern for the lives and dignity of gay people and deems same-sex relationships worthy of constitutional respect.[14] The decision ensured that no longer could sodomy laws continue to be invoked as reasons to fire workers, to deny parents custody of their own children, and to restrict student speech and organizing, among other things. This marked a new era for LGBT Americans by affirming that the constitutional guarantees of liberty and equality apply without regard to sexual orientation.

---

[13] *Romer v. Evans,* 517 U.S. 620 (1996).
[14] *Lawrence v. Texas,* 539 U.S. 558 (2003).

Where We Are Now

The Supreme Court's *Romer* and *Lawrence* decisions, although breakthroughs, did not entirely erase the many prior adverse rulings or the countless court decisions, laws, and policies discriminating against LGBT people. Thus, the movement to reform American law—state by state and at the federal level—continues. The rapid pace of this reform is the reason why this chapter requires a time marker.

Looking forward, then, four features characterize this period of legal and policy reform. *First* is the gulf between parts of the country in which same-sex couples are fully equal, with the same opportunities to create family relationships within marriage as different-sex couples, and other regions in which family recognition is denied through explicit state laws and/or constitutional amendments. Because family law historically has been the province of the states, geographic diversity is not a new phenomenon. What is new is the rapid divergence of states—from a consistent, but largely unconscious, denial of recognition to same-sex couples, to affirmative recognition in some places and emphatic rejection in others.

Second is the resulting uncertainty and confusion that LGBT people may experience when traveling and the vulnerability and anxiety they can face as a result. The United States is one country, and as a modern society it is highly mobile. Ideas are influenced by a dominant national news and entertainment market. Many businesses operate on a national, if not an international, scale and expect employees to travel frequently and sometimes to relocate. Vacation destinations advertise to all corners and try to entice a diversity of travelers. Geographic and cultural distances have seemed to shrink for many Americans. But this is much less true for LGBT people.

Third is that the federal government still largely denies the existence of married gay couples by expressly reserving federal marital benefits and protections, such as Social Security spousal support and equal federal tax treatment, only to heterosexually married Americans, despite the thousands of married same-sex couples in the country.

Fourth is the attention being paid to the needs of LGBT people, and to their families, and the resulting pace of change. The direction of the change process now appears clearly toward inclusion and eventual equality. This means there is pride, optimism, and impatience where once there was mostly shame, fear, and hiding. But with rapid positive change in some places, and backlash in others, many LGBT people are confused, and even overwhelmed, by questions regarding matters most Americans do not think twice about. These can range from whether rental car companies will see a couple as a family or charge them an "extra driver" fee, and whether to complete one or two U.S. customs "family" declaration forms, to whether their state and federal tax returns should be consistent.

These four features characterize family law today, both in the rules recognizing same-sex couples or not and in those governing their parent-child relationships.

What follows are brief descriptions of the systems regulating these relationships, including ways that current law sometimes protects, sometimes excludes, and sometimes creates confusion, depending on where couples are and the issues they face.

The State-by-State Patchwork of Rules Establishing Rights and Responsibilities for Adult Couples

The most visible features of marriage may be those relating to solemnization of a couple's new status. But the rights and duties with respect to each other, relatives, and society can provide essential crisis management for couples and their dependents, including entitlement to financial and other supports. As noted earlier, in the absence of a formal designation of someone, the law determines who can make decisions for a patient and have access to information. The person designated by default may be an estranged blood relative rather than the patient's trusted, day-to-day companion.

Likewise, if a patient's mental health is being affected by relationship problems, it can be helpful for those providing treatment to know whether she or he is stressed because a former partner is breaking a promise of support, or because the patient just realized the law will not enforce the promise. Is the patient feeling betrayed by the former partner, or also by a discriminatory society? Perhaps the patient also is angry at himself or herself for not having understood his or her legal vulnerability. Given how the law is improving in some states and not in others, it is easier than ever for LGBT people to be optimistic that those in authority will treat a same-sex partnership the same way as a heterosexual marriage; yet in many places, such optimism will prove unfounded.

What follows is an overview of issues to be considered, keeping in mind that 1) the legal details are evolving in some parts of the country and not in others at present; 2) federal law has only just started to recognize same-sex couples; 3) many employers have brought their benefit plans in line with their nondiscrimination policies, but a great many have not and are not compelled by law to do so; and 4) the ever-expanding national conversation about marriage equality for same-sex couples can exacerbate the uncertainty and the gulf between the broader rights those couples believe they have and the more limited rights they actually may have.

Marriage And Civil Union: A Comprehensive State Status Created Through a Formal Ceremony

Massachusetts was the first state in the country to require that marriage licenses be issued without regard to the gender or sexual orientation of the applicants. The Iowa Supreme Court reached a similar conclusion, unanimously, in 2009.

In addition, the legislatures of New Hampshire, New York, Vermont, and the District of Columbia all have voted to open marriage to lesbian and gay couples.[15] Connecticut also allows same-sex couples to marry. After that state's legislature created "civil unions" for same-sex couples in 2005, with the same rights and duties as marriage, the Connecticut Supreme Court ruled in 2008 that the separate status was inherently unequal and failed to provide the equality that the state's constitution requires.[16]

The Vermont legislature first coined the term *civil unions* back in 2000, after that state's supreme court ruled that lesbian and gay couples are entitled to equal rights and responsibilities but left open whether that could be accomplished through a separate status or whether marriage must be opened. The New Hampshire legislature followed Vermont's lead, passing a civil unions law in 2008. Both state legislatures then voted in the spring of 2009 to open marriage to same-sex couples and to phase out civil unions. Similarly, in the District of Columbia, the city council created a comprehensive domestic partnership system open to both same-sex and different-sex couples, then opened marriage equally to all couples regardless of gender and sexual orientation, following fast on the heels of Vermont and New Hampshire. Couples in the District can have either partnership or marriage, but not both; if a same-sex couple marries, doing so terminates their domestic partnership.

Of the five states that now allow adult couples to enter into a civil union, Delaware, New Jersey, and Rhode Island offer the status to same-sex couples only, with the same rights and duties as marriage but a separate legal meaning and, as a practical matter, a lesser social status. Hawaii and Illinois, in contrast, offer that separate status without regard to gender or sexual orientation.

Public Registration Systems for Extending Legal Protections and Recording Couples' Commitments

In contrast with the states that have opened marriage or created civil unions, others use a centralized registration system that allows same-sex couples (and

---

[15] In the spring of 2009, the Maine legislature also approved marriage for same-sex couples, and Governor Baldacci signed the bill. But the change was reversed by a voter referendum in November 2009. The Washington State legislature passed a marriage bill and Governor Gregoire signed it in February 2012, although a repeal referendum contest is anticipated. That same week, New Jersey's governor vetoed a similar bill. Lastly, as this chapter is finalized, a bill to allow same-sex couples to marry in Maryland appeared headed for Governor O'Malley's signature.

[16] The Connecticut Supreme Court drew extensively from the May 2008 California Supreme Court decision that, under that state's constitution, lesbian and gay couples must be allowed to marry. An estimated 18,000 same-sex couples married in California between June and November 2008, when voters passed Proposition 8, placing the different-sex-only marriage restriction into the California Constitution.

sometimes different-sex couples) to record the existence of a domestic partnership already formed, without need for a license or solemnization. California was first to take what had been a local registration concept to the state level, in 2000 allowing same-sex couples to file a form with the secretary of state's office and thereby acquire minimal legal rights. In subsequent years, the legislature expanded the rights and obligations of registered couples to nearly those of married couples. Then, in 2009, the California Supreme Court held that the rights offered to gay and nongay couples must be fully equal as a matter of state constitutional law, except for the different-sex requirement for marriage.[17]

Washington and Oregon have followed a similar path, with Washington reaching the goal of complete state rights and duties for registered partners in multiple steps between 2007 and 2009, and Oregon doing so with one law in 2007. Nevada enacted a partnership system with full rights and duties in 2009, with two key distinctions. First, the registry is open to both same- and different-sex couples (like civil unions in Hawaii and Illinois). Second, leaving a blatant and constitutionally suspect discrimination, it excludes equal benefits for state workers with a registered partner rather than a spouse.

Maine and Wisconsin also have state-level partnership registries, but with limited rights similar to the interim protections California and Washington adopted for a time. Since 1997, Hawaii has allowed any two adults of same or different sexes who are ineligible to marry to register as "reciprocal beneficiaries," and thereby acquire limited protections; approval of Hawaii's civil unions legislation in 2011 did not eliminate this registration system. Colorado has created a similar status called "designated beneficiaries," which permits two adults to designate each other for various purposes without attesting to an intimate domestic relationship.

As noted earlier, these state registration systems built on a concept first adopted at the municipal level, starting in the mid-1980s. The local registries have limited ability to convey legal rights, as municipalities generally lack authority over key subject areas, such as spousal and child support, inheritance, medical decision making, torts, tax, and evidence. At the same time, any official recognition of same-sex relationships helps to insist that such relationships be respected. Also, the public recording of couples' intentions—even locally—can be relevant in later disputes with third parties, or if the couple breaks up. In addition, some municipalities use their registries to offer partner benefits to their employees, and some private employers do as well.[18]

---

[17] In *Strauss v. Horton*, 46 Cal. 4th 364 (2009), the California Supreme Court upheld Proposition 8 but also ruled that those same-sex couples who married before its passage remain married, and that the remaining state equality guarantee requires that the rights and duties offered to different-sex couples through marriage and to same-sex couples through domestic partnership registration must be the same.

Agreements Authorizing One to Act or Provide Benefits for Another

Through a formal writing—often called a *power of attorney*—a competent adult may designate another to act on his or her behalf in a range of contexts. These commonly include medical decision making,[19] visitation in a health care setting, or acting with respect to financial or other matters. State laws usually impose requirements to make sure such private documents reflect an individual's free and informed actions.

Often a document designed for health care settings will specify that it acquires force only when the individual is incapacitated or for another reason unable to act for himself or herself. Such documents also may select among blood relatives who otherwise would have equal legal authority to speak, and might disagree. Most important for many LGBT people, such a document can override the legal presumption that a blood or legal relative has authority to make a decision and/or to visit, and instead can authorize any other person or multiple people to do so.

An individual's ability to choose whom he or she wishes to act on his or her behalf does not require that state law allow that individual to enter into any particular form of relationship with the person or persons so designated. Unlike the state's power to create a family status for the range of purposes governed by family law (including rights to receive benefits from third parties and the government), private documents recording individuals' wishes about matters over which they have sole authority should be honored even in states with laws denying legal recognition to same-sex couples as couples.

In addition to a power of attorney for medical decisions, other key documents for giving force to one's choices include a will, trust, or other estate plan; powers of attorney for financial matters; up-to-date beneficiary designations for one's 401(k) or other retirement accounts; life insurance policies; annuities; and other financial planning tools (see Lambda Legal 2010; see also Burda 2004; Clifford et al. 2010). As discussed in the next subsection, options vary among

---

[18] Whether to require public registration of an employee's domestic relationship or to rely on a private affidavit system is the employer's choice. In some places especially, an employee may be deterred from accessing family health insurance by fear of coming out as an LGBT person in the absence of an antidiscrimination law. But employees can be just as worried about revealing their sexual orientation to their employer within a confidential affidavit system. These fears appear to be among the reasons that same-sex partners remain underinsured (Ponce et al. 2010).

[19] These also are called a *health care proxy* and can include an *advance health care directive,* recording an individual's wishes about accepting or refusing life-sustaining treatment if it were to be concluded that the person is sufficiently damaged or in pain, will not recover, and cannot express his or her wishes.

states for protecting parent-child relationships, and an ounce of completing an option is worth many pounds of later attempted cure. Lastly, although family courts do not always enforce relationship contracts as written, such documents can be invaluable evidence of what each party understood about the other, understood both to have agreed, and intended for their relationship.[20]

Same-Sex Couples and Parenthood

The federal and state constitutions protect each person's right to have and raise their own children. That does not, however, entail rights to insist that the government provide parenthood through adoption, fostering, or publicly funded reproductive assistance. In past decades, most lesbians and gay men became parents through a heterosexual relationship and only later came out. Many then faced bias in court if the nongay parent asserted that the child would suffer if raised by a lesbian or gay parent.

As discussed by Barber in Chapter 4 of this book, "LGBT Parenting," however, much has changed. Today, while more same-sex couples are adopting children jointly, more also are having children together, with medical assistance, in ways that leave one of the adults without a legal relationship with the couple's child or children. Just as when a child predated the adults' relationship or when one adult adopts singly, the law considers the other adult a "nonparent" who usually cannot make decisions for the child or provide health or other benefits that depend on a legal bond. Likewise, if the legal parent dies or the adults' relationship fails, the nonlegal parent may have no rights to continue the parent-child relationship, and the child may have no claim for support, intestate inheritance, or other benefits from the "nonparent," even if that adult has been a parent in daily reality since the child's birth.

Parental status often arises from biology (genes and/or gestation) but also can be created by a court order. Adoption is the most common and can be individual, joint, or by a step- or "second" parent. In step- and second-parent adoptions, a parent consents to creation of parental rights in another adult, without relinquishing her own rights.

State law also can presume parental status in specified circumstances, such as when an adult receives a child into his home and holds the child out as his own. Or, if a child is born to a married couple, both spouses may be presumed to be parents even if a third adult donated genetic material or caused the pregnancy through intercourse.

---

[20] Consider especially the discussion of pre- and postnuptial (and analogous pre- and post–domestic partnership registration) agreements in Hertz and Doskow 2011.

These presumptions can be very helpful for same-sex couples who plan for a child together, as they need at least genetic material from elsewhere, if not also a gestational surrogate. But although a presumption may allow both partners to be seen as parents in their home state, they should reduce that presumption to a court order and/or also obtain an adoption judgment if possible. This is because the Full Faith and Credit clause requires states to respect other states' *judgments* even when they disagree with the underlying *laws*. Presumptions, in contrast, commonly lose force when one leaves that state.

Some issues remain unclear as new forms of parentage judgments are used by courts, especially for couples who have had children with medical assistance, because these judgments cost less (but have fewer procedural safeguards) than adoption. Lawyers often recommend second-parent adoption rather than a parentage judgment because it is clearer that adoption judgments should be respected state-to-state. But any form of judgment is better than a presumption, and a legal presumption is better than nothing.

Lastly, even in states without procedures allowing both same-sex parents to secure their parental ties, a legal parent can express her wishes in writing about who should be named guardian of a child or children should that need arise. Courts do not always honor such plans even if formalized, but making such arrangements can help.

Federal Discrimination Against Same-Sex Couples

Whether a same-sex couple is married, in another state relationship status, or not, federal law does not and cannot treat them equally at present. For those legally married, the so-called Defense of Marriage Act (DOMA)[21] restricts the terms *spouse* and *marriage* for federal-law purposes to different-sex partners and their legal union. It also purports to allow states to ignore any interstate-respect duties the federal Full Faith and Credit clause may impose concerning same-sex couples' lawful marriages.

There were no legally married lesbian or gay couples in the United States, or anywhere in the world, when Congress enacted DOMA. But 15 years later, because of that law, tens of thousands of married same-sex couples with full legal obligations under state law cannot file their federal income tax returns jointly, still face federal estate taxes as if they were unrelated, are not recognized for Social Security purposes and some important impoverishment protections in

---

[21] Congress passed DOMA in 1996, after the Hawaii Supreme Court required a trial to test the state's different-sex-only marriage law. That trial—with dueling experts addressing the needs of children—drew national attention and prompted Congress to pass DOMA in record time.

Medicaid, and lack the ability to have a foreign-born spouse immigrate. Married lesbian and gay federal employees still are ineligible for some important benefits, especially spousal health insurance. This unequal treatment of federal workers notably includes military service members, who now can serve openly because the Don't Ask, Don't Tell policy is repealed but remain ineligible for equal benefits for their family members, no matter how lengthy or dangerous their service.

In addition, for public and private sector employees alike, the federal tax laws consider health insurance for an employee's same-sex spouse (or domestic partner) to be taxable imputed income, unlike insurance for an employee's different-sex spouse.

As of this writing, DOMA is being challenged in at least a dozen cases, which are expected to take years. They are boosted by the Obama administration's conclusion that DOMA is unconstitutional and does not deserve a defense by the Justice Department, a role briskly taken by lawyers hired by the House of Representatives. In addition, a bill to repeal DOMA is pending in Congress.[22] While many anticipate that it faces a long, contentious road, support seems to be building among the public and national leaders.[23]

DOMA blocks federal benefits for married lesbian and gay couples based on their marital status, but same-sex couples in civil unions and registered domestic partnerships have a different problem—those statuses do not exist in federal law. Yet, as noted earlier, through new regulations and policy changes *not* barred by existing statutes, the Obama administration has begun recognizing same-sex family relationships of federal employees for a range of employee benefits.[24]

---

[22] The Respect for Marriage Act, S.598, was introduced into the Senate in March 2011 by Senator Dianne Feinstein and had 32 cosponsors as of February 2012. Its companion bill was first introduced in the House in 2009 by Representative Jerrold Nadler and was pending in that chamber as H.R.1116 with 138 cosponsors as of February 2012. President Obama formally endorsed it on July 19, 2011, on the eve of its first Senate hearing. See http://www.whitehouse.gov/blog/2011/07/19/president-obama-supports-respect-marriage-act.

[23] According to an April 2009 Quinnipiac University poll, 54% of voters believe the section of DOMA that denies federal benefits and protections to same-sex spouses should be repealed, while 39% support that part of the law. See http://www.quinnipiac.edu/x1295.xml?ReleaseID=1292.

[24] These include family medical leave, childcare, and relocation benefits. See http://www.whitehouse.gov/the_press_office/Memorandum-for-the-Heads-of-Executive-Departments-and-Agencies-on-Federal-Benefits-and-Non-Discrimination-6-17-09. They do not, however, include family health insurance or certain pension benefits. See, e.g., *Golinski v. U.S. Office of Personnel Management,* with case documents available at http://www.lambdalegal.org/in-court/cases/golinski-v-us-office-personnel-management.html.

In the health arena, the Obama administration also is using the power of the federal purse to insist that facilities receiving Medicaid and Medicare funds respect patient wishes for visitation and decision making. Medical staff must honor private documents expressing patient wishes; however, they may not need to respect family relationships that same-sex couples have formalized under state law. Thus, it remains unclear what protection patients will receive if they have not written such documents or if their loved ones cannot produce them. Yet, President Obama's policy condemns antigay discrimination in this context, and favors liberal visitation for patient comfort, within medical norms given a patient's health needs.[25] That message seems likely to inspire greater recognition of same-sex relationships, and of health professionals' duty to treat all patients with respect.

Similarly, the Obama administration has issued new regulations for programs administered by the Department of Housing and Urban Development, to require greater access and protections for same-sex partners. And the Internal Revenue Service now treats "community income" earned by same-sex spouses in California, and by registered domestic partners in California, Nevada, and Washington, the same as community income of married heterosexual couples.[26] In doing so, the IRS is applying long-standing Supreme Court precedents appropriately and has opened a presumably transitional chapter in which same-sex couples must file their federal and state income tax returns according to different rules. This chapter is necessary if same-sex couples are to reach a future in which federal and state laws all recognize them and their families. But it can be confusing and aggravating now for taxpayers, and probably for IRS agents, too, as these rules are unclear in some respects and are inconsistent with the federal laws that still ignore same-sex couples for the range of other federal tax purposes.[27]

One last example of special relevance to health professionals is "ERISA," the law setting federal standards for employer-provided health and pension plans.[28] Enacted in the 1970s to protect employees against malfeasance by employers

---

[25] See http://www.whitehouse.gov/the-press-office/presidential-memorandum-hospital-visitation.

[26] These are the states in which same-sex couples may enter a broad status and then are presumed to earn wages as "community property" owned equally by both. See http://www.lambdalegal.org/publications/factsheets/fs_the-irs-applies-income-splitting-community-property.html.

[27] Estate taxes are another area of federal taxation where the family relationships of same-sex couples are ignored no matter how long a couple was together, or how intertwined their financial lives may have been. See, e.g., *Windsor v. United States*, Civil Action No. 1:10-cv-8435 (S.D.N.Y. 2011).

[28] ERISA stands for the Employee Retirement Income Security Act. It does not apply to public employee benefit plans and does not preempt state regulation of insurance or medical practice.

and those hired to manage their benefit plans, it now preempts claims against many private employers for equal benefits based on state family laws and/or nondiscrimination laws.

Comparing the Options—What Works, and Why?

A Complete State-Law Package Has Balance and Is Efficient

Marriage, civil unions, and broad domestic partnership laws all offer comprehensive packages of state-law rights and responsibilities that relate to and are in proportion with one another; the rules operate as a balanced system. A duty to pay each other's debts, for example, generally corresponds to a right to receive financial support from each other, to receive damages from a third party who causes the death of the other, and to transfer property from one to the other without taxation. With decision-making authority, these packages include default rules for property ownership and inheritance that apply in the absence of explicit plans. They also include a requirement to end the relationship through a supervised legal proceeding—such as a divorce, dissolution, or termination.

As noted, competent adults can control some of their affairs through private planning. An estate plan and health care proxy can alter some defaults; a "prenuptial" or other relationship agreement can limit disputes and guide a separation (Hertz and Doskow 2011). But, no one can change taxation or tort liability rules with a private contract.

Moreover, for gay and straight alike, preparing such documents can be easier said than done. No one enjoys anticipating sickness, death, or a breakup. So, people procrastinate. Just finding a lawyer can be stressful enough, and then making the decisions about bequests and in case of divorce can be even more so.

The "carrot" of a wedding party and the "stick" of social pressure to marry have long provided incentives inducing heterosexual couples to come within the default system. Marriage and, perhaps to a lesser extent, civil unions now are providing similar incentives for some lesbian and gay couples in a dozen jurisdictions.

Solemnization Is Communication

The ceremony of marriage and civil unions performs functions that can be especially helpful for LGBT people. First is the expressive ritual that can facilitate communication within a couple's network of family, relatives, and friends—an unequivocal "coming out" that invites attendance, not debate. It affirms as it creates in-laws for those who once would have been outlaws. The ritual also confirms clearly for the couple that each is making a full commitment to the other, something often left murky when couples cohabit but cannot—or do not—formalize their relationship legally.

Partnership registration does not include this ritual. While having legal rights is far better than not having them, many couples feel the bureaucratic nature of registration and the withholding of solemnization is stigmatizing; the fewer couples who register compared with those who marry when they can seems to confirm that full equality and the affirmation of a ceremony—plus the security of knowing full legal rights are entailed in the usual way—appeal to many gay couples (Badgett and Herman 2011; Ramos et al. 2009) , though certainly not all (Franke 2011).

Consistently with the research findings, multiple state high courts have concluded that their states' separate, lesser systems of civil unions or domestic partnerships do not satisfy constitutional guarantees of equal protection. One reason is that the lesser status conveys stigma, as noted earlier. In addition, novel, different names connote something alien, which creates confusion and disconnect. Too often, people from rental car agents to paramedics and hospital admitting clerks do not see domestic or civil union partners as family and instead take the view, "when in doubt, don't"—meaning, they do not honor the status as they would that of spouses. Similarly, employers sometimes balk at the (minimal) effort needed to offer domestic partner benefits, but assume that their married gay employees should have the same family benefits as their married heterosexual ones.

Bad Laws Invite Bad Behavior

It sometimes is said that among the strongest arguments for "gay marriage" is the need for "gay divorce." Too often, promises made across pillows, broken after love has waned, prove unenforceable because too vague or otherwise disputed. Similarly, when emotions shift, beneficiary designations can be changed overnight.

If a couple has married or entered another broad status, the family court will have a role in deciding what is fair if the relationship ends. Without such a status to bring disputes into family court, in contrast, an abandoned partner can present contract, fraud, or other claims in civil court. That, however, often is a steep, expensive, uphill climb.

The difference between having a legal status and not can be even more stark and anguishing when parental rights are at stake. If same-sex parents have not secured the parental status of both adults, one likely will have a superior position, if not the *only* protected position. Following the death or incapacity of the legal parent, relatives may get custody instead of a parent-in-fact who lacks legal status.

Moreover, there is nothing new about the legal parent turning against the "nonparent" and denying visitation after a separation if and when antigay laws offer the opportunity. Lawyers who represent LGBT clients in family matters long have discouraged such use of discriminatory laws. But legal texts overflow with cases showing that domestic disputes can bring out the worst in people, regardless of sexual orientation.[29]

Uncertainties Facing Transgender People

When the gender of both adults in a couple determines whether they may enter a legal status, state law controls how each one's gender is ascertained. But few states have clear rules to explain whether or how a person legally may change from the sex assigned at birth and recorded on the birth certificate.[30]

Usually, a marriage that is valid when entered remains valid even if something happens later that would have prevented the marriage had it happened earlier, such as a loss of competence by either spouse. This rule should hold for a gender transition after marriage as well, though few cases have addressed it to date. The lack of explicit gender-definition laws makes things murkier for those who transition *before* marrying. Often it is unclear whether a state respects gender reassignment at all, or whether it matters how much gender-related medical treatment a person has received. Life can be uncertain indeed if a couple does not know what gender their state may deem one of them to be and whether that will invalidate their marriage. For example, courts in Florida, Kansas, and Texas have ruled that gender transitions cannot be recognized (absent future action by the legislature)—voiding marriages the spouses had entered as a heterosexual couple and denying the postoperative transsexual spouses' parental rights, inheritance, and tort claims.

Thus, the private documents and other legal planning discussed earlier can be all the more important for those who cannot be confident what a court might say in a future challenge to a marriage. And again, while courts do not always enforce relationship agreements as written, such documents can record what each party understood about the other and intended for their relationship (Hertz and Doskow 2011[31]). That record can dissuade a nontransgender spouse from later claiming a marriage should be voided because she or he did not know the transgender spouse had transitioned, an assertion that might seem hard to credit, but which divorce courts have heard.

---

[29] The divergence between gay-friendly and gay-unfriendly states now tempts some parents to seek advantage in a new way—by taking a child from the family's home state to one with different policies. Existing laws impede such tactics even when the destination state otherwise might not recognize the second parent's rights as such. But interstate flight adds cost and heartache, regardless of whether it ultimately is unsuccessful.

[30] Many states allow changes of name and the gender markers on identity documents (see, e.g., http://transgenderlawcenter.org/cms/content/id-document-change or http://www.nclrights.org/site/DocServer/fl_namechg_kit.pdf?docID=1281) but still may lack clear rules about how sex is to be determined for gender-restricted purposes, such as marriage.

[31] One example is *Vecchione v. Vecchione,* in which the wife argued that her marriage should be voided because her husband allegedly fooled her into believing he had been born male. The case is discussed in Flynn 2001. See also *Kantaras v. Kantaras,* 884 So. 2d 155 (Fla. App. 2004) (wife persuaded court to void her marriage, and husband's presumed parental rights with it, because Florida law should not recognize his gender transition).

Some Benefits and Costs of Interstate Variation

In our federalist system, the states historically have been laboratories of experimentation, so to speak, especially for family law. They have been free to test no-fault divorce, joint custody, community property, and, more recently, legal recognition for same-sex couples and their parenting relationships.

But variation among states now also poses challenges for same-sex couples. For example, they may visit Cape Cod or Niagara Falls to marry but, unlike heterosexual couples who do the same, later may find themselves unable to divorce. Perhaps paradoxically, many states say they cannot end lesbian and gay couples' out-of-state or foreign-country marriages because they would have to recognize those marriages—contrary to their own policy—in order to terminate them. Further, because in-state residency is *not* required for marriage but *is* required for divorce, gay couples now can find themselves in "wed-*lock*" of a sort heterosexual couples have not experienced for decades.

The Lack of Comprehensive Antidiscrimination Laws

Any discussion of the legal status of same-sex couples must acknowledge the vulnerability that all LGBT people, whether coupled or single, experience due to the lack of comprehensive antidiscrimination laws at both state and federal levels. Although the lack of explicit federal protections is glaring (Lambda Legal 2011), a minority of states now do have laws forbidding discriminatory treatment based on sexual orientation and/or gender identity, and some require equal treatment whether one has, or is, a same-sex spouse or partner rather than one of a different sex. Those rules can apply in employment, housing, and/or public accommodations.[32]

At the federal level, as noted earlier, some new regulations aim to reduce discrimination in programs receiving federal funds. In addition, federal and state laws forbidding sex discrimination in employment and educational programs protect against sexual harassment and also protect against mistreatment due to perceptions that an LGBT person does not conform to gender stereotypes, and, to an evolving extent, due to a gender transition. The U.S. Constitution and state constitutions also offer some protections from government discrimination

---

[32]"Public accommodations" generally means enterprises and organizations offering goods or services to the public for a fee. They can range from local grocery stores to national car rental companies, to regulated services such as banking and insurance, to licensed professional services such as medical care.

against LGBT people, although cases to enforce constitutional protections can be complicated and the doctrines are still evolving.[33]

And yet the lack of express protections against sexual orientation and gender identity discrimination in the federal civil rights laws that apply to employment, housing, education, and public accommodations may be taken as meaning that such discrimination is lawful and consistent with national policy, despite the regulatory changes made by the Obama administration. Especially given how much anti-LGBT discrimination remains (Sears and Mallory 2011), strong federal civil rights protections are overdue.

Such protections would not transform behavior overnight. But they would shift responsibility for controlling bias-motivated abuse from individuals who experience or witness discrimination to those who discriminate or have authority over institutions, as has been done to reduce other prejudice. Moreover, explicit antibias rules encourage LGBT people to expect better treatment, to speak up when treated badly, and thereby to educate those around them who otherwise might remain oblivious about the effects of their behavior or that of others (Frost et al. 2011).

Conclusion

Family law for LGBT people has become complicated. Inconsistency, uncertainty, and change have become the most salient features of how our national legal system treats LGBT people and their families. There now is wide recognition that the law is evolving toward inclusion and protection of same-sex couples. Nevertheless, many high-profile civic, religious, and political leaders oppose these changes.

Even assuming this reform continues apace, the process is erratic. Evolution overall does not dictate the answer in a particular context. Although progress is accelerating, achieving full equality will take time. Many LGBT people, and their loved ones, undoubtedly will experience painful, unjust treatment along the way. The faster the reform process can be, the quicker and deeper the shifts in public attitudes, and the better for everyone who is, or cares about, a lesbian, gay, bisexual, or transgender person.

Key Points

- Some laws governing the family rights of LGBT people are getting better, others worse; the situation is unstable, confusing, and stressful.

---

[33] The most commonly invoked protections are the guarantees of equal protection, due process, liberty and privacy, and the first amendment protections for freedom of speech and association.

- In many states, same-sex partners may not enter any family status—such as marriage, civil union, or registered domestic partnership—with broad protective rules. Even when same-sex couples have entered a status under a state's laws, they remain vulnerable because other states and the federal government do not respect it.

- Whether in a family status under state laws or not, same-sex partners should express their wishes in formal documents regarding matters over which they have control—such as medical decisions, financial affairs, and inheritance—because those documents allow respect for individuals' wishes instead of an assumption in state law and ought to retain their force in interstate travel.

- Wherever they live, same-sex partners raising children should secure all parent-child relationships with court judgments if possible, even if state law recognizes all of the relationships, because judgments are due respect from other states.

- U.S. federal law does not afford equal status to LGBT individuals. It ignores married same-sex couples and so denies rights such as Social Security spousal support, equal federal tax treatment, and the ability to have a foreign-born spouse immigrate.

References

Badgett MVL: The impact of expanding FMLA rights to care for children of same-sex partners. June 2010. Available at: http://williamsinstitute.law.ucla.edu/research/marriage-and-couples-rights/the-impact-of-expanding-fmla-rights-to-care-for-children-of-same-sex-partners-2. Accessed November 6, 2011.

Badgett MVL, Herman JL: Patterns of relationship recognition by same-sex couples in the United States. November 2011. Available at: http://williamsinstitute.law.ucla.edu/wp-content/uploads/Badgett-Herman-Marriage-Dissolution-Nov-2011.pdf. Accessed February 24, 2012.

Badgett MVL, Gates GJ, Hunter ND, et al: Written testimony: S.598, The Respect for Marriage Act: assessing the impact of DOMA on American families. July 20, 2011. Available at: http://williamsinstitute.law.ucla.edu/research/marriage-and-couples-rights/written-testimony-s-598-the-respect-for-marriage-act-assessing-the-impact-of-doma-on-american-families. Accessed November 6, 2011.

Burda JM: Estate Planning for Same-Sex Couples. Chicago, IL, American Bar Association Publishing, 2004

Clifford D, Hertz F, Doskow E: A Legal Guide for Lesbian and Gay Couples, 15th Edition. Berkeley, CA, NOLO Press, 2010

Flynn T: Transforming the debate: why we need to include transgender rights in the struggles for sex and sexual orientation equality. Columbia Law Review 101:392–420, 2001

Franke KM: Marriage is a mixed blessing. The New York Times, June 23, 2011. Available at: http://www.nytimes.com/2011/06/24/opinion/24franke.html. Accessed November 6, 2011.

Frost DM, Lehavot K, Meyer IH: Minority stress and physical health among sexual minorities. Poster presented at the 119th annual convention of the American Psychological Association, Washington, DC, August 4–7, 2011. Available at: http://williamsinstitute.law.ucla.edu/research/health-and-hiv-aids/minority-stress-and-physical-health-among-sexual-minorities-2. Accessed November 6, 2011.

Gates GJ: How many people are lesbian, gay, bisexual and transgender? April 2011. Available at: http://williamsinstitute.law.ucla.edu/research/census-lgbt-demographics-studies/how-many-people-are-lesbian-gay-bisexual-and-transgender. Accessed November 6, 2011.

Gates GJ, Cooke AM: United States Census Snapshot: 2010. 2011. Available at: http://williamsinstitute.law.ucla.edu/wp-content/uploads/Census2010Snapshot-US-v2.pdf. Accessed February 23, 2012.

Hertz H, Doskow E: Making It Legal: A Guide to Same-Sex Marriage, Domestic Partnerships, and Civil Unions, 2nd Edition. Berkeley, CA, NOLO Press, 2011

Human Rights Campaign: The state of the workplace for lesbian, gay, and transgender Americans, 2007–2008. 2009. Available at: http://www.hrc.org/files/assets/resources/HRC_Foundation_State_of_the_Workplace_2007-2008.pdf. Accessed November 6, 2011.

Kaiser Family Foundation and Health Research and Educational Trust: Employer health benefits: 2009 annual survey. 2009. Available at: http://ehbs.kff.org/pdf/2009/7936.pdf. Accessed November 6, 2011.

Lambda Legal: Take the power: tools for life and financial planning. November 10, 2010. Available at: http://www.lambdalegal.org/publications/take-the-power. Accessed November 6, 2011.

Lambda Legal: An unfulfilled promise: lesbian and gay inequality under American law. July 5, 2011. Available at: http://www.lambdalegal.org/publications/factsheets/fs_an-unfulfilled-promise.html. Accessed November 6, 2011.

National Gay and Lesbian Task Force: State nondiscrimination laws in the U.S. June 14, 2011. Available at: http://www.thetaskforce.org/downloads/reports/issue_maps/non_discrimination_6_11_color.pdf. Accessed November 6, 2011.

Obama B: Memorandum for the heads of executive departments and agencies: federal benefits and non-discrimination. June 17, 2009. Available at: http://www.whitehouse.gov/the_press_office/Memorandum-for-the-Heads-of-Executive-Departments-and-Agencies-on-Federal-Benefits-and-Non-Discrimination-6-17-09. Accessed November 6, 2011.

Obama B: Presidential memorandum— hospital visitation: memorandum for the Secretary of Health and Human Services. April 15, 2010. Available at: http://www.whitehouse.gov/the-press-office/presidential-memorandum-hospital-visitation. Accessed November 6, 2011.

Ponce NA, Cochran SD, Pizer JC, et al: The effects of unequal access to health insurance for same-sex couples in California. Health Aff (Milwood) 29:1539–1548, 2010

Quinnipiac University: Gays in the military should be allowed to come out, U.S. voters tell Quinnipiac University national poll. April 30, 2009. Available at: http://www.quinnipiac.edu/x1295.xml?ReleaseID=1292. Accessed November 6, 2011.

Ramos C, Goldberg NG, Badgett MVL: The effects of marriage equality in Massachusetts: a survey of the experiences and impact of marriage on same-sex couples. May 2009. Available at: http://williamsinstitute.law.ucla.edu/research/marriage-and-couples-rights/effects-marriage-equality-masurvey/. Accessed November 6, 2011.

Sears B, Mallory C: Documented evidence of employment discrimination and its effects on LGBT people. July 2011. Available at: http://williamsinstitute.law.ucla.edu/research/workplace/documented-evidence-of-employment-discrimination-its-effects-on-lgbt-people. Accessed November 6, 2011.

White House Blog: President Obama supports the Respect for Marriage Act. July 19, 2011. Available at: http://www.whitehouse.gov/blog/2011/07/19/president-obama-supports-respect-marriage-act. Accessed November 6, 2011.

Questions

3.1   If a competent adult has signed a "health care proxy" or "power of attorney for medical decisions" designating his or her same-sex partner to make decisions, can a legally recognized relative such as a parent or a child override the decisions made by the partner?

> A. No, but only if the patient has confirmed the validity of the document at the start of the treatment relationship.
>
> B. No, the written document controls over legal relatives whether or not state law specifically provides for such documents.
>
> C. No, but only if state law allows the couple to enter some kind of legal status and the couple has done so.
>
> D. Yes, due to the so-called federal Defense of Marriage Act, if the health facility receives federal funding.

The correct answer is B.

In every state, a competent adult can (and should) state his or her wishes in a formal written document, and it will override the default designations of blood or legal relatives, regardless of whether state law confirms this. Such a document has legal effect separately from whether a given state allows same-sex couples to enter a relationship-recognition status.

3.2   If municipalities in State A allow same-sex couples to register as domestic partners, must a hospital in State A honor the relationship of a same-sex couple that married or entered a civil union in State B for visitation, information-sharing, and decision-making purposes after one spouse/partner is injured while traveling in State A?

A. Yes, the Full Faith and Credit clause and Privileges and Immunities clause of the U.S. Constitution require State A to respect the visiting couple's legal status.

B. Probably yes, if the hospital receives federal funding.

C. Probably no, if State A has a broad constitutional amendment prohibiting recognition of same-sex couples' marriages and civil unions and the spouse or partner cannot produce a health care proxy or other documents signed by the patient stating the patient's wishes that the spouse be allowed to visit, receive confidential information, and/or make decisions for the patient.

D. Yes, if the municipalities in State A include hospital visitation, information sharing, and decision-making among the rights of registered domestic partners.

The correct answer is C.

The Full Faith and Credit clause is generally thought not to apply to a legal status, but just to rights confirmed by a court judgment. If a state has passed a law or amended its constitution to deny respect to some out-of-state marriages, the Full Faith and Credit clause probably will not help. In the absence of a power of attorney or other document, the federal regulations may not help a same-sex partner gain access to the spouse's bedside or to information, or make treatment decisions for an incapacitated patient.

3.3   Acme Enterprises, a Fortune 500 company, offers health insurance to its unmarried employees for either a same-sex or a different-sex partner. If Acme operates in a state that bans sexual orientation discrimination in employment but does not recognize any legal status for same-sex couples, may the company eliminate its domestic partner benefits program and offer insurance only for legal spouses?

A. Yes. There is no federal statute requiring equal benefits for lesbian, gay, or bisexual employees with a same-sex partner, or for unmarried employees, and the federal ERISA law blocks any claims based on the state nondiscrimination law.

B. No, as a national company, Acme Enterprises must comply with the federal Equal Protection clause and may not offer its heterosexual workers a way to qualify for family health insurance and no comparable way for its lesbian, gay, or bisexual workers to qualify an equally committed same-sex life partner.

    C. Yes, as long as the elimination of partner benefits is done to contain costs rather than out of prejudice against the company's nonheterosexual employees.

    D. Yes, as long as the company continues to offer spousal health insurance for employees with a same-sex spouse.

The correct answer is A.

The Equal Protection clause does not apply because Acme is a private company and the federal and state constitutions only apply against government. Although doing so would be obviously discriminatory, Acme probably can offer benefits only to its heterosexually married employees and not to its partnered employees and those with a same-sex spouse, because there is no federal law requiring equal benefits regardless of sexual orientation, and the federal ERISA law usually blocks enforcement of state antidiscrimination rights against private employers with respect to employer-provided health insurance.

LGBT Parenting

Mary E. Barber, M.D.

GAY PEOPLE USED TO BE accidental parents. They had children in heterosexual marriages or relationships, then they would come out but continue to be involved in their children's lives when the relationship ended. Sometimes the gay spouse became the primary parent, coparenting with a new same-sex partner.

This was the old story of gay parenting, amusingly told in the French film *La Cage aux Folles* (Molinaro 1978). In the film, Renato, a drag show club owner, and his partner Albin, the club's star performer, have together raised a son: Renato's biological child from a youthful fling with a woman. The film plays into the stereotype of gay men as flamboyantly effeminate and of gay relationships as having stereotypical gendered roles. Renato, the more conventionally masculine partner, plays the father role to their son, while Albin's role is decidedly maternal. When the adult son announces his engagement, his gay parents have the following exchange:

> ALBIN: He's being taken from us, and we won't have any others.
> RENATO: Unless there's a miracle.

Starting in the 1990s, gay people became intentional parents. They came out, met same-sex life partners, and had children together using reproductive technologies or adoption. This new story of gay parenting, sometimes referred to as the gay baby boom or *gayby boom*, is captured in a more contemporary film. In *The Kids Are All Right* (Cholodenko 2010), Nic and Jules are a lesbian couple with two children, Joni and Laser. Both have been conceived by insemination from the same anonymous donor. Nic is the biological mother of Joni, and Jules is the biological mother of Laser. Their symmetrical and seemingly egalitarian way of making a family, where both parents are able to carry a child, is not uncommon and represents a version of the new gay parenting story.

However, reality is a little more complicated than either of these two films. Lesbian, gay, bisexual, and transgender (LGBT) parents have been around for a long time. Some gay couples were planning for children in their relationship even before the 1990s' gay baby boom, and yes, others did come to parenthood accidentally. Today some gay people continue to fall into parenthood in accidental ways, whether through relationships they have before coming out, through meeting someone who already has children from a previous relationship, or through taking in the child of a family member.

In short, as with heterosexual couples, there are many ways to make a family.

Changing Attitudes and Options

What has clearly changed in the last few decades is the visibility of LGBT parents and the options open to same-sex couples or LGBT singles wanting to parent. Sexual- and gender-minority parents previously had realistic and significant fears of losing custody of their children or of not being able to adopt a child if their LGBT identity became known. In the past, reproductive technologies such as donor insemination, in vitro fertilization, and surrogacy were not as accessible to lesbians and gay men as they are now. Discriminatory adoption laws still exist in some states, and in some places laws may not forbid adoption or reproductive assistance, but individual providers can and sometimes do still discriminate. Still, thanks to the pioneering efforts of earlier LGBT parents, LGBT parents today have an easier path to parenthood with more information and support available than ever.

One example of a gay parenting pioneer can be found in the play and film *Torch Song Trilogy* (Fierstein 1983). In the final act, gay drag performer Arnold has taken in 15-year-old David by way of a foster placement and plans to adopt him. The boy is gay, has failed to be accepted in two other foster homes, and has spent some time on the street. Arnold's mother gives voice to what would have been common prejudices of that decade:

ARNOLD: …I try to set an example for him.…
MA: Some example. Arnold, look, you live the life you want. I put my fist in my mouth, I don't say a word. This is what you want. But think about the boy. He likes you. He told me he loves you. He sees you living like this…don't you think it's going to affect him?
ARNOLD: Ma, David is gay.
MA: But he's only been here six months!

ARNOLD: He came that way.
MA: No one comes that way.

Coming out as gay used to mean accepting and potentially mourning the loss of the possibility of becoming a parent, having to "choose between having children and being gay" (Drescher 2001, p. 126). Today, gay men and lesbians coming out do not automatically see a contradiction between being gay and being a parent, and many have the same expectations of partnering and raising children as their heterosexual counterparts.

LGBT Families in the United States

The most recent U.S. Census data have challenged many assumptions about LGBT parenting. Gay couples with children depicted in the media are often affluent, white, and living in the Northeast or California. Yet the most recent census data show that the 581,000 same-sex couples with children in the United States are more likely to be living in the South than in any other U.S. region (Krivickas and Lofquist 2011; Tavernise 2011). Two cities where gay couples are found to be raising children in great numbers are San Antonio, Texas (34% of gay couples have children), and Jacksonville, Florida (32% of gay couples have children). Furthermore, black and Latino gay couples are twice as likely as white gay couples to be raising children.

These data are not perfect. Because the census doesn't ask about sexual or gender identity, these findings do not identify the total number of gay or transgender parents who are raising kids in the United States. The census counts only couples who report the same gender on the census form, who describe each other as either "unmarried partner" or "spouse." Consequently, gay or lesbian single parents do not show up in these counts. It is also likely that this is an undercount because some couples do not check off the "unmarried partner" box, either because they are afraid to come out to government officials or because they do not understand what it means.

Census results also show that about one in every three lesbians has given birth and one in six gay men has fathered or adopted a child (Gates et al. 2007). So LGB parenting is a common phenomenon, and growing.

Little is known about transgender people raising children. Because the census does not ask about transgender identity, transgender parents get lost in the data between single parents, same-sex couples, and opposite-sex couples. Perhaps the most well-known transgender parent is Thomas Beatie, labeled by the media as "the pregnant man." Beatie, a trans man (female to male transgender person) who retained his female reproductive organs, became pregnant because his wife was unable to conceive. His first pregnancy, in 2007, caused a media stir (Goldman 2008); since then, Beatie has gone on to carry and deliver two more children. It is thought that many transgender parents make their gender transition after becoming parents, sometimes after their kids are already grown. However, the very public case of Thomas Beatie does not bear out this assumption, and it is likely that, as with LGB parents, transgender parents follow many paths to raising children.

How Do the Children Do?

Numerous studies of lesbian and gay parents have been published (Biblarz and Stacey 2010; Gartrell and Bos 2010; Perrin et al. 2004; Stacey and Biblarz 2001). These studies have mostly employed small convenience samples, often of affluent white subjects. Factors having to do with family characteristics, such as single- versus two-parent families and whether children were conceived in a heterosexual relationship that preceded the parent coming out or were conceived or adopted in the context of a same-sex-headed family, are mixed across studies. More studies involve lesbian parents than gay male parents as subjects.

Despite some of these limitations, the research consistently shows that children of lesbian and gay parents have no more depression or adjustment, behavioral, or school problems than children raised in heterosexual households (American Psychiatric Association 2002; Biblarz and Stacey 2010; Perrin et al. 2004; Stacey and Biblarz 2001). One longitudinal study (Gartrell and Bos 2010), challenging denigrating cultural stereotypes about LGBT people, showed a remarkable 0% rate of sexual abuse among a sample of adolescent children of lesbians.

Some of the studies found that children of gay and lesbian parents were less rigid in their beliefs about sex roles and more open to same-sex experimentation in adolescence. At least one study suggested that the daughters of lesbians may be more likely to grow up lesbian themselves (Gartrell and Bos 2010), but other analyses found that children of lesbian and gay parents are no more likely to grow up to be lesbian or gay than are children of heterosexual parents (Perrin et al. 2004).

This body of research has been criticized for being "defensive"—setting heterosexual (biological) parenting as the gold standard (Schwartz 2009) and studying whether gay parenting is adequate to meet that standard (Stacey and Biblarz 2001; Volpp and Drescher 2011). If the charge of defensiveness is valid, this approach is also understandable, as much of this research was done while society's (and the law's) views on gay parenting were evolving. Fears of gay and lesbian parents causing harm to children or stigmatizing them at school and with friends, and even fears of gay parents as sexual predators, were common societal attitudes of the past few decades. These homo-ignorant beliefs and fears fueled discriminatory adoption policies and reduced access to reproductive technologies for gay parents. Such prejudicial views are not completely gone now, but they are much less common, in part because of this body of research and the visibility of LGBT parents in neighborhoods, the media, and the literature (Green 1999; Igartua 2009; Savage 1999).

In a growing era of acceptance for LGBT parenting, with a reduction in discriminatory policies and laws, and with greater visibility of LGBT parents, new research is needed. This would focus not on disproving stereotypes about LGBT parents as being harmful to children, but on the specific issues, needs, and potential strengths of those children and their families.

How do LGBT parents help their children as they encounter biased beliefs in school or negative comments from peers? Everyday issues that may come up can often be anticipated and discussed within the family ahead of time. These may include explanations as to how the child with two moms answers the "Who is your dad?" question, or what to do when the other children are making Father's Day cards at school. In the former case, younger children can be equipped to answer matter-of-factly, "I don't have a dad—I have two moms" (see Figure 4–1). For older children and teens, they may want to choose when and to whom to disclose about their family. In the case of the Father's Day cards, the child can choose to make a card for an uncle, grandfather, or family friend, or even for one of his or her mothers. Planning ahead can defuse any number of such issues for a child and even for a teacher perhaps more anxious than the mothers or child about how to deal with such potential minefields. For clinicians treating LGBT parents and their children, it is important to remember that there is no one correct way to navigate these instances of ordinary heterosexism that children will undoubtedly encounter. What is critical is that the parents should discuss them and give the children some options for how to handle them.

What about more serious issues of harassment or bullying that children of LGBT parents may face? As with any bullying, parents need to discuss the incident with the child and try to give the child strategies for how to address it. These may include telling a teacher or principal or getting support from friends. The child may or may not want the parent to intervene with either the school or the parents of the bully. However, if the bullying is serious, is leading to anxiety or other emotional problems for the child, or is physical, the parent may need to intercede. Parents may want to point the school toward resources about LGBT families if the bullying indicates a need for a school-wide educational effort (see "Resources" section later in this chapter).

Perhaps the most important thing LGBT parents can do to buffer their children against heterosexism and antigay bullying is to help connect them to other children of LGBT parents. This can be done through a local LGBT community center, or if no local resource exists, through national organizations (COLAGE, Family Equality Council). Children of LGBT parents can help one another feel less isolated. They can discuss with one another how to cope with ignorant comments and bullying, and how, when, and whether to come out to friends about one's family (Fakhrid-Deen and COLAGE 2010; Garner 2004). Disclosing one's family difference is its own coming out process, and children of LGBT parents may feel that other kids like them understand this even better than their LGBT parent or parents.

Aside from coping with overt antigay bias in the wider world, children of LGBT parents may feel pressure to be models of achievement and good adjustment. They may feel pressure from society and their parents to be successful representatives of gay parenting. In the above-mentioned film *The Kids Are All Right* (Cholodenko 2010), 18-year-old daughter Joni vents to her two moms in a moment of anger:

> JONI: What do you want from me? I did everything you wanted! I got all A's.
> I got into every school I applied. Now you can show everyone what a perfect lesbian family you have!

The pressure to be "perfect" may include the pressure to be straight, to prove to the world that gay parents don't make gay kids. Second-generation LGBTQs, that is, children of LGBT parents who themselves grow up to be LGBT or queer identified, may actually have a hard time feeling comfortable with their identity because of this pressure, which can be vague or explicit, from friends, extended family, and even the parents themselves (Fakhrid-Deen and COLAGE 2010; Garner 2004).

Issues for the Parents

Many of the issues LGBT parents face are comparable to those of the non-LGBT cohort. Gay and lesbian couples who conceive or adopt babies experience the same sleeplessness, worries, and radical changes in lifestyle that new heterosexual parents face. Gay parents who had their children in the context of a heterosexual marriage face many of the same issues as divorced heterosexual parents. Gay people who adopt children experience many of the same questions and feelings as any other adoptive parent would.

Yet LGBT parents may experience these same situations in different ways than their straight counterparts. The sleepless gay couple with the new baby may not have the same support network as their straight neighbors—maybe the couple's parents are not sure they like the idea of their son raising a child with his "roommate," and maybe their gay friends are not interested in helping babysit. The lesbian mom who divorced her husband has an additional task most divorced moms do not: having to come out to her teenage children. If the divorce was not amicable, coming out may be fraught with the risk of losing custody. The gay male couple who choose to adopt may have additional stress in choosing an agency that will work with them as a couple. On the other hand, they do not carry the emotional baggage seen in adopting heterosexual couples who are coping with infertility.

LGBT parents can feel the same pressure to be role models as their children do. Much like an ethnic minority family or immigrant family, as a stigmatized group they may experience a constant sense of responsibility to be a "credit" to

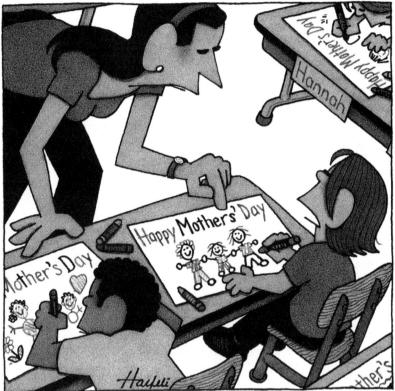

"*I have two mommies. I know where the apostrophe goes.*"

FIGURE 4–1. **Mothers' Day card.**

Source. Cartoon by William Haefeli. Copyright © William Haefeli/*The New Yorker* Collection. Reprinted by permission of The Cartoon Bank/ Condé Nast Publications Inc.

all LGBT families. This sense of being viewed under a judgmental microscope may mean that every problem with a child reflects not only on the child or the issue at hand, but also on their parenting skills as a whole (Fitzgerald 2010).

Although the data come from convenience samples, studies suggest that lesbian mothers may be more likely to end their partnerships than either gay fathers or heterosexual couples with children (Biblarz and Stacey 2010). Speculations about why this might be true include the aforementioned pressure LGBT parents experience. Potentially adding to the sense of needing to be role models in society is the expectation many lesbians place on their relationships being egalitarian. When children are added to a family, differences related to biology (if the birth mother is nursing), parenting styles, interest in spending time with children, work schedules, and income may all make dividing child care and home responsibilities evenly an impossible or even undesirable goal. If one mother has biological ties to the children and one does not, this may potentially lead to jealousy and conflict as well (Glazer and Drescher 2001)—a situation depicted for both lesbian moms and gay dads by Gartrell in Chapter 18 of this book, "Parent-Child Relational Problems." In general, disparities in work allocations or in bonding with the children may lead to strain between the parents if equality was a strong value for one or both (Glazer 2009).

LGBT families are often thoroughly planned. Clarice and Toni, a couple from the long-running comic strip *Dykes to Watch Out For,* illustrate just some of the decisions that go into planning to have a baby through donor insemination (Figure 4–2). The positive sign of all this planning is that children brought or born into LGBT families are both wanted and anticipated. Yet there are also downsides: potential gay parents can overthink every option, falsely believing there is a "right" answer to every decision point, or that they can foresee any potential problem. And when things don't go as expected, as in cases of infertility, miscarriage, or the child having a serious illness or special needs, it can be especially difficult for the parents who thought they had so meticulously "planned" their family (Martin 1993).

LGBT parenting still is not so common, outside major urban centers, that gay parents can easily find other families like theirs in their neighborhood or children's school. Most gay parents find themselves alone among straight parents at the playground, school, and other places they frequent with their children. New LGBT parents typically find a whole cadre of people to whom they never thought they would have to come out—teachers, day care workers, pediatricians, and parents of their children's friends. Further, because they are going through a similar stage of life and have many experiences in common, LGBT parents may find themselves seeking out the company of heterosexual friends and family with children more than that of childless LGBT friends with whom they may have less in common.

Yet ironically, as LGBT parenting becomes more normative and accepted, LGBT parents may increasingly face the same pressure that straight people have had to cope with from time immemorial. Gay and lesbian couples may begin to hear pointed questions from parents about "When will we become grandparents?" and suggestions from friends about starting a family. Gay people who would prefer not to raise children, or gay couples who wish to keep their family planning private, may find such comments intrusive. Those advocating for the ability and rights of gay and lesbian couples to parent have been clear about not making parenting prescriptive for all LGBT people (Martin 1993).

Resources

As with all LGBT patients, LGBT parents presenting for mental health treatment may not be aware of support and educational resources available to them.

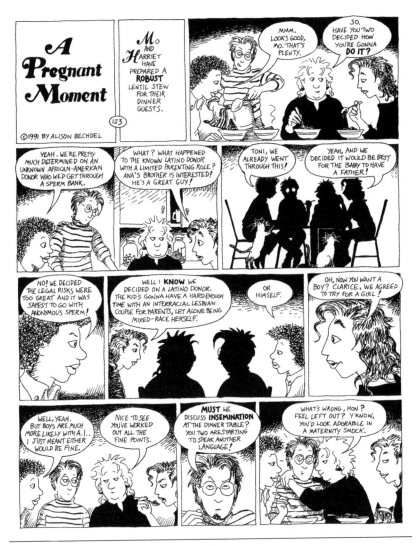

FIGURE 4–2. A pregnant moment.

Clinicians can point parents to organizations (COLAGE [www.colage.org], Family Equality Council [www.familyequality.org]), books about parenting (Martin 1993), children's fiction (deHaan and Nijland 2004; Newman 2009; Newman and Souza 1994; Parnell and Richardson 2005), handbooks written by children of gay parents (Fakhrid-Deen and COLAGE 2010; Garner 2004), and even films (Cholodenko 2010; Wade 2008). Clinicians looking for further resources geared toward treating LGBT parents and their families have a wealth of resources as well (D'Ercole and Drescher 2004; Glazer and Drescher 2001; Group for Advancement of Psychiatry 2011; Martin 1993).

Children of LGBT parents have developed a support network and resources for themselves. COLAGE is a national group of children, youth, and adults with one or more LGBT parents. The group sponsors Family Week, a cross between summer camp and a convention, in different locations throughout the United States and has created resources such as Kids of Trans (COLAGE 2008) and Donor Insemination (COLAGE 2009) guides.

Key Points

- LGBT people have been parenting children for many years, both in the context of heterosexual relationships and after coming out as LGBT. In recent years, LGBT parenting has become more common and more visible.

- The body of research on children of lesbian and gay parents shows that children have no greater mental health or adjustment problems than peers raised by heterosexual parents. However, they may face issues such as heterosexism and antigay bullying and may benefit from support from other children of LGBT parents.

- LGBT parents encounter stressors common to all parents, and they also have unique issues. For example, LGBT parents may feel pressure to serve as role models for all sexual- and gender-minority families, and LGBT parents may need to disclose their sexual or gender minority identity to a new cohort of people they will encounter on behalf of their children.

References

American Psychiatric Association: Adoption and co-parenting of children by same-sex couples: position statement. November 2002. Available at: http://www.psych.org/Departments/EDU/Library/APAOfficialDocumentsandRelated/PositionStatements/200214.aspx. Accessed November 7, 2011.

Biblarz TJ, Stacey J: How does the gender of parents matter? J Marriage Fam 72:3–22, 2010

Cholodenko L (director): The Kids Are All Right (film). Universal Studios, 2010

COLAGE: Kids of trans resource guide. 2008. Available at: http://www.colage.org/resources/kot. Accessed November 7, 2011.

COLAGE: Donor insemination guide. 2009. Available at: http://www.colage.org/resources/for-lgbtq-parents/donor-insemination-guide. Accessed November 7, 2011.

deHaan L, Nijland S: King and King and Family. Berkeley, CA, Tricycle Press, 2004

D'Ercole A, Drescher J (eds): Uncoupling Convention: Psychoanalytic Approaches to Same-Sex Couples and Families. Hillsdale, NJ, Analytic Press, 2004

Drescher J: The circle of liberation: a book review essay of Jesse Green's *The Velveteen Father: An Unexpected Journey to Parenthood.* Journal of Gay and Lesbian Psychotherapy 4:119–131, 2001

Fakhrid-Deen T, COLAGE: Let's Get This Straight: The Ultimate Handbook for Youth With LGBTQ Parents. Berkeley, CA, Seal Press, 2010

Fierstein H: Torch Song Trilogy. New York, Villard, 1983

Fitzgerald TJ: Queerspawn and their families: psychotherapy with LGBTQ families. Journal of Gay and Lesbian Mental Health 14:155–162, 2010

Garner A: Families Like Mine: Children of Gay Parents Tell It Like It Is. New York, HarperCollins, 2004

Gartrell N, Bos H: US National Longitudinal Lesbian Family Study: psychological adjustment of 17-year-old adolescents. Pediatrics 126:28–36, 2010

Gates GJ, Badgett MVL, Macomber JE, et al: Adoption and foster care by gay and lesbian parents in the United States. Washington, DC, The Williams Institute and Urban Institute. March 2007. Available at: http://williamsinstitute.law.ucla.edu/research/parenting/adoption-and-foster-care-by-gay-and-lesbian-parents-in-the-united-states/. Accessed November 7, 2011.

Glazer DF: Discussion of Karine Igartua's "Journey to Parenthood." Journal of Gay and Lesbian Mental Health 13:265–270, 2009

Glazer DF, Drescher J (eds): Gay and Lesbian Parenting. New York, Haworth, 2001

Goldman R: It's my right to have kid, pregnant man tells Oprah. ABC News Online, April 3, 2008. Available at: http://abcnews.go.com/Health/story?id=4581943 andpage=1. Accessed November 7, 2011.

Green J: The Velveteen Father: An Unexpected Journey to Parenthood. New York, Ballantine, 1999

Group for Advancement of Psychiatry: LGBT mental health syllabus. Available at: http://www.aglp.org/gap. Accessed November 7, 2011.

Igartua KJ: Journey to parenthood. Journal of Gay and Lesbian Mental Health 13: 253–264, 2009

Krivickas KM, Lofquist D: Demographics of same-sex couple households with children. U.S. Census Bureau Fertility and Family Statistics Branch, SEHSD Working Paper Number 2011–11. Washington, DC, U.S. Census Bureau, 2011. Available at: http://www.census.gov/population/www/socdemo/Krivickas-Lofquist%20PAA%202011.pdf. Accessed November 7, 2011.

Martin A: The Lesbian and Gay Parenting Handbook: Creating and Raising Our Families. New York, Perennial, 1993

Molinaro E (director): La Cage aux Folles (film). Da Ma Produzione and Les Productions Artistes Associés, 1978; distributed in U.S.A. by United Artists, 1979

Newman L: Mommy, Mama and Me. Berkeley, CA, Tricycle Press, 2009

Newman L, Souza D: Heather Has Two Mommies. New York, Alyson Books, 1994

Parnell P, Richardson J: And Tango Makes Three. New York, Simon & Schuster, 2005

Perrin EC, Cohen KM, Gold M, et al: Gay and lesbian issues in pediatric health care. Curr Probl Pediatr Adolesc Health Care 34:355–398, 2004

Savage D: The Kid: What Happened After My Boyfriend and I Decided to Go Get Pregnant. New York, Dutton, 1999

Schwartz D: Response to Igartua: parenthood as politics. Journal of Gay and Lesbian Mental Health 13:271–281, 2009

Stacey J, Biblarz T: (How) does the sexual orientation of the parent matter? Am Sociol Rev 65:159–183, 2001

Tavernise S: Parenting by gays more common in the South, census shows. The New York Times, Jan 18, 2011. Available at: http://www.nytimes.com/2011/01/19/us/19gays.html. Accessed November 7, 2011.

Volpp S, Drescher J: Point/Counterpoint: what has the lesbian family study taught us about child rearing by gay adults? Clinical Psychiatry News, March 2011, p 7

Wade S (director): Tru Loved (film). Brownbag Productions, 2008

Questions

4.1   Which statement(s) about LGBT parenting is (are) true?

A. Lesbian parenting through donor insemination was unknown before 1990.

B. Because LGBT people come out in early adolescence today, we almost never see instances of gay men having children in the context of heterosexual marriages and later coming out.

C. LGBT people become parents in a variety of ways, such as surrogacy, donor insemination, adoption, having children from heterosexual relationships, or taking in the child of a family member.

D. According to the most recent U.S. Census, the greatest number of same-sex parents are living in the Southeastern United States.

The correct answers are C and D.

Lesbians were using donor insemination to achieve pregnancy before the 1990s gay baby boom. Gay people today can still come out at any age (see Chapters 1 and 2), and some gay men and lesbians still have children in heterosexual relationships before coming out. LGBT people come to parenthood in a variety of ways. The U.S. Census showed that the 581,000 same-sex couples with children were more likely to be living in the Southeast than any other region.

4.2   Which of the following is *not* something LGBT parents can do to help their children cope with heterosexism or bullying?

A. Parents can give their children the scientific literature showing that children of lesbian and gay parents are resilient and well adjusted.

B. Parents can help connect their children with other families like theirs.
C. Parents can read affirming children's books to their children portraying families headed by LGBT parents.
D. Parents can meet with teachers and school administrators about antigay bullying if it occurs.
E. Parents can anticipate questions children may get from peers or adults, and talk to the child about how he or she can respond.

The correct answer is A.

Scientific literature is not age-appropriate for younger children. Even for older ones, it will not reassure the child facing a problem, and it may set up an expectation that the child should be able to cope with heterosexism and antigay attitudes without help. Other children of LGBT parents can help children feel less isolated and can help one another problem-solve how to deal with instances of heterosexism. Similarly, affirmative literature can help decrease feelings of isolation. If bullying is occurring, parents may need to be involved in the child's school and may need to provide education to school leaders. Talking out how to respond to ignorant questions, rude comments, or bullies with other children of LGBT parents or with parents can make facing those scenarios easier.

Sexual Identity in Patient-Therapist Relationships

Petros Levounis, M.D., M.A.
Andrew J. Anson, M.D.

A SUCCESSFUL PSYCHOTHERAPY may depend much more on the connection, chemistry, empathy, and "liking" that develop between a therapist and a patient than on any attribute or characteristic of the therapist. Nevertheless, a therapist's sexual identity often comes into play in the treatment of any patient, including patients who are lesbian, gay, bisexual, and transgender (LGBT). In the past, all therapists were assumed to be heterosexual, and even when they were not, they had to hide their sexual identities in fear of alienating their patients and being ostracized from their profession (Domenici and Lesser 1995; Drescher 1998). In the twenty-first century, at least in the United States, this is less frequently the case. Many LGBT therapists are open about their sexual identities, and LGBT patients often seek such therapists in search of gay-affirmative treatment.

In this chapter we present a clinical vignette with four sexual identity variations that illustrate some of the dynamics and conflicts in patient-therapist therapeutic dyads. We then go on to explore the subject of self-disclosure of a therapist's sexual identity, especially as it relates to the new realities of twenty-first-century social media.

Clinical Case: Therapeutic Dyads

Patient and Therapist

Pablo is a 25-year-old graduate student who comes to the University Mental Health outpatient clinic seeking help for what he thinks may be an anxiety problem. Specifically, Pablo is considering getting married and having children but is not sure if he's ready for the "big leap." "The whole thing is driving me crazy," he says, "to the point that I can no longer perform sexually; I can't even masturbate!" Thomas is a bright and enthusiastic third-year psychiatry resident assigned to the case.

The core themes of the Pablo (patient) and Thomas (therapist) therapeutic dyad in relation to their potential sexual identities are summarized in Table 5–1.

Case 1: Pablo Is Gay, Thomas Is Gay

As soon as they see each other, Pablo and Thomas recognize each other from the "gayborhood." Although they have not met before, at their first meeting both of them feel reasonably certain that the other one is gay. "Great!" thinks Pablo, "At least I did not get stuck with someone who'll judge me for being gay." "Oh no," thinks Thomas, "Now what? Can I effectively treat someone from my 'tribe'?"

If both men are comfortable having a gay identity, then the cultural similarity can be helpful in establishing a rapport quickly. For example, Pablo will likely feel relieved that he won't have to explain in detail—let alone defend—his same-sex attractions, behaviors, relationships, or thoughts on marriage and children and thus can delve into his pressing anxiety problems right away. On the other hand, Thomas's own familiarity with the cultural aspects of being gay may sidetrack him from exploring in depth issues that sound recognizable but, in fact, may have very different meanings for each of them. For example, if Pablo says, "You know how difficult it is to get a surrogate mother," Thomas might be tempted to say, "Yes, of course I do." Avoiding further inquiry by taking this shortcut in the therapeutic process may be not only restrictive, but also misleading: Pablo may be talking about emotional struggles, while Thomas may be assuming he is talking about financial or logistical ones.

Thomas's anxiety about treating someone so close to home—literally and figuratively—perhaps stems from a traditional psychiatric stance that strongly encouraged the therapist to act as a blank screen in order to effectively generate and receive a full spectrum of transferential projections (Drescher 1996/2001). Today, traditional notions of "neutrality" have been significantly revised by "two-person" psychology model of treatments that both assume and make allowances for therapists bringing to the therapeutic dyad much more of their own self, including cultural identities and sensitivities (Mitchell 1988).

Case 2: Pablo Is Gay, Thomas Is Straight

Within seconds of the two men introducing themselves, reasonable assumptions and expectations about each other's sexuality are established: Pablo is wearing a "Silence=Death" T-shirt, whereas Thomas has a picture of his wife and kids on his bookshelf. Pablo is unsure about Thomas's views on homosexuality and cannot stop thinking that despite the American Psychiatric Association's official disapproval of "reparative therapy" (American Psychiatric Association 2000), Thomas may, covertly or overtly, intentionally or unintentionally, try to convert him to heterosexuality. "How do I know that this guy is not one of *those* so-called therapists?" he asks himself. Thomas senses the patient's distrust and toys with the idea of openly declaring his support for gay rights.

In this situation, focusing on developing trust becomes the essential foundation for any subsequent treatment (please also see Chapter 19 of this book, "Partner Relational Problem"). Even in relatively brief psychopharmacology consultations, Pablo is unlikely to openly discuss his concerns or effectively negotiate treatment plans unless he feels that Thomas is sufficiently and appropriately "gay-friendly." If routine psychotherapeutic techniques of establishing a trusting relationship keep hitting a wall of suspicion, doubt, and mistrust from Pablo, Thomas may want to consider a more explicitly gay-affirmative approach, saying, for example, "In my psychiatric training, I learned that homosexuality is neither an illness nor anything that needs treatment."

Beyond the issue of the therapist possibly believing in conversion treatments, Pablo may or may not like the idea of having to explain gay culture to his straight therapist. Drescher (1998) writes: "A curious, beginning therapist who knows little about the lives of gay men will sometimes find patients who are willing to share that information. Other patients may feel that their time should not be used to educate a naive therapist" (p. 228). Furthermore, antigay stereotypes and beliefs are frequently present in the treatment of LGBT patients. Of course, such beliefs can be held by Pablo as well as by Thomas. For example, Thomas could think, "Why would you want to get married anyway, Pablo? Most gay men prefer not to be monogamous, and gay relationships rarely last long." Yet Pablo could have the same stereotypical beliefs that need to be explored in the treatment.

Case 3: Pablo Is Straight, Thomas Is Gay

Pablo is considering marrying Lisa and suspects that his rather effeminate therapist is probably gay. Pablo wonders if Thomas can relate to weddings, families, babies, and in-laws, let alone singles bars and bikini-modeling contests.

Of course, Pablo is justified in questioning whether any human being, man or woman, straight or gay, will be able to understand him. But he also feels the extra burden in trying to be heard by someone he believes "plays for the other team." If Thomas happens to be gay, the cultural differences between the straight and the gay worlds should not deter him from attempting to fully explore Pablo's emotional and sexual anxieties.

This dynamic may seem similar to and somewhat symmetrical with the gay patient–straight therapist dynamic described above in Case 2, but there are two fundamental differences: First, minorities have more familiarity with majority values, and thus gay therapists usually know more about the straight world than straight therapists usually know about the gay world. Second, because of societal homophobia and heterosexism, and the accompanying internalized homophobia, the gay therapist treating a straight patient may feel not only uneasy and inadequate about his work but also ashamed—a countertransference unlikely to be experienced by a straight therapist treating a gay patient.

Case 4: Pablo Is Straight, Thomas Is Straight

Pablo openly talks about his fear of not being able to be faithful to his girl-friend—soon to be wife—because he finds himself constantly checking out and fantasizing about other women. He sees that Thomas is wearing what looks like a wedding ring on his left hand and says, "Is it possible for a man to stay with the same woman for the rest of his life? Are you monogamous? I really need to know." In the course of the conversation that follows, Thomas says in passing, "Your relationship with Lisa will likely be different than my relationship with my wife." And just like that, the two men have established their sexual identities to each other.

What is this therapeutic dyad doing in an LGBT book? First, straight patients and straight therapists are not isolated from LGBT people, who may play very important roles in their lives. Pablo perhaps has difficulty accepting a lesbian soon-to-be sister-in-law, and perhaps Thomas questioned his own sexuality in the past in the context of his admiration for his gay male psychotherapist. Furthermore, just because Pablo and Thomas innocently and expediently "came out" to each other as straight, they cannot and should not be assumed to be locked in their respective sexual orientation labels. Did their initial revelations actually express their actual identities—or their eventual identities? What is to be made of Pablo's intense feelings for his tennis partner, Ben? Bisexuality is rarely considered as a possibility and often not accepted as an honest sexual identity (Rosenthal et al. 2011). The more we study human sexuality, the more we appreciate the myriad facets of sexual identity, orientation, behavior, fear, and fantasy that transcend strict boundaries, including the labels in the LGBT acronym. Both Pablo and Thomas will have a lot to learn from each other by keeping an open mind and attending to transferential and countertransferential feelings that at times may involve same-sex warmth, respect, hatred, jealousy, love, and sexuality.

Should Therapists Disclose Their Sexual Identity?

There is no consensus about whether and how a therapist should disclose her or his sexual orientation (Drescher and Byne 2009). Some assert that in most cases, it doesn't matter to the patient who the therapist is sexually attracted to or is having sex with. Gay, lesbian, and heterosexual therapists will all enter into a variety of transference relationships with patients, regardless of their own and their patient's orientation or even gender. Moreover, the question of transference may be even less relevant in psychiatric settings centered on psychopharmacology, where the transferences are more limited.

On the other hand, not disclosing one's homosexual orientation, in a hetero-normative culture, frequently implies that one is heterosexual (Isay 1991). This both misrepresents the LGBT therapist and perpetuates this distortion for lesbian, gay, bisexual, or questioning patients. Advantages and disadvantages of matching patients with therapists who are open about their sexual orientation

TABLE 5–1. Sexual identity core themes in therapeutic dyads

		Pablo (patient)	
		Gay	Straight
Thomas (therapist)	Gay	Rapport vs. Overidentification	Understanding vs. Shame
	Straight	Trust vs. Mistrust	Openness vs. Closure

were discussed in the previous section, but if there is one thing that can be learned from the literature and the trends of social media in the last few decades, it is this: people are curious about the intimate lives of others, and patients (at least some) will be curious about those of their therapists.

One familiar scenario in the psychoanalytic literature describes the patient who, in the context of a psychotherapy session, addresses her curiosity about her therapist. Is the therapist married? Does she have a husband and children who live with her in a big house in the suburbs? The therapist, only after a skilled and detailed exploration of the patient's feelings, fears, and fantasies about the possible answers to these questions, must decide if it would be therapeutically useful to disclose her sexual identity at this point in their work. Disclosing one's sexual identity, in such instances, must be weighed against the implications of withholding this information from the patient. Magee and Miller (1997), for example, have posited that nondisclosure in this scenario would be the equivalent of a "breach in the therapeutic fabric of trust" (p. 208). Table 5–2 provides some examples of circumstances when disclosing one's sexuality may be helpful and when it may not.

Regardless of one's approach to self-disclosure, it is increasingly common for patients to learn their therapist's orientation in other ways, by indirect inquiries and indirect disclosures.

The Patient's Indirect Inquiries

The indirect inquiry can happen within a session. Guthrie (2006) gives the example of a patient who remarks, "I hope you and your wife have a good vacation" (p. 66). He posits that these indirect inquiries often feel safer, as they allow patients to disavow their curiosity about the therapist's sexuality. For patients struggling with a homosexual orientation, acknowledging curiosity to a therapist might feel particularly scary or revealing. Likewise, such inquiries might signal an invitation for *indirect disclosure,* which may also feel safer for the patient who is not yet ready to "know," in a direct way, the therapist's identity.

However, other writers have pointed out that inquiries within the therapy session need not be as overt or conscious. Magee and Miller (1997) believe that "most analysands know a great deal about their analysts" and point out that "day after day, season after season, year after year, patients consciously and unconsciously register changes in their analyst's office, clothing, moods, levels of attentiveness, qualities of silences" (p. 206).

Patients think of this concept of "knowing," in much less technical language, as "gaydar," a portmanteau of "gay" and "radar:" Wikipedia defines *gaydar* as

> [T]he intuitive ability to assess someone's sexual orientation as gay, bisexual, or straight. Gaydar relies almost exclusively on nonverbal clues. These include (but are not limited to) the sensitivity to social behaviors and mannerisms; for instance, acknowledging flamboyant mannerisms, overtly rejecting traditional gender roles, a person's occupation and grooming habits.
> (http://en.wikipedia.org/wiki/Gaydar)

Patients exercise intuition about the intimate lives of their therapists in a manner somewhat similar to the way their therapists are constantly using intuition and nonverbal cues to understand what their patients have and have not said. The idea that patients may be observing their therapists by using methods similar to those therapists use to observe patients goes back to Ferenczi's (1933) early work in mutual analysis and is taken up by modern interpersonal and relational analysts (Hoffman 1983). While this concept applies to both gay and straight patients, there is reason to believe that some LGBT people have sophisticated gaydar. Research suggests that LGBT people may be better able to correctly identify other people's sexual orientation by viewing silent videos or pictures than are their heterosexual counterparts (Lawson 2005; Shelp 2002).

Russell (2006) adds that "clients—at least those who are able to stand enough outside the solipsism of their own pain—know a great deal about their therapists and their political and social beliefs," and states that without the therapist directly disclosing anything, patients are able "to extrapolate from how therapists are in the session to how they are in their larger worlds" (p. 80).

Increasingly, however, patients have access to other information that forms their picture of their therapists "in their larger worlds." The literature contains several case studies in which patients learned of or began to suspect their therapist's identity from a comment by a friend, from a name or listing in a gay or lesbian publication, or from encountering the therapist at a specific event, in a certain part of town, or with a same-sex partner (Isay 1991; Magee and Miller 1997). It is worth noting that social media are changing exponentially the number of ways this is happening and will happen in the future. It is the increasingly rare patient who does not enter his or her psychiatrist's name into a search en-

TABLE 5–2. Considerations for self-disclosure of sexual identity

Consider direct disclosure when…	Consider holding off disclosure when…
• Therapeutic work is just beginning and patient feels comfortable asking therapist directly about orientation.	• Indirect inquiries communicate a discomfort with knowing about therapist's identity in a direct way.
• Patient has identified "coming out" or normalizing homoerotic thoughts and feelings as a therapeutic goal, and therapist is lesbian, gay, bisexual, or transgender.	• Patient's fantasies about the therapist produce material that warrants further exploration.
• Patient indirectly expresses continued curiosity about therapist's orientation.	• Patient is particularly defended against exploring questions of his or her own sexuality.
• Therapist or clinic advertises as LGBT-oriented.	• Patient expresses particularly violent views against homosexuality, and therapist is lesbian, gay, bisexual, or transgender.
• Not disclosing would undermine the patient-therapist alliance.	• Therapist has significant unresolved feelings about her or his own orientation.
• Patient's misinterpretation of the therapist's orientation reinforces patient's feelings of self-hatred.	

gine for "hits" or search for the clinician's page on Facebook. Market research by Harris Interactive (2010) demonstrated that gay and lesbian Americans are significantly more likely to read blogs, belong to social networking sites such as Facebook and MySpace, log in, and frequent these sites more times a day than heterosexual cohorts. The result is the evolution of gay and lesbian online "communities" where patients are as likely to find their therapists today as they are to bump into them at the gym (Levounis 1999).

The Therapist's Indirect Disclosures

Today, therapists have many ways in which they might disclose their sexual identity without ever talking about it in a session with a patient. Some would argue that disclosure happens at every point of therapy (Cole 2002), and others have pointed out therapists disclose much about themselves by choosing the neighborhood where they work, the way they decorate their offices, whether they wear a wedding ring, and so forth.

Indirect disclosures in a session can be nuanced, as Guthrie (2006) illustrates in his above-mentioned patient who comments on the therapist "vacationing with his wife:"

> [B]y encouraging the patient to explore the fantasy that I have a wife, I open up a dialogue that may well lead to discussing my sexual orientation. On the other hand, a patient's indirect approach may allow a therapist to avoid the topic of his or her sexual orientation altogether. A patient, sensing the therapist's discomfort, may collude in silence to protect the latter from a potentially uncomfortable discussion. (p. 66)

Therapists not only make indirect choices about disclosure in deciding whether to be silent, but also in their manifest familiarity (or not) with the cultural references that patients bring into their sessions (movies, slang, pop culture, porn sites, sexual positions, etc.).

As mentioned in the previous section, social media is a vehicle through which patients can indirectly inquire about their therapist's personal life. However, consciously or unconsciously, mental health professionals may also indirectly "disclose" information about themselves and their sexual identities through the Internet. Even with standard privacy settings, it is relatively easy for patients to access a psychiatrist's wall posts or pictures or stumble upon a therapist's profile on a gay or lesbian dating site. In a culture where, increasingly, the personal is public, some patients will recognize their therapist in a "Millionaire Matchmaker" episode or in an "It Gets Better" video on YouTube.

Technological changes create challenges for present and future professionals striving to keep their private and professional lives separate. In the past, the challenges might have been limited to managing scenarios like "What if you, a gay therapist, discover that your gay patient attends the same gym or frequents the same gay bar?" Therapists today are confronted with other scenarios: "Do we let friends of friends see our Facebook photos? What should one do if a patient sends a friend request? What if a single therapist discovers a patient is using the same dating website? What if a patient frequents and posts to the same blogs?"

Although it is unclear whether therapists are obligated to separate their personal and professional lives to a greater degree than other professionals, keeping one's sexual identity completely out of the public domain has become nearly impossible. Ultimately, direct or indirect disclosure of sexual identity for therapists today is determined by 1) their training and theoretical beliefs, 2) their anxiety or comfort with their own sexual identity, and 3) their own solutions to integrating their sexual identity into their public identities, both as professionals and as individuals in the private sphere.

Key Points

- An LGBT therapist treating an LGBT patient frequently finds rapport, familiarity, and understanding to be helpful in the treatment, but the therapist should also be careful not to overidentify with the patient's problems.

- A straight therapist treating an LGBT patient often has to familiarize herself or himself with gay culture, be cognizant of antigay stereotypes and beliefs, and gain the patient's trust.

- Self-disclosure of an LGBT therapist's sexual identity can help patients who struggle with coming out and would like to normalize homoerotic thoughts and feelings. In some cases, nondisclosure may undermine the patient-therapist alliance.

- Directly or indirectly, patients regularly inquire about their therapist's sexual identity. In the age of social networking, it is relatively easy to find personal information about one's therapist.

References

American Psychiatric Association, Commission on Psychotherapy by Psychiatrists: Position statement on therapies focused on attempts to change sexual orientation (reparative or conversion therapies). Am J Psychiatry 157:1719–1721, 2000

Cole G: Infecting the Treatment: The Experience of an HIV-Positive Psychoanalyst. Hillsdale, NJ, Analytic Press, 2002

Domenici T, Lesser RC (eds): Disorienting Sexuality: Psychoanalytic Reappraisals of Sexual Identities. New York, Routledge, 1995

Drescher J: Across the great divide: gender panic in the psychoanalytic dyad (1996), in Sexualities Lost and Found: Lesbians, Psychoanalysis and Culture. Edited by Gould E, Kiersky S. Madison, CT, International Universities Press, 2001, pp 91–109

Drescher J: Psychoanalytic Therapy and the Gay Man. Hillsdale, NJ, Analytic Press, 1998

Drescher J, Byne W: Homosexuality, gay and lesbian identities, and homosexual behavior, in Kaplan and Sadock's Comprehensive Textbook of Psychiatry, 9th Edition. Edited by Sadock BJ, Sadock VA, Ruiz P. Baltimore, MD, Lippincott Williams & Wilkins, 2009, pp 2060–2090

Ferenczi S: Confusion of tongues between the adult and the child. Int J Psychoanal 30:225–230, 1933

Guthrie C: Disclosing the therapist's sexual orientation: the meaning of disclosure in working with gay, lesbian, and bisexual patients. Journal of Gay and Lesbian Psychotherapy 10:63–77, 2006

Harris Interactive: Gay and lesbian adults are more likely and more frequent blog readers: social networks, blog popularity remain high for gay Americans over past three years. July 13, 2010. Available at: http://www.harrisinteractive.com/NewsRoom/PressReleases/tabid/446/mid/1506/articleId/435/ctl/ReadCustom%20Default/Default.aspx. Accessed November 8, 2011.

Hoffman I: The patient as interpreter of the analyst's experience. Contemp Psychoanal 19:389–422, 1983

Isay AR: The homosexual analyst: clinical considerations. Psychoanal Study Child 46:199–216, 1991

Lawson W: Queer eyes: blips on the gaydar. Psychology Today Magazine, November/December 2005

Levounis P: Gay patient—gay therapist: a case report of Stephen. Journal of Gay and Lesbian Psychotherapy 3:11–22 1999

Magee M, Miller DC: Lesbian Lives: Psychoanalytic Narratives Old and New. Hillsdale, NJ, Analytic Press, 1997

Mitchell SA: Relational Concepts in Psychoanalysis: An Integration. Cambridge, MA, Harvard University Press, 1988

Rosenthal AM, Sylva D, Safron A, et al: Sexual arousal patterns of bisexual men revisited. Biol Psychol 88:112–115, 2011

Russell GM: Different ways of knowing: the complexities of the therapist disclosure. Journal of Gay and Lesbian Psychotherapy 10:79–94, 2006

Shelp SG: Gaydar: visual detection of sexual orientation among gay and straight men. J Homosex 44:1–14, 2002

Questions

5.1 A 65-year-old lesbian teacher, Patty, says her lesbian therapist, Theresa, is "the best" because she understands her like no one else in the world. Patty explains: "Very often I don't even have to finish my sentences, Theresa does it for me and she's always right! It's great having a gay doc." Which of the following themes is most central to this therapeutic dyad?

    A. Openness vs. isolation.
    B. Rapport vs. overidentification.
    C. Understanding vs. shame.
    D. Trust vs. mistrust.

The correct answer is B.

While Patty and Theresa have established excellent rapport, in part related to their shared sexual identity, it is possible that the two women have overidentified on a number of issues. One risk of this treatment is of the therapist's providing answers for her own life as solutions for the patient's problems.

5.2   Marc, a college sophomore, asks for a gay therapist at the student health center. He is assigned to Paul, who is openly gay. During their first encounter, Marc asks Paul: "Are you gay?" What is the most appropriate response?

   A. Yes.
   B. No.
   C. Maybe.
   D. Why do you ask?

The correct answer is A.

As Marc has explicitly asked for a gay therapist, there is little need to be coy about answering the question. While Paul may want to explore Marc's desire to have a gay therapist as treatment unfolds, lying or avoiding the question would likely undermine the patient-therapist alliance.

5.3   A psychopharmacology patient sends you a Facebook "friend request." What is the best next step?

   A. Accept the request and bring up the issue during the next session.
   B. Ignore the request, bring it up during the next session, and then decide whether to accept the "friend request."
   C. Ignore the request, bring it up during the next session, and let your patient know that you don't accept "friend requests" from patients.
   D. Ignore the request and discuss it with your patient only if she brings it up.

The correct answer is C.

Facebook exchanges between patients and physicians are not covered by the Health Insurance Portability and Accountability Act of 1996 (HIPAA) privacy and security rules, and as such are not permitted.

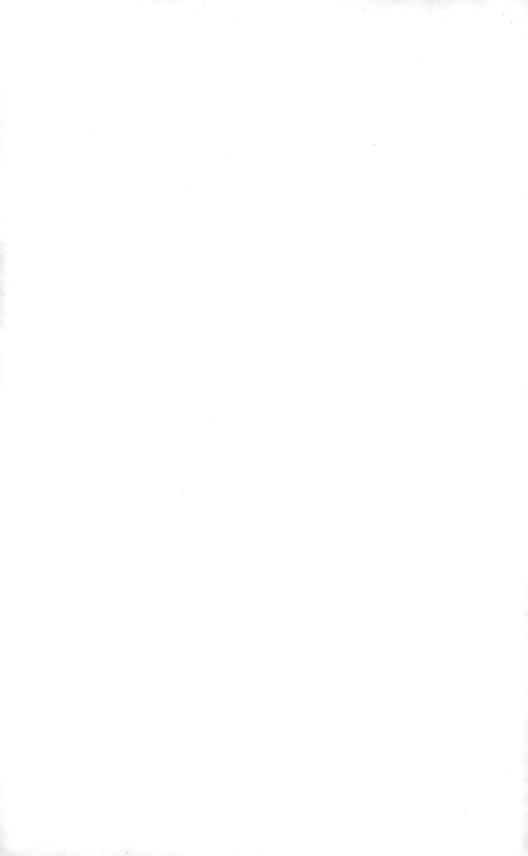

PART II

CASE STUDIES

Attention-Deficit/Hyperactivity Disorder

Distraction and Attraction: ADHD Diagnosis and Treatment in LGBT Patients

John K. Burton, M.D.

ATTENTION-DEFICIT/HYPERACTIVITY DISORDER (ADHD) affects executive function, the higher-level brain circuits that determine which responses to competing stimuli will be inhibited and which will be acted on. Executive function is crucial for organizing and planning ahead; it is the "CEO" of the brain. ADHD thus affects a wide variety of cognitive functions, not only learning and memory, but also social judgment and emotion regulation.

Approximately two-thirds of individuals with the disorder have impairment lasting into adulthood, but up to 80% have never come to clinical attention (Newcorn et al. 2007). This lack of appropriate diagnosis creates numerous problems, including mood, anxiety, and substance abuse comorbidities, and impairments in social, occupational, and romantic spheres. Individuals with ADHD are also vulnerable to problems in psychodynamic function. Anxiety about self-control, misattunement in relationships with others, and difficulties processing internal emotional states can lead to a pattern of reliance on maladaptive defense mechanisms (Gilmore 2000). In lesbian, gay, bisexual, and transgender (LGBT) individuals, many of whom already feel anxiety about their self-worth or the expression of their sexual identity, the symptoms of ADHD can create a complex clinical picture that requires sensitivity to the interrelationship between sexuality and executive function.

Case Example: Cain

Chief complaint: Cain was a 30-year-old man living alone in an apartment he owned in a trendy downtown neighborhood. He had a history of short stints working for others but had started his own company consulting to television advertisers a few years prior. His novel approach and fresh solutions to old problems earned him rapid success and accolades in the field. He had recently sold the company, though he continued to stay as its chief executive officer. Cain had dated women and men as a young adult but felt that he was "mostly" gay. Cain summarized his chief complaint as, "I'm a little lost."

History of presenting problem: Despite the significant increase in his income and job security, Cain was dissatisfied with his daily routine since he had sold his company. He was increasingly frustrated with the perceived inability, on the part of both the parent company executives and his new team of employees, to "get" what his company was about. No longer being his own boss also meant that he had more free time. Cain was now confronted by a feeling of deep loneliness that he had avoided in his entrepreneurial 24/7 work schedule. As a young and successful businessman, he was a "catch," but in trying to date, he was unable to follow through beyond a few superficial encounters. He described a pattern of quickly losing interest after the initial excitement of meeting someone new.

Appearance: Cain presented as a slim man with freckles and a forelock of bright red hair that repeatedly fell in front of his eyes, giving him a boyish appearance incongruent with his executive position. He wore a tailored blue oxford shirt with the top three buttons undone, jeans, scuffed Gucci loafers, and no socks. In our first meeting, he answered questions thoughtfully but often seemed to give more information than was necessary. He was friendly, but moved about in his seat frequently, giving the impression of being uncomfortable. His pale blue eyes darted about the room as he talked, multitasking, as if he were taking a mental inventory of my office. My initial countertransference to Cain was to feel drawn to his many strengths, yet I felt a parallel discomfort, not sure that he was "getting" what I was trying to convey to him.

Review of symptoms: Cain denied feelings of depression or episodes of elevated mood. He also denied problems with panic attacks, obsessions, or social anxiety. Cain did describe often feeling restless and struggling to complete projects. He also noted that he often lost track of conversations, though he made sure he never gave the impression that he was not listening at work. However, in his social life his friends would sometimes comment that he seemed uninterested or bored. We reviewed each of the 18 symptoms listed in the DSM-IV-TR diagnostic criteria for ADHD and found Cain met criteria for 7 out of 9 symptoms of inattention and 4 out of 9 symptoms of hyperactivity/impulsivity, though he had a history of at least 6 out of 9 hyperactivity symptoms in childhood (see Table 6–1).

Cain also acknowledged that he was often worried and anxious about a variety of things that would occur throughout the day, whether they were related to

---

**TABLE 6–1.   DSM-IV-TR diagnostic criteria for attention-deficit/
hyperactivity disorder**

A.   Either (1) or (2):

(1)   six (or more) of the following symptoms of **inattention** have persisted for at least
6 months to a degree that is maladaptive and inconsistent with developmental
level:

Inattention

(a)   often fails to give close attention to details or makes careless mistakes in
schoolwork, work, or other activities

(b)   often has difficulty sustaining attention in tasks or play activities

(c)   often does not seem to listen when spoken to directly

(d)   often does not follow through on instructions and fails to finish schoolwork,
chores, or duties in the workplace (not due to oppositional behavior or
failure to understand instructions)

(e)   often has difficulty organizing tasks and activities

(f)   often avoids, dislikes, or is reluctant to engage in tasks that require sustained
mental effort (such as schoolwork or homework)

(g)   often loses things necessary for tasks or activities (e.g., toys, school
assignments, pencils, books, or tools)

(h)   is often easily distracted by extraneous stimuli

(i)   is often forgetful in daily activities

(2)   six (or more) of the following symptoms of **hyperactivity-impulsivity** have
persisted for at least 6 months to a degree that is maladaptive and inconsistent
with developmental level:

Hyperactivity

(a)   often fidgets with hands or feet or squirms in seat

(b)   often leaves seat in classroom or in other situations in which remaining
seated is expected

(c)   often runs about or climbs excessively in situations in which it is
inappropriate (in adolescents or adults, may be limited to subjective feelings
of restlessness)

(d)   often has difficulty playing or engaging in leisure activities quietly

(e)   is often "on the go" or often acts as if "driven by a motor"

(f)   often talks excessively

Impulsivity

(g)   often blurts out answers before questions have been completed

(h)   often has difficulty awaiting turn

(i)   often interrupts or intrudes on others (e.g., butts into conversations or
games)

B.   Some hyperactive-impulsive or inattentive symptoms that caused impairment
were present before age 7 years.

TABLE 6–1.   DSM-IV-TR diagnostic criteria for attention-deficit/ hyperactivity disorder *(continued)*

C.   Some impairment from the symptoms is present in two or more settings (e.g., at school [or work] and at home).

D.   There must be clear evidence of clinically significant impairment in social, academic, or occupational functioning.

E.   The symptoms do not occur exclusively during the course of a pervasive developmental disorder, schizophrenia, or other psychotic disorder and are not better accounted for by another mental disorder (e.g., mood disorder, anxiety disorder, dissociative disorder, or a personality disorder).

Code based on type:

> **314.01   Attention-deficit/hyperactivity disorder, combined type:** if both Criteria A1 and A2 are met for the past 6 months
>
> **314.00   Attention-deficit/hyperactivity disorder, predominantly inattentive type:**   if Criterion A1 is met but Criterion A2 is not met for the past 6 months
>
> **314.01   Attention-deficit/hyperactivity disorder, predominantly hyperactive-impulsive type:**   if Criterion A2 is met but Criterion A1 is not met for the past 6 months

Coding note: For individuals (especially adolescents and adults) who currently have symptoms that no longer meet full criteria, "in partial remission" should be specified.

Source.   Adapted from *Diagnostic and Statistical Manual of Mental Disorders,* 4th Edition, Text Revision. Washington, DC, American Psychiatric Association, 2000. Used with permission. Copyright © 2000 American Psychiatric Association.

---

work or to social interactions. He felt anxiety throughout the day most days, with attendant muscle tension, had occasional difficulty sleeping, and often felt short-tempered. Comorbidity is the rule with ADHD; nearly half of ADHD-diagnosed patients also carry a diagnosis of an anxiety disorder (Kessler et al. 2006) (see Figure 6–1).

Cain described drinking socially and had never used alcohol to excess. He had tried marijuana once and found the effect unpleasant. He had tried cocaine in college and did use it somewhat regularly for a period of time, though not since he had started his company. He had also used stimulants in college to complete papers or to cram for an exam. He described them as effective for these purposes and denied feeling a need to use them regularly or to get high.

Past and family history: Cain had a brother who had had learning difficulties in high school and a nephew with ADHD. There was no other significant past psychiatric, family, or medical history.

Impression: Cain presented with symptoms of ADHD, as well as comorbid generalized anxiety disorder, but before we could make the diagnosis, we needed to explore Cain's development. The current DSM criteria for ADHD (American

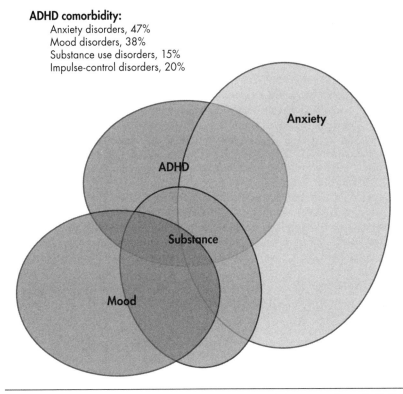

ADHD comorbidity:
Anxiety disorders, 47%
Mood disorders, 38%
Substance use disorders, 15%
Impulse-control disorders, 20%

FIGURE 6–1. Overlapping comorbidities with attention-deficit/ hyperactivity disorder (ADHD), especially anxiety, depression, and substance abuse.

Psychiatric Association 2000) require evidence of symptom impairment going back to at least age 7. Reviewing the history of inattention and hyperactivity going back to childhood is not only useful for diagnostic purposes, but also is the beginning of an exploration of the effect of ADHD on the patient's development. In Cain's case, we found evidence of symptoms at each stage of life: preschool, latency, adolescence, and young adulthood. This was a crucial step in helping Cain address the challenges that he faced, especially the development of his homosexual desire and his gay identity.

Developmental history: Cain was the youngest of three boys born to married parents in a middle-class suburban community. Cain's father was a busy and well-respected physician, and his mother began to work managing his father's office when Cain entered preschool. Cain recalls that he often felt lonely in early childhood. A painful memory involved being nicknamed "The Tasmanian Devil" by his preschool teacher. His impulsivity was an obstacle to making friends, and he described always feeling like "the weird kid." Cain recalled a humiliating episode when his brothers tricked him into playing hide and seek, only to go off together while he was hiding. Cain increasingly retreated into television, a coping mechanism that restricted his social life but also foreshadowed his later career success. Parents often deny the diagnosis of ADHD in their children by saying, "He can't have ADHD, he can pay attention to the TV [computer, Internet, video games, a 700-page Harry Potter book, etc.] all day. In fact, I have to yell to get him away from it!" It is important to remember that ADHD is not a deficit of attention but a problem with attention *regulation,* in that attention is drawn to the most intense stimulus. Children with ADHD often can focus for hours on an activity if it is highly stimulating to them.

Cain described an absence of overt homophobia in both his household and his community. His father had a gay brother who was a respected member of the family, and there were a few openly gay students in his high school. Nevertheless, Cain felt confused by his own early adolescent homoerotic feelings and kept them to himself. In elementary school, Cain had been at the top of his class academically, despite continuing to get in trouble for talking out of turn and not sitting still. He had also become active in the school's drama department. With the onset of puberty, he made an effort to avoid attention, stopped doing theater, and retreated into academics. He rationalized that he was more academic and more ambitious than his brothers, who had more active dating lives. He acknowledged, however, that in order to do well in school he had to spend three times as long on homework and study as his peers seemed to require.

In college, Cain experienced a series of frustrating sexual encounters with both men and women. He denied dating women for the purpose of appearing straight; he genuinely had attraction to women and was confused about his sexual feelings in general. However, he also acknowledged that he wished he could be straight, since that made him feel less like "the weird kid" (Corbett 2001). Ultimately, Cain realized that his attraction to men was more "visceral," and he self-identified as gay his senior year of college. It was only then that he came out to his parents. He did not come out to his brothers until after his company became successful.

After college, before he started his company, Cain had a period of time when he was very sexually active. He recalls being able to walk into a bar and immediately find an attractive man whom he would take home. "It was like *The Matrix,*" he said. "I could see all the guys like they was just those streaming numbers. I just took a minute to take the whole thing in and then honed in on the right code. It was easy back then. Too easy maybe." This history contrasted completely with Cain's current sexual life, but it helped us to appreciate the intensity of Cain's sexual impulses and how they might feel frightening as well as exciting.

Treatment

Psychoeducation

The first step in treating any individual with ADHD should be to help the patient understand how DSM symptoms apply to him or her as an individual. Psychoeducation also includes discussing the role of medication and psychotherapy. The meaning of the diagnosis should be explored even if the physician is only prescribing medication, because discussing it will certainly affect adherence to treatment. Cain resisted medication initially because it concretized his fears about himself that he was not in control if he needed medication. Understanding these fears allowed me to empathize with Cain's anxiety. "You really work so hard to keep everything under control," I told him. "It must be exhausting to perform up to your own high demands." Cain became tearful when he replied, "No one has ever recognized that before, but it's true. I don't allow any room for slipping up, because I'm afraid that if I slipped up, it would be very bad." Although this discussion began in the context of making a diagnosis, it was the beginning of a psychodynamic exploration of its meaning to Cain. This allowed us to consider rational pharmacotherapy. Later, we would understand how the diagnosis also resonated with a deep sense of deficit that related to his identity as a gay man.

Medication

The decision to use medication to treat ADHD is one that should come out of a collaborative understanding with the patient of his or her individual target symptoms. Target symptoms are essentially the patient's specific version of DSM symptoms; that is, instead of following relatively abstract constructs of "sustained attention," "disorganization," or "restlessness," we look for readily identifiable behaviors or experiences in the patient's daily life. Defining Cain's target symptoms helped us focus on what we expected medication would change. We also looked at the way Cain's target symptoms had a negative impact on his romantic life. For example, his difficulty following a conversation and his subjective sense that he was not listening had an obvious negative impact on his experience of dating.

Choosing a medication to treat adult ADHD requires consideration of several factors. Although adult studies do not show the same high effect size that studies in children do, the psychostimulants are overall very effective in adults (Newcorn et al. 2007). Other medications that have been used to treat ADHD are atomoxetine, bupropion, desipramine, and others. Although these have been shown to be more effective than placebo, and should be used when patient characteristics or preference indicates, overall they are second-line treatments.

There has been concern that use of stimulant medication in individuals with ADHD leads to greater substance abuse. In fact, the opposite has been found in many studies; stimulant medication has even been successfully used in active cocaine abusers with no increase in substance abuse and no redirection of the controlled medication (Riggs et al. 2004). Given the high rate of substance abuse in the LGBT community, particularly stimulant-like substances such as cocaine and crystal meth, it is important to realistically assess the patient's drug use. Nevertheless, an LGBT patient with well-documented ADHD should not be deprived of the benefit of stimulant therapy in the interest of excess caution or prejudice. Although Cain had used cocaine in the past, he was not an active user. He did not have a pattern of stimulant abuse, though he had used these drugs without a prescription. There has also been concern about the rate of sudden death in patients who have been prescribed stimulant medication. Subsequent review of all available research data found that the concern about cardiac events with stimulants was unfounded. The current recommendations include screening to obtain a cardiac history, a family history of cardiac disease, and a cardiac examination. There is no need for an electrocardiogram if these are negative, as was the case with Cain. If there are positive findings, a referral to a cardiologist is warranted, but stimulants may still be used with caution in patients with some cardiac abnormalities.

Although we considered atomoxetine because it is often the treatment of choice with comorbid anxiety, we chose a trial of a long-acting form of methylphenidate. A stimulant has the advantage of immediate assessment of the effect of medication. Despite Cain's symptoms of worrying and irritability, he did not notice a worsening of his anxiety. In fact, on a moderate dose achieved within 2 weeks of titration, he noted a significant improvement in his target symptoms. His symptoms of anxiety lessened and did not require further medication treatment. This suggested that the diagnosis of generalized anxiety disorder was secondary to his ADHD symptoms—both a consequence of and a compensation for his chronic sense of not being completely in control of input from his environment. Once he was able to attend better and his life was more organized, the need for constant vigilance decreased significantly. He became less irritable at work, more easygoing in general, and more approachable in social situations.

Psychotherapy

Although medication alone is adequate to treat the core symptoms of ADHD, there is a role for psychotherapy. Distraction and impulsivity can take a toll on all aspects of development, including the ability to form relationships, to work with others, and to develop a secure and stable identity. Behaviorally oriented interventions, such as ADHD "coaching," can help the patients develop organizational habits that they did not develop earlier in life and can have a profound benefit on functioning. Psychodynamic psychotherapy can also be helpful. The LGBT patient in particular benefits from the exploration of these issues in a psychodynamic psychotherapy.

ADHD and LGBT Development

The diagnosis of ADHD provided a developmental lens through which we could understand Cain's developing sexual desires. At the oedipal stage when longings for male identification are present in both heterosexual and homosexual boys, Cain's feeling of being the "weird" kid affected his sense of value as a boy but also gave meaning to his desire for other men that arose later in adolescence. In adolescence, anxiety about bodily control normally intensifies and centers on sexuality. Cain already had a heightened sense of anxiety about his ability to control his body and his interactions with the environment. He had had a brief respite during latency and was able to sublimate his natural tendency for spontaneity, but puberty brought about an intensification of his anxiety about self-control and the need to restrict his self-expression.

Recognizing how ADHD can affect the transference can allow for important therapeutic work. In the initial phase of treatment, when Cain would come late to a session he would apologize profusely, revealing the harshness of his superego. Cain, as an intelligent and psychologically savvy man, expected me to interpret his lateness as passive-aggressive. While Cain likely did harbor unconscious aggression, such an interpretation in this phase of treatment would only validate his sense of being out of control of his drives. Instead, I empathized with the real impact that Cain's organizational and attentional difficulties had on his life, including in getting to our sessions. Gradually, Cain began to feel more secure as he got used to the benefit of medication and trusted that I would not be judgmental. This allowed him to accept the profound role that ADHD had played in his life. The harshness of his superego and his need for vigilance lessened. We were then able to look at the ways in which Cain did use forgetting and distractibility as ready-made defense mechanisms aimed at avoiding awareness of his drives, such as by not noticing the interest of an attractive man.

Conclusion

Cain's case illustrates the unique challenges that confront the LGBT person with ADHD. Cain found a highly successful solution to the problem of his undiagnosed ADHD in his career, but his self-esteem and his romantic life suffered. A thorough psychiatric assessment was crucial for recognizing the diagnosis of ADHD. Exploration of his past history led to a better appreciation of the impact of his symptoms on each phase of his development. Treatment began with psychoeducation and a collaborative discussion about the role of medication in treating ADHD. Improvement in attention and overall executive function led to greater awareness of the defensive uses of inattention and disorganization in Cain's psychosexual development. This was a central theme in Cain's psychotherapy that led to greater self-awareness and improvement in his relationship functioning.

Jensen and colleagues (1997) have theorized that ADHD could be considered an evolutionarily determined variant in the human species. They speculate that a rapidly shifting attention and high motor activity would be beneficial in hostile environments. Individuals with ADHD can perform well in modern environments that are suited to their unique cognitive style. A higher proportion of ADHD has been found in creative people and entrepreneurs like Cain. Similarly, LGBT people grow up with a conflicted perspective on themselves and their place in the world. This creates problems with self-esteem, yet many LGBT people find a healthy use for this "outsider" perspective, especially when value is placed on creativity and self-expression. For the LGBT person with ADHD, this conflict is heightened. The sense of not fitting in and the anxiety about self-control are concentrated in one's sexual and relationship experience. Acknowledging the role that ADHD plays in this conflict can help the individual find the most successful balance in all areas of his or her life.

Key Points

- A diagnosis of ADHD should be considered in the presentation of adults with impairment in work or romantic relationships, even if there is no obvious impairment in their educational history.

- Diagnosis and treatment of the adult with ADHD is enriched by exploring impairment in childhood caused by the symptoms of inattention and/or impulsivity and hyperactivity.

- Even when an LGBT patient has not experienced overt homophobia, ADHD can cause significant impairment in self-esteem and in comfort with self-expression. The identification and treatment of ADHD in an LGBT individual can be of substantial benefit in the psychotherapeutic work of consolidating a healthy, adult self-representation that integrates an LGBT identity.

- Psychostimulants should be considered as a first-line treatment in adults with ADHD who are appropriately monitored, even if there is a history of substance abuse, although active substance abuse should be treated first.

References

American Psychiatric Association: Diagnostic and Statistical Manual of Mental Disorders, 4th Edition, Text Revision. Washington, DC, American Psychiatric Association, 2000

Corbett K: Faggot=loser. Studies in Gender and Sexuality 2:3–28, 2001

Gilmore K: A psychodynamic perspective on attention-deficit/hyperactivity disorder. J Am Psychoanal Assoc 48:1259–1293, 2000

Jensen PS, Mrazek D, Knapp PK, et al: Evolution and revolution in child psychiatry: ADHD as a disorder of adaptation. J Am Acad Child Adolesc Psychiatry 36:1672–1679, 1997

Kessler RC, Adler L, Barkley R, et al: The prevalence and correlates of adult ADHD in the United States: results from the National Comorbidity Survey Replication. Am J Psychiatry 163:716–723, 2006

Newcorn JH, Weiss M, Stein MA: The complexity of ADHD: diagnosis and treatment of the adult patient with comorbidities. CNS Spectr 12 (suppl 12):1–14, 2007

Riggs PD, Hall SK, Mikulich-Gilbertson SK, et al: A randomized controlled trial of pemoline for attention-deficit/hyperactivity disorder in substance-abusing adolescents. J Am Acad Child Adolesc Psychiatry 43:420–429, 2004

Questions

6.1   A 35-year-old gay man presents with difficulty keeping organized at work and stress about his job security. He notes worrying about what his superiors think of him and anxiety about whether he will be able to progress in his current company. At times he has difficulty sleeping, and he occasionally experiences stomach upset on workdays. A thorough psychiatric assessment reveals symptoms of inattention and impulsivity going back to childhood. The patient is otherwise healthy and has no family history of cardiac problems. He and his partner have a weekend house in a gay community that is known for its open sexual attitude and active social life. He drinks alcohol on weekends but denies other drug use. In this patient, a trial of a stimulant medication is

   A. Contraindicated because the addition of a stimulant will worsen the patient's anxiety disorder.
   B. Contraindicated because stimulants are not effective in a patient of this age.
   C. Not contraindicated.
   D. Contraindicated because crystal meth use is too prevalent in the gay community to safely prescribe a Class II controlled substance that could cause sudden cardiac death.

The correct answer is C.

The psychostimulants are the most effective class of medication for the core symptoms of ADHD with an effect size of approximately 90% in some studies. Although the effect size is less in adults, stimulants should still be considered as first-line treatment once the diagnosis is made. Stimulants can cause agitation or anxiety, but they can be used successfully in patients with anxiety disorders, and in some cases, the anxiety may actually improve if it is related to the impairment caused by ADHD.

Stimulants are Class II controlled substances, and it is important to educate the patient about their abuse potential, but appropriate treatment should not be withheld. There is no concern about sudden cardiac death in a patient with no cardiac history.

6.2   Exploring the developmental and psychodynamic effects of ADHD with an LGBT patient is

   A. Not useful because medication is the most effective treatment for the core symptoms of ADHD regardless of a patient's sexual orientation.
   B. Useful because it helps the clinician reassure the patient that problems with organization and inattention are separate from relationship and identity issues.
   C. Useful because it is necessary for making the diagnosis of ADHD.
   D. Useful because acknowledging the role that ADHD plays in conflicts about sexual desire and identity formation can help the LGBT patient find the most successful solutions to problems in relationships and self-esteem.

The correct answer is D.

Medication alone has been shown to be the most effective treatment for the core symptoms of ADHD, but most patients, including LGBT patients, also need to deal with the secondary effects of their symptoms. These include not only work and academic success but also managing relationships and developing a sense of self-worth. In the LGBT patient, this can be particularly important, as deficits in executive function can worsen conflict about sexual desire and feelings of inferiority. It is true that evidence of symptom impairment going back to childhood is necessary to make the diagnosis, but a psychodynamic understanding of these symptoms goes beyond what the DSM requires.

Substance Dependence

Methamphetamine: Dionysus Versus the Good Little Boy

Steven Joseph Lee, M.D.

METHAMPHETAMINE IS A POWERFULLY ADDICTIVE drug with broad appeal that cuts across different age groups, genders, ethnicities, and socioeconomic lines (Halkitis 2009). The prevalence of methamphetamine use among men who have sex with men is markedly higher than in the general population. According to 2009 data from the National Survey of Drug Use and Health, lifetime prevalence of methamphetamine use among the general U.S. population is 5.1%, and the prevalence of past year use of methamphetamine is 0.5% (U.S. Department of Health and Human Services 2010). In contrast, various studies of methamphetamine use among gay men estimate between 7.4% (Stall et al. 2001) and 10.4% (Halkitis and Parsons 2002) of gay men have used methamphetamine in the recent past. This drug has an appeal to gay men who use it as a compelling but maladaptive coping tool, particularly around sexual issues (Lee 2006). The following case illustrates how one gay man used methamphetamine to address multiple areas of psychological conflict over his sexual orientation.

DSM-IV-TR criteria for substance dependence (American Psychiatric Association 2000) are shown in Table 7–1.

TABLE 7–1.   DSM-IV-TR diagnostic criteria for substance dependence

---

A maladaptive pattern of substance use, leading to clinically significant impairment or distress, as manifested by three (or more) of the following, occurring at any time in the same 12-month period:

(1) tolerance, as defined by either of the following:

  (a) a need for markedly increased amounts of the substance to achieve intoxication or desired effect

  (b) markedly diminished effect with continued use of the same amount of the substance

(2) withdrawal, as manifested by either of the following:

  (a) the characteristic withdrawal syndrome for the substance (refer to Criteria A and B of the criteria sets for withdrawal from the specific substances)

  (b) the same (or a closely related) substance is taken to relieve or avoid withdrawal symptoms

(3) the substance is often taken in larger amounts or over a longer period than was intended

(4) there is a persistent desire or unsuccessful efforts to cut down or control substance use

(5) a great deal of time is spent in activities necessary to obtain the substance (e.g., visiting multiple doctors or driving long distances), use the substance (e.g., chain-smoking), or recover from its effects

(6) important social, occupational, or recreational activities are given up or reduced because of substance use

(7) the substance use is continued despite knowledge of having a persistent or recurrent physical or psychological problem that is likely to have been caused or exacerbated by the substance (e.g., current cocaine use despite recognition of cocaine-induced depression, or continued drinking despite recognition that an ulcer was made worse by alcohol consumption)

Specify if:

  With physiological dependence: evidence of tolerance or withdrawal (i.e., either Item 1 or 2 is present)

  Without physiological dependence: no evidence of tolerance or withdrawal (i.e., neither Item 1 nor 2 is present)

Course specifiers:

  Early full remission

  Early partial remission

  Sustained full remission

  Sustained partial remission

  On agonist therapy

  In a controlled environment

Case Example: Carlos

Carlos is a 54-year-old gay Colombian American man who works as a senior partner at a New York law firm. He presented for treatment of methamphetamine dependence after a recent relapse following an inpatient rehabilitation. Carlos emigrated to the United States with his family when he was 5 years old. His family had been affluent in Colombia, where both parents had been university-educated professionals. Carlos's family sought political asylum and moved to Miami, Florida, leaving behind most of their wealth. Carlos's father started a business and soon was able to move the family into an upper-middle-class neighborhood. Carlos grew up hearing stories of the family's former wealth, and despite living a comfortable life in Miami, he always had a sense of financial deprivation.

Carlos's father was a conservative Catholic with "strict but fair morals," and Carlos's memories of him were idealized and almost exclusively positive: educated, hard-working, and proud, with a strong sense of traditional Latino values. His mother encouraged Carlos to develop intellectual pursuits by spending time with him reading literature and history books. Both parents allowed Carlos wide latitude in developing autonomy, trusting him to behave well when outside of their supervision. Carlos vacillated between feeling pride that his parents had confidence in him and wondering if their lack of involvement in his life was a lack of caring.

It was vitally important to Carlos to maintain an image of being "the perfect little boy," to maintain his parents' trust and assure himself of their approval and love. He earned excellent grades in school, and he was well liked by teachers and other students. When he began feeling attraction to other boys in high school, he was deeply ashamed and fearful of discovery by his parents and his peers. His first sexual encounter was a drunken episode at age 16 with his best friend. They remained friends for years afterwards, but that single incident was never discussed or repeated. Carlos did not continue to explore his sexual feelings until he moved away from home to start college. His father died from lung cancer when Carlos was 24. Carlos came out to his siblings the following year, and a year later to his mother. His mother was supportive and told him that she loved him no matter what his sexual orientation was.

Carlos first started using methamphetamine at the age of 49. At the time, his long-term relationship was falling apart, and he had an anonymous sexual encounter with a man who introduced him to the drug. Prior to that, Carlos would occasionally drink small quantities of alcohol, and he had no experience with other recreational substances because of a disapproving attitude. Methamphetamine made the sexual experience exhilarating, a dramatic contrast from the passionless and dwindling physical contact of his existing relationship. Carlos began using methamphetamine with increasing frequency, using it almost weekly by the end of his first year.

Initial concern by Carlos's partner turned into silent indifference when the partner, financially dependent on Carlos, felt unable to challenge him. Carlos took advantage of this silence to allow himself to continue using methamphetamine despite his partner's full knowledge. He told himself that his partner's indifference was a reflection of the emptiness of their relationship, and he used this as a rationalization to continue to seek methamphetamine-fueled sex with other men.

During his second year of using methamphetamine, Carlos transitioned from intranasal use to smoking to injecting. Drug use was always associated with sexual activity, either with hired escorts or sex partners he found on the Internet. Initially, methamphetamine use would begin on Friday night and end by Saturday night or Sunday morning. However, weekend use began spilling into his work week, and Carlos started missing work on Mondays, showing up for work on Tuesdays feeling tired and depressed. By the time he fully recovered on Thursday, he had intense cravings to use methamphetamine again on Friday. When Carlos's drug use began to take a serious toll on his ability to work, he admitted himself to a drug rehabilitation program. After rehab, Carlos lived for 2 months in a sober-living house while he returned to work, and he became heavily involved in 12-step programs, eventually settling on Alcoholics Anonymous (AA) as his meeting of choice. Carlos struggled with the principles of AA, alternating between feeling like a failure for his inability to embrace its philosophy and arguing against AA principles using the doctrine of his Catholic faith. He grew increasingly alienated from AA, and after 18 months of sobriety he relapsed on methamphetamine. He continued attending AA meetings, but repeated slips using methamphetamine intensified his feelings of being a failure in AA. His reaction was to argue even more fervently against the 12-step principles. The distress Carlos felt at being a failure in AA led him to use methamphetamine even more. Now feeling that AA was worsening his drug use, he stopped attending meetings completely.

The experience of failure and inability to control his emotions and behavior was foreign to Carlos. As he saw himself quickly resuming his destructive pattern of drug and sex binges, he presented himself for individual therapy, desperate to find some way to regain a sense of control and sobriety.

During the course of therapy, a number of themes emerged that shed light on how Carlos used methamphetamine to address his psychological needs. The most apparent function that methamphetamine served was to enhance sexual experiences: he used it exclusively in sexual situations. Sexual pleasure was so much better with methamphetamine that eventually Carlos stopped having sober sex altogether. Under the drug's influence, Carlos's sexual drive was dramatically intensified, and his sex/drug binges would last from 7 hours to 3 days. The pursuit of sexual pleasure led Carlos, for whom barriers to sexual pleasure became intolerable, to neglect his usually scrupulous use of condoms to protect himself from HIV.

With further exploration, it became clear that the overwhelming sexual drive caused by methamphetamine helped Carlos overcome his strong unconscious prohibitions against gay sex. Carlos learned from an early age that homosexuality was condemned by his family's conservative Catholic religion. As an adult, he rationalized a loophole in his beliefs, telling himself that God could not condemn a man for loving another human being, regardless of gender. This intellectualized remedy convinced Carlos that he fully embraced his sexual orientation. However, it became clear in therapy that Carlos harbored deep feelings of guilt and shame about being gay. In addition to his religious beliefs, Carlos recalled adolescent fantasies of his parents discovering that he was gay and reacting with profound disappointment and rejection. As a child, Carlos had a tenuous sense of security regarding his parents' love. Their lack of involvement in his life during his adolescence caused him to doubt their love and affection for him.

In order to maintain the sense of being loved, he had to uphold for them the image of being the "perfect little boy," and perfection included being heterosexual.

Prior to using methamphetamine, Carlos had been able to have sex with men, but his unconscious guilt limited his ability to fully experience sexual pleasure. In contrast, when using methamphetamine, his drive to have sex was so much greater than his reservations that for the first time, Carlos experienced a pleasure that was relatively unconflicted and unambiguous. This was a powerful experience that drew him to use methamphetamine repeatedly.

In therapy, Carlos explored his feelings and beliefs about being gay. Initially he believed that he had no negative beliefs about homosexuality. However, over time he became more aware of his feelings of guilt and the belief that he had failed his parents. With this greater awareness, Carlos was better able to recognize when these feelings arose, and he began to work at correcting these cognitive distortions. He began to reconcile his adolescent fears with the reality that his mother accepted his sexual orientation and continued to love him.

Another major appeal of methamphetamine for Carlos was the cathartic experience of transgression. Carlos was a hard-working perfectionist with strict Catholic morals and a fervently antidrug attitude. He worked hard during his childhood and adult years to maintain the "perfect little boy" image to please his parents. The experience of breaking free of his constraints by committing the forbidden act of using drugs, in conjunction with the euphoria induced by methamphetamine, was a dramatic relief from the intense pressure of his rigid perfectionism. Under the influence of methamphetamine, he was able to experience a sense of freedom that he had never allowed himself.

In addition to using drugs, the activities that Carlos engaged in while high contributed to the powerful experience of transgression. Methamphetamine commonly causes a strong desire to seek novel experiences and to push psychological limits. This drug effect led Carlos to continually try new activities that had been considered forbidden. Sex without condoms became a way to ignore the rules of "proper" sex. Carlos began to experiment with extreme sex with new forms of "anal play" and sadomasochistic fantasy. He met other methamphetamine users who enjoyed engaging in "race play," in which participants would act out forbidden racial stereotypes in sexual situations. He became fascinated by men he met who incorporated Satan worship into their methamphetamine-fueled sex, representing the pinnacle of cathartic relief from the restrictions of his Catholic morals, though this was a boundary that Carlos was too frightened to cross. At the height of Carlos' methamphetamine use, during episodes of drug-induced paranoid psychosis, Carlos's guilt about his drug use and sexual activities manifested in the belief that he was being followed by demonic signs and messages when he searched for sex.

In therapy Carlos worked on easing the perfectionist demands he put on himself. Gradually he was able to tolerate a greater degree of experiencing himself as imperfect, with less of a threatening sense that he was worthless or unlovable. While this remains a significant challenge for Carlos, his increased ability to be less stringent has attenuated some of the need for the cathartic relief that methamphetamine provided him.

As Carlos explored his experiences with methamphetamine, he realized that through his drug use, he had become part of a social network that helped him to feel part of a community. During his childhood, Carlos had a sense that he was different from other children, and as his sexual feelings intensified during adolescence, Carlos felt a growing sense of separation from his peers. Though he was well-liked by other students, he considered only two students to be close friends. In high school Carlos played varsity sports and maintained a façade of being a part of the popular crowd. He was voted "most likely to succeed" by his classmates, but his popularity felt like a sham. Even with the two friends that he considered close, Carlos never confided in them his true feelings because he feared rejection for being gay.

After coming out in his early adult years, Carlos had no difficulty in meeting men for sex or dating, though he never developed what he considered to be real friendships with gay men. In addition to his devout Catholic faith, Carlos's conservative social and political views often set him apart from most gay men. When he attended social gatherings with gay men, he often withheld his genuine opinions on topics of conversation, imagining he would be angrily rejected by others for his conservative views. When he did speak, he began with a defensive tone that invited antagonism and often pushed others away. Carlos realized that he feared being rejected by others, and he used his social and political conservatism to instigate arguments and turn his fear of rejection into a self-fulfilling prophecy. Although being gay began as the source of Carlos's isolation, he continued his pattern of keeping a distance from his peers, even within the gay community.

When Carlos started using methamphetamine, he became familiar with escorts and other gay men who used methamphetamine regularly. They all shared the experience of being renegades who used an illegal drug that was looked down on by the gay mainstream, and he felt that this shared experience created a bond between them. He fantasized that this group camaraderie is what teenagers felt when sitting among friends smoking marijuana, and he felt that this was his opportunity to experience that adolescent bonding.

Carlos maintained relationships only with the escorts he hired, not with other gay men. He became friends with those escorts, and together they would seek other gay men on the Internet with whom they could use methamphetamine and have sex. By paying the escorts, Carlos was able to guarantee that he would not be rejected, a risk he was not able to take with sex partners he did not pay. Carlos fantasized that the escorts truly liked him and wanted his friendship, though he had nagging doubts that they were only interested in his money and though he did realize that these financial relationships placed a limit on how deep these "friendships" could become.

Carlos developed a relationship with one escort in particular, whom he considered a real friend. That escort taught Carlos how to inject methamphetamine, showing him "safe" ways to use clean needles and syringes, and instructing him with rules of how much to use and how to go about having sex while high. When Carlos broke the rules, the escort would become angry and chastise him and would try to correct his behavior to maintain some sense of safety. Through this mentoring relationship, Carlos felt nurtured. On several occasions, the two lay in bed having intimate and revealing discussions about how they were both addicted to methamphetamine and how they needed to stop. However, Carlos often returned to this escort's home to use methamphetamine, coming to a place where he felt cared for during times when he needed support. In therapy, Carlos associated this relationship to fantasies of how he wished his parents could have cared for him differently, being more involved in his life, mentoring him, and chastising him when he did wrong.

The initial work with Carlos involved standard relapse prevention techniques, such as identifying triggers for methamphetamine use and practicing strategies for managing cravings. While alcohol was not a primary substance of abuse, it was an important trigger because it made Carlos want to act out sexually, and its disinhibiting effect frequently led Carlos to call his drug dealer for methamphetamine. An important part of Carlos' relapse prevention treatment was to abstain from all mood-altering substances, in addition to methamphetamine.

As Carlos's relapse prevention progressed, various psychological issues relating to methamphetamine use revealed themselves, and Carlos moved into a more exploratory therapy to address the underlying needs that were only transiently addressed by methamphetamine use. Carlos identified an unconscious guilt about his sexual orientation that made it difficult for him to fully satisfy his sexual needs. His guilt also drove his need to maintain the persona of the "perfect little boy," which kept him under constant pressure that needed release. He also identified longtime feelings of alienation and difficulty allowing himself to bond socially with people in a nonsexual way. Carlos was able to maintain sobriety for 11 months before relapsing. After that, he maintained longer periods of sobriety with relapses that were short-lived, and he is currently 2 years sober. Rather than using methamphetamine to address the symptoms of his psychological conflicts, Carlos has been able to work in therapy at addressing the underlying issues directly.

Key Points

- Methamphetamine is a powerful stimulant that markedly increases interest in and pleasure derived from sex.

- In addition to the pharmacological properties of a drug, associated characteristics, such as activities performed while intoxicated and people with whom drugs are used, can be strong behavioral reinforcers.

- Drugs are often used to self-medicate psychological or physical discomfort. In addiction treatment, it is important to identify the underlying problems for which a drug is being used as a maladaptive coping tool.

References

American Psychiatric Association: Diagnostic and Statistical Manual of Mental Disorders, 4th Edition, Text Revision. Washington, DC, American Psychiatric Association, 2000

Halkitis PN: Methamphetamine Addiction: Biological Foundations, Psychological Factors, and Social Consequences. Washington, DC, American Psychological Association, 2009

Halkitis PN, Parsons JT: Recreational drug use and HIV-risk sexual behavior among
    men frequenting gay social venues. Journal of Gay and Lesbian Social Services
    14:19–38, 2002

Lee S: Overcoming Crystal Meth Addiction: An Essential Guide to Getting Clean. New
    York, Marlowe & Company, 2006

Levounis P, Ruggiero JS: Outpatient management of crystal methamphetamine depen-
    dence among gay and bisexual men: how can it be done? Prim Psychiatry 13:75–80,
    2006

Stall R, Paul JP, Greenwood G, et al: Alcohol use, drug use and alcohol-related problems
    among men who have sex with men: the Urban Men's Health Study. Addiction
    96:1589–1601, 2001

U.S. Department of Health and Human Services, Substance Abuse and Mental Health
    Services Administration, Office of Applied Studies: National Survey on Drug Use
    and Health, 2009. Ann Arbor, MI, Inter-university Consortium for Political and
    Social Research, 2010

Questions

7.1   A 26-year-old man is brought in to the emergency room by police, who
       were called by his landlord. They found the man's apartment filthy, with
       rotten half-eaten food on the floor, pieces of electronic equipment lying
       in piles on various tables, and black sheets covering the windows. The
       man is agitated, stating that people have been watching him through his
       windows and trying to listen to him through bugs in his television and
       stereo. He threatened his landlord, whom he believes to be part of a con-
       spiracy to report his activities to the FBI. The man's face and arms are
       covered with small scabs, and he has a skin infection on his right arm.
       The best intervention is to

       A. Administer an intramuscular injection of an antipsychotic
          and admit the patient to the psychiatric unit for treatment of
          schizophrenia.
       B. Return the patient to police custody because this is a criminal
          issue not appropriate for the emergency room.
       C. Discharge the patient to home with an appointment to see the
          hospital clinic psychiatrist in one week.
       D. Collect urine for a toxicology screen to rule out psychosis sec-
          ondary to stimulants.

       The correct answer is D.

       Symptoms of methamphetamine intoxication can mimic symptoms of
       schizophrenia, with paranoid delusions and hallucinations. In addition,
       this patient has multiple skin lesions, which are the result of skin picking

in response to tactile hallucinations of bugs crawling under his skin, a common symptom of methamphetamine intoxication called *formication*. The skin infection on the man's arm may be from a site where he injected methamphetamine or other drugs. It is important to differentiate psychotic symptoms from methamphetamine from schizophrenia, a psychiatric illness that requires long-term treatment with antipsychotic medication. Psychosis from methamphetamine may respond to antipsychotic medications, but the course of treatment is usually brief. It is inappropriate to discharge the man from the emergency room because he is currently paranoid and threatening.

7.2   A 35-year-old gay man was recently discharged from his third admission to a 4-week residential drug treatment program. After previous discharges, he lasted 3–4 weeks before using methamphetamine again and finding sex partners on the Internet. Which of the following should be considered in this man's drug counseling sessions?

   A. Counsel the man about the risks of HIV and other sexually transmitted diseases, and emphasize the importance of using condoms during sex.
   B. Advise the man against having any sex for the next 6 months.
   C. Advise the man not to use the Internet.
   D. All of the above.

The correct answer is D.

For many gay men, methamphetamine use is intimately connected to sexual activity, and many men cannot imagine having sex without methamphetamine (Lee 2006). Sex itself, as well as sexual fantasies, can trigger intense cravings for methamphetamine (Levounis 2006). One strategy used by many therapists is to advise against sexual activity for 6–12 months while the patient accumulates abstinent "clean time" and develops relapse prevention skills that will protect him from strong triggers. When the patient is ready, sexual activity is gradually reintroduced, with discussion about how the patient experiences sex. The therapist should examine how the patient deals with emerging thoughts about methamphetamine and focus on the positive aspects of sober sex to help the patient recover some sense of pleasure from sex without methamphetamine. For some gay men, Internet sex sites are an integral part of their search for methamphetamine-fueled sex, and the websites themselves can be strong triggers that lead to drug relapses. If the Internet cannot be completely avoided, restricting use of any sex sites should be considered. Because of the disinhibited sexual activity associated with methamphetamine use, condom use, as well as not sharing needles with others, should be addressed to minimize harm that may occur in the event of a relapse. Language used in these discussions should focus on the serious medical consequences of HIV and other sexually transmitted diseases, because overly graphic discussions of sex can be triggering for those in early recovery from methamphetamine abuse.

Schizophrenia

Diagnosis or Difference?

Ronald E. Hellman, M.D.
Helene Kendler, L.C.S.W.

THE SUBJECT OF THIS CASE STUDY is a woman with schizophrenia who sought treatment at her current outpatient clinic when she concluded, after several years, that her former mental health providers did not understand her needs. She was referred to the clinic by a support program for lesbian, gay, bisexual, and transgender (LGBT) people with major mental illness, because of the clinic's subspecialization in LGBT issues. The LGBT program is one of several culturally specific offerings at the clinic, providing a full range of core psychiatric services in a culturally sensitive and affirmative environment for LGBT-identified patients. It provides an affirming and comfortable environment for LGBT patients within an otherwise mainstream, primarily heterosexual, cis-gendered setting (Hellman 2011; Hellman et al. 2010) (see Figure 8–1).

At the time of intake, Alexis did not clarify what her unaddressed needs were. Only after seeing her therapist for several months did she disclose that she did not feel comfortable or safe discussing her sexual orientation and gender identity issues with her former providers, and so she had remained silent about these. The case illuminates her concerns while challenging the clinician to discern what is pathological and what is merely different.

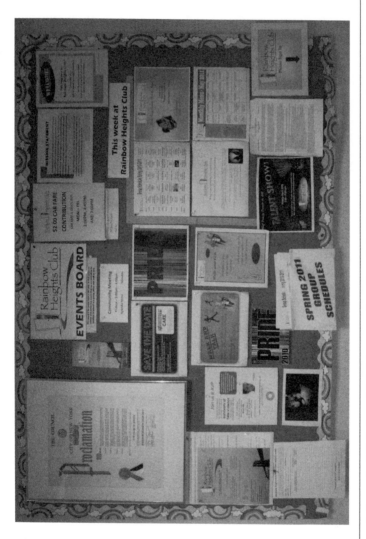

FIGURE 8–1.   **Events board at Rainbow Heights, a sociocultural clubhouse for LGBT people with major mental illness.**

Source.   Photograph by Ben Davis, 2011. http://www.rainbowheights.org.

Case Example: Alexis

Alexis is a 44-year-old Hispanic lesbian born and raised in New York City, where she still lives. She initially identified as "questioning," rather than as gay, bisexual, or transgender. As time went on, she revealed issues of gender identity. She maintained a short haircut but only sparingly allowed herself to wear men's clothing and pass as a man, despite wanting to do so on a more frequent basis. Eventually, she described herself as "a transgender butch lesbian" and increasingly sought out safe opportunities to dress and act like a man during social activities in the LGBT program.

Alexis presented as gentle, cooperative, and well related. She was well groomed and casually dressed. At the time of her admission to the clinic, thought disorder was present in most of her verbalizations, with words and phrases mixed up, vagueness, occasional thought blocking, and general disorganization in which she found herself unable to coordinate activities of daily living. She would become confused about when to shower, or she would forget to shower at all. She was unable to make a shopping list for a meal, or if she succeeded in making a list, she would buy the wrong ingredients.

During periods of decompensation, Alexis would hear voices that seemed to come both from her external environment and from her teeth, stomach, and tonsils. She described the voices as belonging to men and women of different races and ethnicities. Usually they denigrated her. Sometimes they talked about "the devil and blood." In a recent episode, she believed they were the voices of her roommate's family members.

Alexis is diagnosed with schizophrenia, undifferentiated type (Tables 8–1 and 8–2) (American Psychiatric Association 2000). She has a history of more than 20 psychiatric hospitalizations beginning in her late teens. Many of these were precipitated by nonadherence to medication. Some hospitalizations occurred because she felt well, stopped her medication, and relapsed. One resulted when she felt too sedated on chlorpromazine and discontinued taking it. Several hospitalizations were precipitated by the stress of independent living, and one followed the death of her mother.

Alexis often felt anxious, lonely, and bored. She professed a desire to pursue gainful employment but became overwhelmed when thinking about how to accomplish this. Years earlier, she had worked as a hairdresser after completing a year of college. She stopped because of the stress of adhering to a regular work schedule, which had caused her to decompensate. She lives on Social Security Disability.

Over the years, Alexis attended various outpatient programs, including day treatment and partial hospitalization programs, before beginning treatment in 2007 at her current community mental health clinic. She did not have a wide social support system before joining the LGBT support program, where she made several acquaintances.

Alexis is the second oldest of four sisters. She described her childhood as "happy and normal." Her father did maintenance work at a nearby office building where her mother did clerical work. She had a fair relationship with her father, who died from a heart attack when Alexis was 20 years old. Her mother then moved to the Dominican Republic but died shortly thereafter. Alexis had been very close to her mother, who was a major source of emotional support, and her death was a significant loss. Alexis continues to have a close relationship

---

TABLE 8–1.   DSM-IV-TR diagnostic criteria for schizophrenia

A. *Characteristic symptoms:*   Two (or more) of the following, each present for a significant portion of time during a 1-month period (or less if successfully treated):

    (1) delusions

    (2) hallucinations

    (3) disorganized speech (e.g., frequent derailment or incoherence)

    (4) grossly disorganized or catatonic behavior

    (5) negative symptoms, i.e., affective flattening, alogia, or avolition

    Note: Only one Criterion A symptom is required if delusions are bizarre or hallucinations consist of a voice keeping up a running commentary on the person's behavior or thoughts, or two or more voices conversing with each other.

B. *Social/occupational dysfunction:*   For a significant portion of the time since the onset of the disturbance, one or more major areas of functioning such as work, interpersonal relations, or self-care are markedly below the level achieved prior to the onset (or when the onset is in childhood or adolescence, failure to achieve expected level of interpersonal, academic, or occupational achievement).

C. *Duration:*   Continuous signs of the disturbance persist for at least 6 months. This 6-month period must include at least 1 month of symptoms (or less if successfully treated) that meet Criterion A (i.e., active-phase symptoms) and may include periods of prodromal or residual symptoms. During these prodromal or residual periods, the signs of the disturbance may be manifested by only negative symptoms or two or more symptoms listed in Criterion A present in an attenuated form (e.g., odd beliefs, unusual perceptual experiences).

D. *Schizoaffective and Mood Disorder exclusion:*   Schizoaffective disorder and mood disorder with psychotic features have been ruled out because either (1) no major depressive, manic, or mixed episodes have occurred concurrently with the active-phase symptoms; or (2) if mood episodes have occurred during active-phase symptoms, their total duration has been brief relative to the duration of the active and residual periods.

E. *Substance/general medical condition exclusion:*   The disturbance is not due to the direct physiological effects of a substance (e.g., a drug of abuse, a medication) or a general medical condition.

F. *Relationship to a pervasive developmental disorder:*   If there is a history of autistic disorder or another pervasive developmental disorder, the additional diagnosis of schizophrenia is made only if prominent delusions or hallucinations are also present for at least a month (or less if successfully treated).

Source.   Reprinted from *Diagnostic and Statistical Manual of Mental Disorders,* 4th Edition, Text Revision. Washington, DC, American Psychiatric Association, 2000. Used with permission. Copyright © 2000 American Psychiatric Association.

TABLE 8–2. DSM-IV-TR diagnostic criteria for schizophrenia subtypes

---

Paranoid type

A type of schizophrenia in which the following criteria are met:

   A.   Preoccupation with one or more delusions or frequent auditory hallucinations.

   B.   None of the following is prominent: disorganized speech, disorganized or catatonic behavior, or flat or inappropriate affect.

Disorganized type

A type of schizophrenia in which the following criteria are met:

A.   All of the following are prominent:

   (1)   disorganized speech

   (2)   disorganized behavior

   (3)   flat or inappropriate affect

B.   The criteria are not met for catatonic type.

Catatonic type

A type of schizophrenia in which the clinical picture is dominated by at least two of the following:

   (1)   motoric immobility as evidenced by catalepsy (including waxy flexibility) or stupor

   (2)   excessive motor activity (that is apparently purposeless and not influenced by external stimuli)

   (3)   extreme negativism (an apparently motiveless resistance to all instructions or maintenance of a rigid posture against attempts to be moved) or mutism

   (4)   peculiarities of voluntary movement as evidenced by posturing (voluntary assumption of inappropriate or bizarre postures), stereotyped movements, prominent mannerisms, or prominent grimacing

   (5)   echolalia or echopraxia

Undifferentiated type

A type of schizophrenia in which symptoms that meet Criterion A are present, but the criteria are not met for the paranoid, disorganized, or catatonic yype.

Residual type

A type of schizophrenia in which the following criteria are met:

   A.   Absence of prominent delusions, hallucinations, disorganized speech, and grossly disorganized or catatonic behavior.

   B.   There is continuing evidence of the disturbance, as indicated by the presence of negative symptoms or two or more symptoms listed in Criterion A for Schizophrenia, present in an attenuated form (e.g., odd beliefs, unusual perceptual experiences).

with her youngest sister. She denied any psychiatric history in her immediate family but thought there was a history in distant relatives.

Alexis had periods of homelessness in the past, during which she slept with men in return for money and temporary shelter. She has had three intimate relationships with women, the last ending 2 years prior to her admission to this clinic. She continues to feel the loss of these relationships.

She currently shares an apartment with another woman in a supportive housing program. She is Catholic and prays in the privacy of the apartment. She stopped attending church years ago because of its teachings that homosexuality is a sin.

She does not currently use drugs or alcohol, except beer on rare occasions. She had a history of alcohol abuse that ended when she was 24 years old. There is no history of suicidal or homicidal ideation.

Alexis is prescribed risperidone. On admission to the outpatient clinic risperidone was increased, with improvement in her symptoms.

Alexis sees her psychiatrist once a month and a psychotherapist biweekly for 30 minutes. Both participate as staff members of the clinic's LGBT-affirmative program. Alexis often presents concrete dilemmas related to organizing and maintaining activities of daily living and medication adherence. Interpersonal conflicts, primarily with roommates, have periodically emerged as a focus of treatment. Therapy focused on examining her tendency to avoid or delay conflict. For example, Alexis would cover for a roommate who failed to help clean the apartment. She would do all of the roommate's chores for months until she could no longer suppress her anger and a loud verbal argument would ensue. Her case manager often intervened to restore order.

With therapy, Alexis was able to express her needs earlier on and negotiate more effectively with roommates. Her LGBT peer support group helped buffer stress regarding issues of stigma, stereotyping, and marginalization by roommates. She became more confident, asserting her sexual orientation and gender identity while learning how and when to confront stereotyping at her residence. On two occasions, however, she felt it was too risky to address such issues, and she was ultimately moved to a different supportive apartment.

Emotional safety remains elusive. Alexis has repeatedly stated, "I don't fit in any group" and "Nobody understands me." She has expressed shame about her cross-gender identity. Her therapist continues to explore Alexis's feelings regarding gender, encouraging her to express her needs without fear of rejection or judgment. She has become more assertive of her gender within the LGBT environment and in other situations where it was unlikely that she would be subjected to physical violence. Psychoeducation was provided about the common fears among transgender individuals and the reality that they are a response to the transphobia that exists within mainstream culture. Although Alexis is now better able to tolerate explorations of her need to "sometimes be a man," she continues to avoid the topic for periods of time.

Discussion

Alexis presented with a history of distressing and functionally disabling symptoms that had occurred over many years, including hallucinations, delusions, and disorganized speech and behavior associated with marked impairment in social and occupational functioning—symptoms typical of schizophrenia. There was no medical condition, substance abuse history, or significant mood presentation to suggest another diagnosis.

Alexis is a natal woman in her mid-40s who initially questioned her sexual orientation and arrived at a level of comfort identifying as a woman attracted to women, but also questioned her gender identity, taking tentative steps to explore living and identifying as a man. She did not fit the traditional notion of transsexualism with its characteristic intense desire to be a member of the other sex from an early age, with associated requests for hormones and genital surgery. Her exploration in later life of a possible cross-gender identity is characteristic of those who identify along the diverse transgender spectrum. She was initially reluctant to take on this label and has not identified as a transgender man (trans man).

The tentative nature of her gender exploration could be understood within the context of the intense stigma that gender-nonconforming individuals face in society and perhaps the subsequent pressure to feel a part of at least one of the LGBT subgroups (the lesbian community). Her confusion, ambivalence, and tentativeness could evoke similar feelings in her clinicians, who may wonder if the questioning of her gender identity is related to her psychotic illness.

Alexis had the impression that her previous therapist assumed when Alexis spoke of being "different," Alexis was referring to the signs and symptoms of schizophrenia and the ways in which her illness had isolated her and compromised her ability to develop meaningful relationships with others. She became reluctant to explore issues related to her sexual orientation and gender identity. Sensing that her previous therapist was unfamiliar with concepts and terminology related to nonconforming gender identities exacerbated her discomfort in sessions. As rapport developed in the first 2 months of treatment with her current therapist, Alexis went into further detail about her fear of discussing her concerns with her previous therapist. She said, "I was still a little in the closet to myself about being a lesbian, but I was even more afraid to say that I felt sometimes like a man. He never asked me anything about it, and I don't think he wanted to know."

One of the most stigmatized of human characteristics in our culture is an atypical gender presentation. Mainstream society's gender paradigm is binary: biologically male infants are considered to be boys who will grow up to become men; anatomically female newborns are considered to be girls who will grow up to become women, typically with characteristics, roles, behaviors, dress, and mannerisms molded within a social framework. Despite lessening in the rigidity of gender roles and behaviors in our society, the binary paradigm remains dominant and is intergenerationally reinforced through child-rearing practices shaped by cultural expectations and peer pressure.

People who live "outside the box" of gender conformity face rejection by their families and society. They may also be at greater risk for marginalization by mental health providers. As children and adolescents, they are more likely to be ostracized, bullied, scapegoated, and physically assaulted. They can experience isolation without recourse to avenues of support and acceptance. Developmental milestones, when acquiring social skills and the ability to form and maintain friendships and intimate relationships, may be disrupted. As adults, they may be denied employment, having to endure reduced socioeconomic status.

The deleterious effects of society's attitudes toward gender-nonconforming individuals are magnified in the lives of people with schizophrenia. In rural areas of the United States, there are few safe places in which to be "out" about a nonconforming gender identity. Even in more diverse urban settings such as New York City, where this patient lived, the dual stigma associated with gender nonconformity and a psychotic disorder kept Alexis indoors much of the time. In public, she reported incidents of being spat on by strangers, being shoved on the subway, and being the object of epithets regarding her gender presentation. A history of insults, threats, and assaults is commonly reported by transgender people. Because of its visibility, Alexis, like many other transgender patients at the clinic, identified her nonconforming gender presentation as creating more danger for her on the street than her status as a person with mental illness.

When the gender-atypical person also has a psychotic disorder, it can sometimes be difficult to differentiate paranoia from real instances of abuse and discrimination. While it can be helpful to estimate the plausibility of the reported frequency and nature of these experiences, and to obtain corroborating information where possible, it is essential to acknowledge the frightening and traumatic aspects of these experiences, ensure the safety of the individual, provide support, and provide symptom relief where appropriate.

A casual clinical understanding regarding measures of a "successful" gender transition can read like a list of stereotypes of the opposite gender (American Psychiatric Association 1994). Nevertheless, many gender-atypical individuals reject expectations of "passing" in a binary-gendered world, accepting personal definitions of gender that fall outside of or in between the categories of male and female. This variability has given rise to a wide spectrum of transgender expression.

Even though the term *transgender* has never constituted a classification within the psychiatric nomenclature (Drescher 2010), there may be a tendency to view those less able to conform to traditional expectations of gender as clinically troubling, and the presence of a psychotic disorder can notch up the clinical confusion and lead to incorrectly pathologizing some patients.

Cross-gender phenomena, in rare circumstances, can be manifestations of psychosis. When they are not a psychotic manifestation, the individual is aware of having been born as a member of a biological gender, and of not being actually a biological member of the other sex, but has an intense desire to identify and live as a member of the other sex. This conviction is a persistent trait, rather than a state-based one that only manifests itself at times of psychotic decompensation. In contrast, cross-gender presentations as psychotic phenomena tend to be implausible—for example, using bizarre rationales to "explain" why they have the genitals and physical appearance of their natal gender (Baltieri and De Andrade 2009).

True cross-gender requests to alter physical appearance differ from the requests seen in those with body dysmorphic disorder, where a specific body part, independent of gender, is the focus, and there is a perception of a deformity and not a desire to conform in physical appearance to the other sex. Sometimes, "alter" personalities in dissociative identity disorder are of the opposite sex to the patient. Here, other distinct personalities suddenly and recurrently take control of behavior and identity, often with an extensive lack of recall. A transgender person has a consistent understanding of their dilemma, and there is no sudden change in gender as would be associated with a personality "alter."

This case illustrates some of the issues that psychiatry has confronted, and continues to encounter, regarding how clinicians distinguish between diagnosis and difference. Alexis has a diagnosis of schizophrenia, has a lesbian sexual identity, and wrestles with her gender identity. In all three domains, she is outside of society's conventional box, and her deviations from society's norms risk (or carry) pathological designations.

The debate that led to the declassification of homosexuality in DSM-III (American Psychiatric Association 1980) spurred an overall effort to rigorously define the boundaries of what constitutes a mental disorder (Spitzer 1981). It was discovered that, at most, guidelines could be established—such as impaired functioning and clinically significant distress that is not due to social stigma—but there could not be a precise definition of mental disorder because concepts of illness are socially constructed and influenced by cultural values.

The guidelines for determining whether a mental disorder is present are, nevertheless, powerful. They illuminate why Alexis's constellation of distressing psychotic symptoms and functional impairment would be classified as a psychiatric diagnosis that we call schizophrenia, even when it remains for the future to know how well the diagnostic category reflects a specific underlying disorder (etiology).

Alexis enjoyed her erotic and romantic relationships with women and came to define herself as a lesbian. When distress is related to sexual orientation, it typically derives from conflicts with, for example, family, peer, or religious expectations, but sexual orientation is not in itself a source of innate distress, nor does it impair functioning. By these criteria, the guidelines tell us that homosexuality is a difference, not a diagnosis.

By contrast, Alexis experienced significant distress as she struggled to explore and define her gender identity. Even here, her struggle was clearly associated with stigma, both within the sexual minority community and in the community at large. It is possible that this difficulty became somewhat conflated with paranoia from schizophrenia. At this stage in her presentation, her distress was not focused on any incongruence between her gender identity and anatomical characteristics (she defines herself as a masculine-acting, lesbian woman), and she was not requesting medical procedures, such as hormones and surgery, to resolve incongruence—characteristics typical of those diagnosed with gender identity disorder in DSM-IV-TR (American Psychiatric Association 2000). Alexis's distress was due to social condemnation and challenges with social identification rather than anatomical incongruence, and her gender issues appear to have more to do with difference than diagnosis. The gender identity disorder categories have undergone a considerable evolution (Drescher 2010) and are again being reconsidered for the fifth edition of the *Diagnostic and Statistical Manual of Mental Disorders* (DSM-5) in order to better ensure appropriate diagnosis and access to care that enhances comfort with gender (Lev 2004).

Key Points

- The binary view of gender is oversimplified. There is a spectrum of gender identities. Clinicians need to be able to differentiate between gender differences and aspects of gender that contribute to DSM diagnoses.

- Stigmatization related to sexual orientation and gender nonconformity can be exacerbated when mental illness is present. Even in LGBT-affirmative environments, sexual minority patients need time to develop trust.

- Issues with gender, sexuality, and psychosis should be viewed within the larger context of a person's life, not just through the narrow lens of symptoms and diagnoses, in order to best promote recovery from mental illness and the pain of oppression and alienation.

References

American Psychiatric Association: Diagnostic and Statistical Manual of Mental Disorders, 3rd Edition. Washington, DC, American Psychiatric Association, 1980
American Psychiatric Association: Gender identity disorder, diagnostic features, in Diagnostic and Statistical Manual of Mental Disorders, 4th Edition. Washington, DC, American Psychiatric Association, 1994, pp 576–577
American Psychiatric Association: Diagnostic and Statistical Manual of Mental Disorders, 4th Edition, Text Revision. Washington, DC, American Psychiatric Association, 2000

Baltieri DA, De Andrade AG: Schizophrenia modifying the expression of gender identity disorder. J Sex Med 6:1185–1188, 2009

Drescher J: Queer diagnoses: parallels and contrasts in the history of homosexuality, gender variance, and the diagnostic and statistical manual. Arch Sex Behav 39:427–460, 2010

Hellman RE: Institutional aspects of the initial interview, in The Initial Psychotherapy Interview: A Gay Man Seeks Treatment. Edited by Silverstein C. Boston, MA, Elsevier, 2011, pp 97–115

Hellman RE, Huygen C, Klein E, et al: A study of members of a support and advocacy program for LGBT persons with major mental illness. Best Pract Ment Health 6:13–26, 2010

Lev AI: Transgender Emergence: Therapeutic Guidelines for Working With Gender-Variant People and Their Families. New York, Haworth, 2004

Spitzer RL: The diagnostic status of homosexuality in DSM-III: a reformulation of the issues. Am J Psychiatry 138:210–215, 1981

Questions

8.1   Which statement is true?

A. Cross-gender identification satisfies the definition of a mental disorder.

B. Transsexualism was not a psychiatric diagnosis prior to DSM-III, but homosexuality was.

C. A cross-gender disorder would be the correct diagnosis for a man attempting to pass as a woman in public who is assaulted by a group of teens and now has clinically significant distress.

D. A married woman, erotically attracted to her husband, increasingly resents that he treats her as a woman when they have sex. She realizes that she has always felt that her true gender is male, and she is now able to acknowledge a long-standing desire to be rid of female anatomical characteristics. She seeks help. The clinician would be correct in diagnosing a gender-related disorder.

E. Hormonal and surgical sex reassignment is ruled out when a patient is diagnosed with schizophrenia.

F. B and D.

The correct answer is F.

Mental disorders require the presence of clinically significant distress that is not due to social stigma. Such distress did exist for the married woman due to incongruence between her gender identity and anatomical gender. Distress in a transgender person due to violence is not a gender disorder (other diagnoses, such as acute stress disorder, may apply). Transsexualism was considered to be a manifestation of neurosis or psychosis but did not receive a separate classification in DSM-I or DSM-II. If evaluation of cross-gender phenomena in a person with schizophrenia is determined to be trait-related and not a state-related manifestation of psychosis, and they have the capacity and insight to understand their gender status and the risk and benefits of hormonal and surgical interventions, they may be considered for an anatomical transition.

8.2   In patients with schizophrenia:

   A. The desire to be a member of the other sex is considered a delusional manifestation of the psychotic disorder.
   B. A homosexual orientation is considered a manifestation of the psychotic disorder.
   C. The conviction of a female patient that her parents had her penis removed at birth and that she really is a man is considered a delusional manifestation of the psychotic disorder.
   D. A male presenting in female clothing and a wig should be considered psychotic.
   E. A, C, and D.

The correct answer is C.

Transgender expression and same-sex concerns may derive from a psychotic process or co-occur with it. Careful evaluation over time, rather than premature diagnostic conclusions, should lead the clinician to the correct diagnosis.

Major Depressive Disorder

The Unhappy Ad Man: Major Depression in a Gay Man

ROBERT M. KERTZNER, M.D.

DEPRESSION IS A MAJOR clinical and public health concern of lesbians, gay men, and bisexual (LGB) persons, with elevated rates of lifetime and current depression reported in this population (King et al. 2008). A leading reason for which LGB persons seek mental health care, depression is associated with other morbidities, such as substance use disorders and suicide, and is linked to lower quality of life. Given the prevalence of depression among LGB persons and its multiple effects on well-being, depression constitutes a significant problem for clinicians treating sexual minority patients.

The assessment and treatment of depression in LGB persons rests on basic psychiatric skills common to all patient care, strengthened by a familiarity with the developmental dynamics of forming a sexual minority identity and the social and cultural context of sexual minority lives. While the treatment of depression in LGB persons bears many similarities to working with patients in the general population, the life experiences of LGB persons shape factors related to the risk for, presentation of, and treatment of depression.

No single case can illustrate the range of depressive phenomenology in LGB persons, which encompasses multiple cultural, religious, ethnic/racial, class, health-related, and age-cohort factors. Gender introduces specific risk factors in addition to more generic risk factors common to LGB persons; lesbians, for instance, contend with both sexism and heterosexism and are more likely to live in poverty than heterosexual women and heterosexual and nonheterosexual men (Albelda et al. 2009). Bisexual men and women experience additional stressors that increase risk for depression, such as encountering bi-phobia from lesbians and gay men, and may have difficulty finding supportive bisexual communities. With these considerations in mind, the following case discussion, although focused on a gay man, includes observations that pertain to LGB persons in general.

Case Example: Michael

Initial impressions: Michael is a single Caucasian 34-year-old graphic arts designer with a recent history of depressed mood, decreased capacity to experience pleasure, early-morning awakening with pronounced anxiety, impaired concentration, feelings of worthlessness, and pessimism about his prospects of advancement in work and of finding a long-term partner. Over the past several months, he has increasingly felt that his life is empty, but he has not had suicidal thoughts. Although he has not missed work, he has missed several important deadlines for the completion of tasks. He has also withdrawn from friends and has been spending evenings and weekends at home by himself, "vegging out" on what he calls mindless television. Michael contacted me after speaking with a close friend who encouraged him to get help.

In his initial appointment, Michael provided the following history: he experienced two prior depressive episodes; the first, during his sophomore year in college, was characterized by several months of sadness, social withdrawal, early-morning awakening, and marked anxiety about academic assignments. He eventually sought help at the student health service and received a course of counseling and escitalopram treatment that he took for 6 months, with significant diminishment of his symptoms. He reported a second depressive episode after graduating from college and moving to the large city in which he currently resides; Michael attributed this depression, again characterized by anxiety, insomnia, and social withdrawal, to rejection by a romantic partner and his concern that he wasn't attractive enough to be "competitive" in the dating world of young gay men composing his peer group. His internist prescribed venlafaxine that relieved his depressive symptoms, although he disliked the sexual side effects and insomnia caused by this medication and wondered if the venlafaxine made him a little "speedy." He stopped the medication after 6 months and received no mental health care subsequently.

At the time of our first meeting, Michael reported being in good physical health with no significant medical conditions. Michael last tested HIV negative a year ago. He describes drinking "socially," by which he means one to two drinks a night, several times a week, when out with friends; over recent months, this has shifted to one or two glasses of wine at home most evenings. In his late twenties, he used Ecstasy regularly on weekends; he discontinued this because of the recurrence of sad feelings several days after Ecstasy use. Michael has smoked cigarettes since his early twenties; he is now down to less than one pack per day.

When I asked about his family history, Michael reported that his father drank excessively at times and become irritable and verbally abusive; his mother has seen a therapist and been prescribed medication for depression; and a paternal cousin has been diagnosed with bipolar disorder.

My initial diagnostic impressions of Michael were major depressive episode, recurrent (moderate level of intensity, nonpsychotic) (Table 9–1) and no clear Axis II diagnosis (American Psychiatric Association 2000). A family history of bipolar disorder and certain aspects of Michael's presentation—such as prominent anxiety, serotonin-norepinephrine reuptake inhibitor (SNRI)–induced activation, and onset of first depressive episode at an equivocally young age—indicated a need for further assessment to rule out a bipolar spectrum mood disorder. The significance of comorbid substance use needed to be assessed, including whether alcohol use was greater than reported and if it was confounding Michael's clinical presentation (for instance, contributing to his early-morning awakening and anxiety). It would be important to explore his motivations for alcohol use, including whether drinking was intended to blunt feelings of shame over sexual orientation, reduce sexual inhibitions, or treat social anxiety or dysphoric mood. Similarly, in anticipation of possible interventions to reduce nicotine use, I was interested in exploring his motivations for smoking, such as weight maintenance or stress management.

Michael was born and raised in the suburbs of a small Midwestern city, the middle child of three (he has a brother 2 years his senior and a sister who is 5 years younger). He recalls his mother being sad much of his childhood and his father being inebriated many evenings and making disparaging remarks about his mother. Michael felt his father favored his brother, a highly competitive athlete, with whom he shared an interest in sports. The birth of his sister and subsequent course of her childhood developmental disabilities created additional stress at home. Michael felt close to his mother and maternal grandmother, who lived nearby; the latter encouraged his interest in drawing and reading. He sensed that his father pulled away from him and from his family around the time his sister was born.

Michael was raised in the Catholic church, although his family stopped attending Mass after his sister's birth. He briefly considered entering seminary training in his teen years but now considers himself to be a lapsed Catholic.

He describes his childhood as basically happy, although recalls feeling "different" in early childhood, preferring to play alone rather than with male peers with whom he felt uncomfortable. On a few occasions in middle school, he remembers being taunted for his dressy clothes, but later in high school he fell in with an "arty" crowd and experienced a sense of belonging.

Michael was aware of attractions to boys at age 9. At 14, he developed a crush on a neighborhood friend that culminated in several episodes of mutual masturbation, followed by this friend's abrupt withdrawal of interest in Michael (and subsequent involvement in heterosexual dating and peer groups). This was a devastating experience for Michael; he remembers feeling humiliated, but felt he could not discuss this experience with anyone, compounding his sense of rejection and isolation. Michael subsequently tried to ignore his attraction to other boys, hoping that this was a passing phase. It took several years for Michael to accept an identity as a gay man; this occurred after he left home for college and he joined a campus organization for sexual minority students. He came out to his mother during sophomore year; she said that she had suspected that he was gay for a long time and that this didn't change her love for him. She also asked Michael not to tell his father, at least for the time being.

After several short-lived relationships with men, Michael met his first serious boyfriend during junior year in college and described a great sense of relief

---

TABLE 9–1. DSM-IV-TR diagnostic criteria for major depressive episode

---

A. Five (or more) of the following symptoms have been present during the same 2-week period and represent a change from previous functioning; at least one of the symptoms is either (1) depressed mood or (2) loss of interest or pleasure.

   Note: Do not include symptoms that are clearly due to a general medical condition, or mood-incongruent delusions or hallucinations.

   (1) depressed mood most of the day, nearly every day, as indicated by either subjective report (e.g., feels sad or empty) or observation made by others (e.g., appears tearful).   **Note:** In children and adolescents, can be irritable mood.

   (2) markedly diminished interest or pleasure in all, or almost all, activities most of the day, nearly every day (as indicated by either subjective account or observation made by others)

   (3) significant weight loss when not dieting or weight gain (e.g., a change of more than 5% of body weight in a month), or decrease or increase in appetite nearly every day.   **Note:** In children, consider failure to make expected weight gains.

   (4) insomnia or hypersomnia nearly every day

   (5) psychomotor agitation or retardation nearly every day (observable by others, not merely subjective feelings of restlessness or being slowed down)

   (6) fatigue or loss of energy nearly every day

   (7) feelings of worthlessness or excessive or inappropriate guilt (which may be delusional) nearly every day (not merely self-reproach or guilt about being sick)

   (8) diminished ability to think or concentrate, or indecisiveness, nearly every day (either by subjective account or as observed by others)

   (9) recurrent thoughts of death (not just fear of dying), recurrent suicidal ideation without a specific plan, or a suicide attempt or a specific plan for committing suicide

B. The symptoms do not meet criteria for a mixed episode.

C. The symptoms cause clinically significant distress or impairment in social, occupational, or other important areas of functioning.

D. The symptoms are not due to the direct physiological effects of a substance (e.g., a drug of abuse, a medication) or a general medical condition (e.g., hypothyroidism).

E. The symptoms are not better accounted for by bereavement, i.e., after the loss of a loved one, the symptoms persist for longer than 2 months or are characterized by marked functional impairment, morbid preoccupation with worthlessness, suicidal ideation, psychotic symptoms, or psychomotor retardation.

Source. Reprinted from *Diagnostic and Statistical Manual of Mental Disorders,* 4th Edition, Text Revision. Washington, DC, American Psychiatric Association, 2000. Used with permission. Copyright © 2000 American Psychiatric Association.

in experiencing sexual and emotional intimacy with him. The relationship ended when the partner graduated and moved to a distant city. Over ensuing years Michael has had a series of short-term relationships, meeting partners in bars or via Internet sites; in recent years he has become disillusioned with the quality of these connections and is increasingly concerned about finding a long-term partner. In addition, there have been several occasions when Michael has become markedly anxious about possible HIV exposure after instances of unprotected receptive anal sex.

Michael is a talented graphic arts designer who has worked at two advertising agencies since receiving a master of fine arts degree. He laughingly refers to himself as "aiming to please" at work, which, in most respects, has made him a valued employee. Yet he sometimes feels that he is not taken seriously enough. He was recently upset when a younger colleague was promoted instead of him.

Michael maintains close friendships with several colleagues from work and fellow alumni from college; it was one of these friends, with whom Michael usually has dinner once a month, who became concerned about his depression and urged him to seek help. His relationship with his parents has improved over recent years. His father has "mellowed" with age and is now very solicitous, encouraging him to bring a "friend" home for the holidays, although Michael is anxious about this prospect.

Michael's additional developmental history raises several themes that are common to LGB persons and are thought to increase risk for psychiatric morbidity. The expectation and experience of rejection because of one's sexual identity; concealment of sexual identity, experience of discrimination, and internalization of negative attitudes about homosexuality are thought to constitute a type of minority stress experienced by LGB persons (Meyer 2003) that is associated with an increased risk for depression and other disorders. Many if not most LGB adults experience these stressors in childhood or adolescence, often related to nonconforming gender role behaviors or an emerging awareness of homosexual or bisexual interests. Not being able to talk with anyone about being harassed or bullied may be particularly injurious to the self-esteem of children and adolescents and often compounds the experience of victimization.

Michael's experience of feeling different as a child, being teased in middle school, and feeling humiliated by a teen love interest exemplify such stressors and sense of social isolation. Although the topic was not mentioned by Michael in his initial history, I wondered about the possibility of childhood abuse, given the history of his father's verbal abusiveness (directed towards his mother) and reports of elevated rates of physical, emotional, and sexual abuse in the childhood and adolescence of sexual minority adults, which increase risk for depression in adulthood.

A critical question is the extent to which Michael has internalized negative societal attitudes toward homosexuality, given that internalized homophobia and its resultant sense of shame have implications for the capacity to tolerate emotional intimacy, sustain a sense of self-worth, and manage risks associated with substance use or sexual behavior in adulthood. In this regard, one factor underlying Michael's alcohol use and occasions of unprotected sex may be underlying problems with his self-regard as a gay man.

Now in his mid-thirties, Michael regards the prospect of remaining single as an increasing source of anxiety and self-doubt. In the context of gay men's lives, difficulties accepting dependency needs, often equated with a disparaged sense of femininity, is an important dynamic that can undermine the establishment of long-term intimate partnerships (Isay 2006). Isay suggests that some gay men are anxious about "contaminating" would-be romantic partners with a sense of shame over not being masculine enough or a perception that their sexual needs and desires are transgressive. To the extent that being in a relationship can promote greater self-acceptance as a gay man, provide a bulwark against stress associated with negative life events, and lessen concerns about the aging process, Michael's difficulties in finding a long-term partner can be seen as both a consequence of earlier adversities and an ongoing risk factor for depression.

First meeting: Michael arrives early for the initial interview and enters the consultation room casually and neatly dressed. He seems mildly anxious but appears eager to discuss his difficulties. He establishes good eye contact, carefully surveys the room, and speaks thoughtfully with an underlying sense of sadness. At times, he becomes tearful, such as when discussing his sense of isolation, loneliness, and hopelessness about relationships. Michael says that he occasionally thinks that if he were to develop a fatal illness or be killed in an accident, this wouldn't be the worst thing in the world, but he denies any specific suicidal thoughts. There is no evidence of psychosis or neurocognitive difficulties.

Michael displays good insight into his difficulties (he has been reading about depression on the Internet) and realizes his friend was correct in urging him to seek care. He is hesitant about having to go back on antidepressant medications that might cause weight gain and sexual side effects. In addition, he has mixed feelings about prior psychotherapy, sometimes feeling that he wasn't an interesting enough patient and at other times realizing that he was withholding information for fear of being judged by his therapists. Michael says he is now interested in getting help with his depression and examining what might be holding him back from more fulfilling romantic relationships and greater recognition at work. He seems relieved when I recommend that we work together on a weekly basis.

Treatment course: My initial treatment recommendations for Michael were to 1) resume antidepressant medication and 2) begin a course of weekly psychotherapy with the explicit aim of addressing long-standing concerns about his self-confidence and desirability to others, with goals of work advancement and finding a partner. I also considered several other aims common to psychotherapy with many gay men: fostering self-acceptance as a gay man, addressing issues of shame related to sexuality, and strengthening motivation toward healthier behaviors (e.g., moderation of sexual risk and substance use behaviors).

I suggested that Michael resume antidepressant medication, and after discussing his concerns about weight gain and sexual side effects, he agreed to begin bupropion. After 2 weeks on medication, Michael noticed an improvement in mood and a decreased sense of hopelessness. Whereas a selective serotonin reuptake inhibitor (SSRI) or SNRI medication might have been more helpful for anxiety, Michael preferred to try bupropion because of its side-effect profile. I recommended that Michael stay on the medication indefinitely, given his history of three depressive episodes. Michael was able to discuss his ambivalence about taking an antidepressant medication, recalling his father's derisive comments about his mother's use of psychiatric medication.

Early in treatment, we discussed Michael's ambivalence about psychotherapy itself. Although he was eager to explore the issues we formulated together, Michael cancelled or rescheduled several sessions. Michael admitted he felt anxious that he wasn't going to do something "right" and would be a displeasing patient. I understood this in terms of his specific anxieties about attachment and intimacy, but also with an awareness that sexual minority persons such as Michael bring to treatment expectations, hopes, and fears about the treatment experience. Although therapies that aim to change sexual orientation are no longer practiced by mainstream therapists, many LGB patients still have a sense of apprehension about whether a therapist will be familiar with or nonjudgmental about their sexual identity.

I came to understand the psychological aspects of Michael's depression as a hybrid of psychodynamics specific to his personal history and common to the process of developing a minority sexual identity. For instance, while Michael's experience of feeling different is typical of the childhood of many gay men, the *meaning* Michael attached to this feeling can be understood as shaped by elements of his history: a depressed mother, a father who abused alcohol, a developmentally disabled sister, and a favored brother. This environment led Michael to develop a perception of the world as populated by the vanquished and the victorious, and this influenced his emerging sense of self, particularly as someone growing up "different," which felt, at times, like being "a loser."

As psychotherapy progressed, I began to appreciate Michael's coping strategies and resources that helped protect him against depression. His close relationship with a grandmother who encouraged his creative pursuits and his identification with a peer group in high school helped to support a positive sense of being "different" and to minimize a sense of being an outlier. In general, loving relationships with parents, the availability of social support, a sense of connectedness to an LGB community, and being able to safely be "out" about sexual orientation are factors associated with decreased risk for depression in sexual minority persons.

In psychotherapy, Michael spoke of his sense of shame about not living up to his father's expectations and of a complicated identification with his mother, who was experienced as a highly imperfect ally during childhood and adolescence. Eventually, as he became more comfortable discussing his feelings about me, Michael was able to acknowledge that sometimes I disappointed him (rather than thinking that he disappointed me), and he came to understand that this did not negate the value of treatment or his own sense of worth. We explored why he assumed I would be critical of him, particularly if he expressed angry or competitive feelings towards me. This transference-based work allowed Michael to feel a greater sense of legitimacy about his grievances and a diminished fear that he would be rejected for stating his needs and opinions.

These changes, in conjunction with improvement in mood from medication treatment, helped Michael counter his disparaging feelings about being undesirable, needy, and not "competitive," which he associated with being gay. Treatment enabled Michael to be more comfortable being assertive, to better tolerate conflict, and to be more confident at work. By facilitating these gains, treatment supported his well-being by increasing opportunities for adult developmental experience. In the second year of treatment, he was promoted at work to a position that was more challenging and fulfilling, and he began a promising love relationship. He looked forward to introducing his partner to his parents.

It is true of many patients that developmental gains protect against recurrence of depression. For LGB patients, broadened developmental opportunities in childhood, adolescence, and young adulthood that help consolidate a positive sense of identity and strengthen intimate bonds have preventive mental health value. A response to depression in LGB persons thus warrants more than clinical interventions; it warrants social interventions to create more favorable environments for LGB persons. These social interventions include programs to help families accept their homosexual children, anti-bullying curricula, the provision of social and community support, and the repeal of discriminatory laws that preclude full participation in civic life by lesbians and gay men.

At present, the developmental impact of being stigmatized in early life because of gender nonconformity or perceived sexual orientation continues to cast a long shadow over the mental health of many LGB persons. In addition, sexual orientation discrimination, despite an improving legal and social climate for LGB persons, continues to increase risk for psychiatric morbidity. For these reasons, depression is likely to remain a leading clinical and public health issue for sexual minority persons. Clinicians familiar with the developmental and environmental context of LGB lives can bring to their practice a clinical and psychosocial savvy that helps treat depression and promote well-being in this population.

Key Points

- Depression is a major clinical and public health concern of LGB persons.

- The risk of depression in LGB persons is increased by experiences of childhood abuse, harassment and victimization due to gender nonconformity or sexual orientation, concealment of sexual identity, internalized homophobia, and discrimination related to homosexuality or bisexuality.

References

Albelda R, Badgett MVL, Schneebaum A, et al: Poverty in the lesbian, gay, and bisexual community. The Williams Institute, 2009. Available at: http://williamsinstitute.law .ucla.edu/wp-content/uploads/Albelda-Badgett-Schneebaum-Gates-LGB-Poverty -Report- March-2009.pdf. Accessed February 27, 2012.

American Psychiatric Association: Diagnostic and Statistical Manual of Mental Disorders, 4th Edition, Text Revision. Washington, DC, American Psychiatric Association, 2000

Isay RA: Commitment and Healing: Gay Men and the Need for Romantic Relationships. New York, Wiley, 2006

King MK, Semlyen J, Tai Sharon S, et al: A systematic review of mental disorder, suicide, and deliberate self harm in lesbian, gay and bisexual people. BMC Psychiatry 8:70 doi:10.1186/1471-244X-8-70, 2008

Meyer IH: Prejudice, social stress, and mental health in lesbian, gay, and bisexual populations: conceptual issues and research evidence Psychol Bull 5:674–697, 2003

Questions

9.1   Which of the following is associated with depression in LGB persons?

    A. Substance abuse.

    B. Internalized homophobia.

    C. HIV sexual risk behavior.

    D. A and C.

    E. All of the above.

The correct answer is E.

Substance abuse, internalized homophobia, and HIV sexual risk behavior are all associated with depression in LGB persons. Substance abuse is associated with depression in the general population, but in LGB persons may also reflect the historical role bars and clubs played as venues for LGB socialization and the disinhibiting effects of alcohol and drugs on sexual expression. Internalized homophobia interferes with self-acceptance of LGB personal identity and prevents LGB persons from affiliating with LGB communities that offer valuable social support. The relationship between HIV risk behaviors and depression is bidirectional, as exemplified by dysthymia and moderate levels of depression undermining a sense of personal efficacy to maintain safer sex behaviors and, on the other hand, depression resulting from the stress associated with becoming HIV-infected or living with HIV.

9.2   Which interventions can be helpful in reducing or preventing depression
      in LGB persons?

     A. Psychotherapy.
     B. Anti-bullying curricula in schools.
     C. Advocacy to combat sexual orientation discrimination.
     D. Helping persons change their sexual orientation.
     E. All of the above.
     F. A, B, and C.

The correct answer is F.

Psychotherapy, anti-bullying curricula in schools, and advocacy to combat sexual orientation discrimination can all be helpful in reducing or preventing depression in LGB persons, whereas efforts to change sexual orientation are likely to be associated with harmful psychological effects. Psychotherapy lessens depression in LGB persons by helping patients examine negative attitudes about homosexuality and exploring shame related to sexuality. Anti-bullying curricula establish norms of zero tolerance of harassment for would-be perpetrators, victims, and bystanders, with the intent of decreasing the incidence of bullying and psychological distress experienced by victims. Efforts to combat sexual orientation discrimination remove an important source of minority stress and depression; conversely, social and public policy that supports equal opportunity and social inclusion for LGB persons promotes their well-being. In contrast, interventions to change sexual orientation are likely to retraumatize LGB persons by making their same-sex desires ego-dystonic and interfering with their ability to sustain relationships of sexual and emotional intimacy.

Dysthymic Disorder

The Psychological Long-Term Nonprogressor

PHILIP A. BIALER, M.D.

DYSTHYMIC DISORDER OR DYSTHYMIA is most commonly defined as a chronic depressed mood for most of the day, for more days than not, as indicated by subjective account or observation by others, for more than two years. In addition, no major depressive episode was present during the first two years of the disturbance, and the disturbance is not better accounted for by a chronic major depressive disorder (Table 10–1) (American Psychiatric Association 2000).

Case Example: Jim

Jim is a 55-year-old man with HIV/AIDS who was referred for psychopharmacological treatment in 1997 because of a worsening depression. At that time he was already a long-term survivor, having been treated for what turned out to be his first HIV-related illness in 1982 when he was found to have idiopathic thrombosis purpura. His HIV-seropositive serostatus was confirmed in 1985, at which time he was told he would probably die within 2 years. By the time of our first visit, he had suffered additional HIV-related medical problems, including peripheral Kaposi's sarcoma in the late 1980s and then a non-Hodgkin's lymphoma diagnosed in 1995. Both of these problems were successfully treated, although the chemotherapy regimen for the lymphoma had been particularly debilitating. Since then he has been stabilized on a regimen of highly active antiretroviral therapy (HAART); his viral load has been undetectable and a

TABLE 10–1.   DSM-IV-TR diagnostic criteria for dysthymic disorder

A.   Depressed mood for most of the day, for more days than not, as indicated either by subjective account or observation by others, for at least 2 years.   **Note:** In children and adolescents, mood can be irritable and duration must be at least 1 year.

B.   Presence, while depressed, of two (or more) of the following:

   (1)   poor appetite or overeating

   (2)   insomnia or hypersomnia

   (3)   low energy or fatigue

   (4)   low self-esteem

   (5)   poor concentration or difficulty making decisions

   (6)   feelings of hopelessness

C.   During the 2-year period (1 year for children or adolescents) of the disturbance, the person has never been without the symptoms in Criteria A and B for more than 2 months at a time.

D.   No major depressive episode has been present during the first 2 years of the disturbance (1 year for children and adolescents); i.e., the disturbance is not better accounted for by chronic major depressive disorder, or major depressive disorder, in partial remission.

   Note: There may have been a previous major depressive episode provided there was a full remission (no significant signs or symptoms for 2 months) before development of the dysthymic disorder. In addition, after the initial 2 years (1 year in children or adolescents) of dysthymic disorder, there may be superimposed episodes of major depressive disorder, in which case both diagnoses may be given when the criteria are met for a major depressive episode.

E.   There has never been a manic episode, a mixed episode, or a hypomanic episode, and criteria have never been met for cyclothymic disorder.

F.   The disturbance does not occur exclusively during the course of a chronic psychotic disorder, such as schizophrenia or delusional disorder.

G.   The symptoms are not due to the direct physiological effects of a substance (e.g., a drug of abuse, a medication) or a general medical condition (e.g., hypothyroidism).

H.   The symptoms cause clinically significant distress or impairment in social, occupational, or other important areas of functioning.

   Specify if:

         Early onset: if onset is before age 21 years

         Late onset: if onset is age 21 years or older

   Specify (for most recent 2 years of dysthymic disorder):

         With atypical features

functional immunological status restored. Although he has had several other significant medical problems over the years, none of them have been HIV-related and none have been life-threatening.

When I first started seeing him, Jim was severely depressed and inpatient treatment was being considered. He was tearful during most of the initial evaluation, expressed hopelessness and helplessness, and questioned why he had survived so much physical distress only to suffer from so much emotional pain. Both his primary care physician and his therapist said that during times of medical crises he seemed to do better emotionally but when he was medically stable, his underlying issues would overwhelm him.

Although I was only supposed to manage his medications, Jim came to see me weekly; he felt that as we were both gay men, he could identify with me, saw me as a role model, and felt more comfortable talking about sexual issues than he did with his female therapist. In fact, he often stated that he had a much stronger emotional response in our sessions. To minimize splitting, I was in frequent contact with his therapist, who in many ways was relieved that he was also seeing me because she was feeling so frustrated by his lack of progress.

From the beginning of the treatment, Jim focused on how little he had achieved in his life despite his potential. He was a talented artist, very creative and a graduate of one of the best university arts programs in the country. He had a difficult time acknowledging that he had suffered from very severe medical problems, which would have impeded almost anyone's career, and that his lack of accomplishment did not reflect his being "a damaged person," as he so often put it.

Developmentally, Jim still sees himself as a 22-year-old college graduate with much potential. He frequently ruminates about his childhood and adolescence and how little emotional support he received from his parents, especially from his father. He admits he probably had had low-level depression since childhood, but this was not the kind of thing that could be talked about in his family. He feels this depression made it more difficult for him to achieve anything after he graduated from college and that it still acts as an impediment to progress in his life.

Jim has become more sexually confused and has been unable to maintain a long-lasting intimate relationship for at least 15 years. He has retreated into a fantasy world of what he calls his "alter ego": using a woman's name, he meets men online who are interested in having encounters with a cross-dresser. Many of these encounters involve the use of cocaine, although he minimizes the drug issue because he only does it "once in awhile and only if the other person brings it," ignoring that men who have cocaine are usually the ones he looks to for hookups. He still talks about the idea of having a "normal" relationship but then dismisses whatever this might mean on the grounds that no one would want him because he has AIDS. He has also continued to have medical problems, including two surgeries for bilateral mastoiditis, a severe episode of gout precipitated by one of his antiretroviral medications (which required inpatient treatment followed by rehabilitation), and a stress fracture. He also suffered the loss of his sister, who died of kidney failure, and subsequently of his father, who succumbed to Alzheimer's disease.

And yet Jim goes on. He attends classes at an art school as a scholarship student and he has won several awards. He has been involved in groups that support people with HIV, such as Gay Men's Health Crisis (GMHC) and Friends In Deed. A combination of venlafaxine and bupropion has been moderately helpful in ameliorating some of Jim's depressive symptoms such as low mood and hopelessness, especially when he dips into full-blown major depression. However, the underlying dysthymia never totally abates. He switched his therapists to try a cognitive-behavioral therapy (CBT) approach to see if this could help reform his negative thoughts and his focus on the past. He started attending Sexual Compulsives Anonymous and other 12-step meetings to address his sex and drug issues. There have been hints of possible career options in that he designed, hand-lettered, and drew all the wedding invitations for a friend's wedding and served as a creative director for an old college friend's startup.

However, after periods of seeming improvement and activity, the resentment and despair return because, as he is on disability, he cannot be legally paid for doing any work or he would lose his benefits. Jim constantly compares himself to his friends and where they are in their lives: married with families, financially successful with nice homes, and starting to think about retirement. Ironically, where I once served as a role model, now I also am an envied object, representing the success that has eluded him. He is angry about still living in the same walk-up apartment he first moved into soon after arriving in New York almost 30 years earlier. He says: "How can I get a job now? Who would hire me? It's too late."

Jim says he just doesn't fit in anymore. He does not like going to GMHC because, instead of the young gay men who were banding together to fight the disease 25 years ago, the clientele now represents the current face of AIDS: people of color, women, and drug users. He does not fit into the gay world any more with its emphasis on youth and gym bodies—he is older and has a body disfigured by lipodystrophy. Instead of feeling welcomed into the community, he feels shunned. "They just don't have any appreciation for what people my age have been through. I'm like a dinosaur."

However, part of his problem is that he still thinks like a man in his twenties or thirties and recalls how easy it used to be for him to attract people. He does not know many people his own age any more.

Discussion

This is a complex case that highlights many issues that are relevant for and can affect the mood of gay men, and gay and bisexual men with HIV/AIDS in particular (see Table 10–2). Many of the HIV-related issues may also apply to lesbians who are seropositive, but their numbers are relatively small. Although Jim feels that his HIV issues are no longer relevant to other gay men, the epidemiological statistics indicate that HIV/AIDS remains a very important medical and psychological factor affecting this population. Recent figures from the Centers for Disease Control and Prevention (CDC) reveal that through 2009, more than a half-million men who have sex with men (MSM) had been diagnosed with AIDS since the beginning of the epidemic and about half of these men had died. Currently there are approximately a half-million MSM living with HIV. MSM account for 53% of all new HIV infections, and this is the only risk group in the United States in which new HIV infections are increasing (Centers for Disease Control and Prevention 2009).

TABLE 10–2.   Factors that can affect mood in gay men with HIV/AIDS

- Cognitive effects of HIV
- Central nervous system opportunistic infections
- Central nervous system neoplasms
- HIV medications
- HIV-related medical problems
- Stigmatization
- Loss/bereavement
- Lipodystrophy/body image problems
- Disability
- Substance use

Jim does represent a subgroup of long-term AIDS survivors, adding another dimension to his treatment. Some of these long-term survivors have been further characterized as long-term nonprogressors and have suffered few HIV-related medical problems and no immunological decline. While Jim does not strictly meet these criteria, like several men I have seen in my clinical practice, he does seem to be in many ways a psychological long-term nonprogressor who has made little psychological growth in the 30 years he has been living with HIV/AIDS. How much of this arrested growth can be attributed to his serious medical issues and how much to his underlying psychiatric issues, including the chronic underlying dysthymia that predates the HIV infection, is an open question. And finally, how does this all relate to his identity as a gay man? It is impossible to separate one aspect from the other, and all of these issues will affect the treatment approaches.

Pharmacotherapy

The first treatment approach to consider is the indication for antidepressant medication for a patient like Jim. The effectiveness of antidepressant medication for the treatment of dysthymia has been studied in multiple trials, and meta-analyses of the use of antidepressants in major depression, minor depression, and dysthymia indicate a benefit superior to psychotherapy alone (Cuijpers et al. 2008; Imel et al. 2008; Markowitz et al. 2005). Most authors recommend the use of low doses of selective serotonin reuptake inhibitors (SSRIs) for the treatment of dysthymia with dosage modification during episodes of full-blown major depression. When choosing a specific medication in gay men who are also being treated for HIV/AIDS, however, one must be aware of the potential for drug-drug interactions.

With this in mind, a comprehensive medication history takes on greater importance and should include any nonprescribed or over-the-counter medications, supplements, and drugs obtained from buyer's clubs or clinical trials that the patient may be taking. Of the medications that may be included in a HAART regimen, the protease inhibitor ritonavir may present the most problems. Ritonavir is a potent inhibitor of cytochrome P450 (CYP) 2D6, which is a major metabolic enzyme for many of the SSRIs as well as other psychotropic medications. Therefore, choosing an SSRI that is metabolized by multiple enzymes may help avoid toxicity caused by ritonavir-induced metabolic inhibition. Citalopram and escitalopram, as well as the selective norepinephrine inhibitors venlafaxine and duloxetine may be good choices. Fluoxetine, which is mainly metabolized by CYP2D6, should probably be avoided in patients taking ritonavir. Any psychiatric medication that is a potent inhibitor of CYP3A4 should also be avoided. This is because CYP3A4 is the main metabolic enzyme for all of the protease inhibitors, and inhibition of their metabolism can lead to severe, debilitating toxicity.

Efavirenz is another medication that has become a common component of HAART regimens. Its pharmacokinetic profile is similar to ritonavir, and choosing an antidepressant for patients taking efavirenz should probably be similar to those for patients taking ritonavir. Neuropsychiatric side effects are a bigger problem for patients taking efavirenz. While the potential for vivid, sometimes disturbing dreams has been well documented, there are some anecdotal reports that this medication can worsen depressive symptoms among patients who already have depressive disorders such as dysthymia. These patients must be carefully monitored, and if their depression cannot be adequately treated, then coordination of care with their primary HIV physician takes on additional importance and modification of the HAART regimen should be considered.

One final and important cautionary note concerning the medical management of dysthymia: Some patients and clinicians may feel that the supplement St. John's wort is an acceptable alternative treatment for minor depression. However, St. John's wort is absolutely contraindicated for any patient with HIV taking a protease inhibitor or a non-nucleoside reverse transcriptase inhibitor because it can induce the metabolism of these HIV drugs, resulting in decreased serum levels and thus decreased effectiveness.

The potential for drug-drug interactions among gay men and women with HIV/AIDS is a complex subject, and a fuller review is beyond the scope of this chapter. Websites such as www.aidsmeds.com or www.hiv-druginteractions.com can be helpful when choosing an antidepressant for the treatment of dysthymia.

Psychosocial Issues

This case highlights several psychosocial issues that must be acknowledged regardless of the form of therapy used. One important issue for many of the gay men who are long-term survivors of HIV/AIDS is that they have suffered multiple losses. These men often came of age and adopted their sexual identities in the late 1970s and early 1980s when the AIDS epidemic was raging unchecked. After going through their own personal process of coming out and accepting their sexual attractions, their sexual activity, and their relationships as normal, they now were facing what felt to many of them like punishment for their hard-fought lifestyle. Many lost friends, lovers, and entire support networks. For many of these men and women, rebuilding a network has been close to impossible. Many of the community-based organizations (CBOs) that were founded by gay men to provide the support and advocacy still exist, but many of these men now complain that they no longer are comfortable seeking services from these organizations. As the epidemic grew to encompass populations beyond gay men, the CBOs' missions grew to provide services for all of those affected. Nevertheless, the enormous losses have had lasting effects on those who already have depressive disorders, including dysthymia. Individual and group treatment is still the mainstay of addressing the loss with proven efficacy, and efforts should be made to engage patients in these treatments (Goodkin et al. 1999; Sikkema et al. 2004).

Concerns about body image may also need to be addressed with the dysthymic gay patient, and once again this may be a particular problem among gay men with HIV/AIDS. Many of the medications in the HAART regimen can cause lipodystrophy, a redistribution of body fat, which leads to a characteristic and sometimes stigmatizing appearance. The cheeks and temporal areas on the face can appear sunken and wasted, the arms and legs lose fat and become very thin, and much of the fat then becomes redistributed to the abdomen and behind the neck, a so-called buffalo hump. When patients become aware of how their body has changed, they sometimes isolate themselves, leading to worsening depression. Sometimes a modification of the HAART regimen may help. Some patients seek out plastic surgery to have fat substitutes and other fillers injected into their face or liposuction to have the hump reduced. An improved self-image may have a beneficial effect on a patient's mood. The synthetic growth hormone releasing factor tesamorelin (Egrifta) has recently been approved for the treatment of lipodystrophy.

Disability is another issue with a profound impact on the management of dysthymia among gay men who are also long-term HIV survivors. Although the HIV/AIDS may be well controlled, with laboratory tests indicating good health—and many of these men may appear healthy—many of them remain on long-term disability. Either too sick and weak when they initially stopped working, or having chosen to go on disability because they did not expect to live very long, these men now depend on their benefits to pay for the treatment that keeps them alive. Many complain of feeling trapped, and this adds to their sense of stunted psychological development. They are at an age when they should be at the peak of career productivity but have no career at all. The feelings of low self-worth and lack of accomplishment, as well as the lack of the structure and iden-tification that a job can provide, are all major issues to discuss with the dysthy-mic patient. Not all long-term HIV survivors have remained on long-term disability. Some have found personal meaning in their survivorship that has allowed them to forge new careers and lead extremely productive lives. One then has to consider whether dysthymia has contributed to some patients' inability to become more functional.

Finally, the ability to develop and maintain long-lasting intimate relation-ships becomes complicated for the gay man dealing not only with a chronic de-pression but also a stigmatizing, potentially infectious disease, a poor self body image, and low self-worth due to lack of career accomplishments. Once again, a vicious cycle of low levels of support due to lack of an intimate relationship can lead to worsening of the depression, which leads to further isolation.

Psychotherapy

Which psychotherapeutic approaches are most effective for the dysthymic pa-tient? CBT can help the patient identify negative irrational thoughts about self, situation, and the future. The therapist can then work with the patient to exam-ine these thoughts, weigh the evidence, and restructure and challenge these thoughts instead of believing and acting on them. Interpersonal therapy (IPT) has also been shown to be effective in studies evaluating the treatment of de-pression in people with HIV/AIDS, as well as for the treatment of dysthymia in general (Markowitz et al. 1998, 2005). IPT helps the patient relate changes in mood to events in the environment and changes in social roles. IPT also strives to address interpersonal deficits and help the patient mourn life's challenges while encouraging the finding of new life goals. Both CBT and IPT are relatively brief forms of therapy and, along with medication, can help "kick-start" the pa-tient's recovery from a depressed mood. Long-term supportive therapy has been less studied but may be helpful in supporting the patient's strengths and resilience that allows the individual to make difficult concrete changes in dys-functional patterns, leading to longer-lasting improvement. In fact, a 10-year study looking at the naturalistic course of dysthymia revealed that the mean in-terval to recovery from entry into the study was greater than 5 years, supporting the need for long-term treatment of the dysthymic patient (Klein et al. 2006).

Conclusion

Jim's therapist and I continue to check in with each other frequently. Jim tells us that the only reason he goes on is because his mother still depends on him. However, she just turned 90. What will happen after she dies? It is possible he might kill himself. However, Jim is a real survivor who, despite a tragic life story, keeps rebounding despite his continued depression. Even for the dysthymic HIV-positive long-term survivor, hope can spring eternal.

Key Points

- Psychosocial issues that may contribute to depressed mood in gay men with HIV/AIDS include AIDS-related illness, medications, poor body image, disability, and lack of intimate relationships.

- Pharmacotherapy may be more effective for treating dysthymia in the short term. Psychotherapy or combination treatment may be more helpful in the long term.

- When prescribing antidepressants to an HIV-infected patient, there is a potential for drug-drug interactions when ritonavir and possibly efavirenz are part of a HAART regimen. Always check available resources for potential medication interactions when treating patients with HIV.

References

American Psychiatric Association: Diagnostic and Statistical Manual of Mental Disorders, 4th Edition, Text Revision. Washington, DC, American Psychiatric Association, 2000

Centers for Disease Control and Prevention: HIV Surveillance Report, Vol 21, 2009. Available at: http://cdc.gov/hiv/topics/surveillance/resources/reports/. Accessed November 9, 2010.

Cuijpers P, van Straten A, Oppen P, et al: Are psychological and pharmacological interventions equally effective in the treatment of adult depressive disorders? A meta-analysis of comparative studies. J Clin Psychiatry 60:1675–1685, 2008

Goodkin K, Blaney NJ, Feaster DJ, et al: A randomized controlled clinical trial of a bereavement support group intervention in human immunodeficiency virus type 1-seropositive and -seronegative homosexual men. Arch Gen Psychiatry 56:52–59, 1999

Imel ZE, Maltever MB, McKay KM, et al: A meta-analysis of psychotherapy and medication in unipolar depression and dysthymia. J Affect Disord 110:197–206, 2008

Klein DN, Shankman SA, Roose S: Ten-year prospective follow-up study of the naturalistic course of dysthymic disorder and double depression. Am J Psychiatry 163:872–880, 2006

Markowitz JC, Kocsis JH, Fishman B, et al: Treatment of depressive symptoms in human immunodeficiency virus-positive patients. Arch Gen Psychiatry 55:452–457, 1998

Markowitz JC, Koscis JH, Bleiberg KL, et al: A comparative trial of psychotherapy and pharmacotherapy for "pure" dysthymic patients. J Affect Disord 69:167–175, 2005

Sikkema KJ, Hansen NB, Kochman A, et al: Outcomes from a randomized controlled trial of a group intervention for HIV positive men and women coping with AIDS-related loss and bereavement. Death Stud 28:187–209, 2004

Questions

10.1   Meta-analyses have shown which treatment to be the most effective for dysthymic disorder?

    A. Cognitive-behavioral therapy.
    B. Pharmacotherapy.
    C. Interpersonal therapy.
    D. Supportive psychotherapy.

The correct answer is B.

Several meta-analyses of studies comparing the effectiveness of medication and different psychotherapeutic methods for the treatment of dysthymia have consistently demonstrated pharmacotherapy to be more effective. However, some of these authors also point out that the studies included in the meta-analyses generally look at treatment response for relatively short time periods and suggest that psychotherapy may be helpful in the long-term management of patients with dysthymic disorder.

10.2   What psychosocial issues can contribute to depressed mood in gay men with HIV/AIDS?

    A. Lipodystrophy and poor body image.
    B. Dependence on disability benefits.
    C. Lack of intimate relationships.
    D. All of the above.

The correct answer is D.

In addition to biological contributors to mood disorders in patients with HIV/AIDS, there are multiple psychosocial stressors faced by gay men, and in particular long-term survivors of HIV/AIDS, that can contribute to depressed mood and must be addressed in their treatment. The above list is not exhaustive, and individual coping with a debilitating chronic illness should be explored.

Bipolar Disorder

Identity Crisis

CHRISTOPHER A. MCINTOSH, M.D.

THE "CHIEF COMPLAINT" in medicine is characterized by the opening words the patient uses to describe why he or she has come to the doctor for help. The chief complaint may or may not be congruent with the "reason for referral" (RFR) outlined by the referring health professional.

Case Example: Jean-Paul

"I am a 35-year-old divorced, French-Canadian, Catholic, alcoholic homosexual. Need I say more?" Jean-Paul pronounced dramatically when I asked him why he had come to see me. I looked down at the note provided by Jean-Paul's most recent inpatient psychiatrist. It read, "RFR—Management of bipolar disorder, type I." (See Tables 11–1 and 11–2 [American Psychiatric Association 2000].)

Jean-Paul's chief complaint was both appropriate and ironic. It was appropriate because identity issues would be central in our work together to sort out Jean-Paul's many life problems. It was ironic because a reluctance to "say more" was not one of those problems.

In fact, on our first meeting Jean-Paul displayed pressured speech, grandiosity, increased psychomotor activity, and elevated mood, all classic signs and symptoms of a manic episode (see Table 11–1). I was able to get enough questions in edgewise to establish that rehospitalization was not immediately necessary. Seeing that the referral note indicated a history of noncompliance with mood-stabilizing medication, I reached into my filing cabinet to retrieve a lab requisition to obtain a lithium level as well as a toxicology panel.

TABLE 11–1.   DSM-IV-TR criteria for manic episode

A. A distinct period of abnormally and persistently elevated, expansive, or irritable mood, lasting at least 1 week (or any duration if hospitalization is necessary).

B. During the period of mood disturbance, three (or more) of the following symptoms have persisted (four if the mood is only irritable) and have been present to a significant degree:

   (1) inflated self-esteem or grandiosity

   (2) decreased need for sleep (e.g., feels rested after only 3 hours of sleep)

   (3) more talkative than usual or pressure to keep talking

   (4) flight of ideas or subjective experience that thoughts are racing

   (5) distractibility (i.e., attention too easily drawn to unimportant or irrelevant external stimuli)

   (6) increase in goal-directed activity (either socially, at work or school, or sexually) or psychomotor agitation

   (7) excessive involvement in pleasurable activities that have a high potential for painful consequences (e.g., engaging in unrestrained buying sprees, sexual indiscretions, or foolish business investments)

C. The symptoms do not meet criteria for a mixed episode.

D. The mood disturbance is sufficiently severe to cause marked impairment in occupational functioning or in usual social activities or relationships with others, or to necessitate hospitalization to prevent harm to self or others, or there are psychotic features.

E. The symptoms are not due to the direct physiological effects of a substance (e.g., a drug of abuse, a medication, or other treatment) or a general medical condition (e.g., hyperthyroidism).

   Note: Manic-like episodes that are clearly caused by somatic antidepressant treatment (e.g., medication, electroconvulsive therapy, light therapy) should not count toward a diagnosis of bipolar I disorder.

Source.   Reprinted from *Diagnostic and Statistical Manual of Mental Disorders,* 4th Edition, Text Revision. Washington, DC, American Psychiatric Association, 2000. Used with permission. Copyright © 2000 American Psychiatric Association.

"Is that *really* necessary, doctor?" Jean-Paul asked archly.

"Humor me," I shot back with a smile, recognizing a familiar, playful countertransference response to patients with euphoric mania.

At our next meeting we reviewed Jean-Paul's bloodwork results. The toxicology panel result was negative, and the lithium level was subtherapeutic. Neither was a surprise to Jean-Paul.

"I'm high on life, doctor, don't you see?"

Another familiar feeling flooded me: reluctance. Here I was about to appeal to Jean-Paul to give up feeling on top of the world and take his medication properly to terminate his manic episode. Who really wants to be the buzz kill, the strait-laced goody-two-shoes blowing the whistle on the party?

TABLE 11–2. DSM-IV-TR criteria for bipolar I disorder, most recent episode manic

---

A.   Currently (or most recently) in a manic episode.

B.   There has previously been at least one major depressive episode, manic episode, or mixed episode.

C.   The mood episodes in Criteria A and B are not better accounted for by schizoaffective disorder and are not superimposed on schizophrenia, schizophreniform disorder, delusional disorder, or psychotic disorder not otherwise specified.

If the full criteria are currently met for a manic episode, *specify* its current clinical status and/or features:

   Mild, moderate, severe without psychotic features/severe with psychotic features

   With catatonic features

   With postpartum onset

If the full criteria are not currently met for a manic episode, *specify* the current clinical status of the bipolar I disorder and/or features of the most recent manic episode:

   In partial remission, in full remission

   With catatonic features

   With postpartum onset

Specify:

   Longitudinal course specifiers (with and without interepisode recovery)

   With seasonal pattern (applies only to the pattern of major depressive episodes)

   With rapid cycling

Source.   Reprinted from *Diagnostic and Statistical Manual of Mental Disorders,* 4th Edition, Text Revision. Washington, DC, American Psychiatric Association, 2000. Used with permission. Copyright © 2000 American Psychiatric Association.

Background: Oddly enough, "goody-two-shoes" would have once been an apt description of Jean-Paul. Growing up in a devout, well-off Catholic family in Quebec, he was faithful to the church and to school and eager to please his parents in every possible way. He was a star pupil, a leader in student government, and a promising tennis player. The third youngest in a line of nine siblings, he experienced intense competition for attention from parents who were excellent providers of instrumental support but were not emotionally demonstrative. "What do you need?" was their most common response to a child coming to them for help, and it was tacitly understood that they were not referring to emotional needs.

Jean-Paul's religious outlook was uncompromisingly Catholic. Active in the Catholic youth movement, he disdained moral relativism and held papal authority in the highest esteem. While many young people of his age in Quebec were turning away from the Catholic Church, he embraced its comforting rituals and traditions.

Yet compromises were indeed necessary for Jean-Paul as he dealt with internal psychic conflict over his homosexuality. Unable to contain his distress over a series of sexual experiences with a manipulative older neighbor boy, he let his marks tumble uncharacteristically in middle school. When called before his father to account for this, he grasped desperately for any other possible explanation and blamed his competitive tennis lessons. Sacrificing a sport he adored was the price to be paid to keep the secret and have a chance at regaining his father's esteem.

Through high school and university, an idealized conventional heterosexual life continued to be his dream and goal. He experienced frequent bouts of depressed mood and had chronic sleep problems, but he let no one in on his true feelings and maintained a façade of driven, focused hypercompetence. A chaste relationship with a good Catholic girl led to marriage just after university graduation, and this is where the façade crumbled.

Jean-Paul experienced his first full-blown manic episode soon after getting married. He was eventually hospitalized by his family after leaving a trail of relational destruction that included alienated work colleagues and a baffled wife who proceeded to divorce him after he admitted in a couples-therapy session that "I think I'm probably gay."

Jean-Paul was well for a time after discharge from the hospital. Like many individuals with bipolar disorder, after a period of wellness he decided to stop taking his maintenance mood stabilizer. In many respects he now experienced significantly less social pressure, since with the odious stain of divorce he could no longer maintain the illusion of an idealized Catholic life. He had a period of several years of mostly euthymic mood as he put his former career on hold and found low-stress work that paid the bills and allowed him to just get by.

Eventually, though, the ambitious part of him resurfaced, and he took a high-stress job in the advertising industry. He managed the stress this time not only with defensive denial but also with alcohol, a vice with a degree of social acceptance among his new work colleagues.

Feeling a degree of renewed confidence in his life, he decided that this was the time for his "coming out." Since he had already come out to his family at the time of his last hospitalization, this coming out was more like the original meaning of the expression, as when debutantes would "come out" into society at a debutante ball (Chauncey 1994).

Jean-Paul later told me: "If I was going to do gay, I was going to do it right!", and after connecting with some gay colleagues at work, he spent a few months analyzing exactly how to do just that. He came to the conclusion that it was all about parties and access to them, and so he dove into the gay "circuit party" subculture with all the drive he had previously devoted to Catholicism. Within a year he had parlayed his considerable social skills to become a "scene queen." If there was a party happening anywhere in the city of Montreal, Jean-Paul could tell you where it was, who was deejaying, how to get on the guest list, and where to buy your drugs.

Alcohol was supplemented over this period by a variety of illicit drugs, especially cocaine, which helped him chase or extend the manic highs that enabled him to party four nights a week and still function at work on Monday. He disliked ecstasy (methylene dioxymethamphetamine; MDMA) because it promoted a "lovey-dovey" intimacy that made him uncomfortable. In fact, despite placing himself at the center of a highly sexualized scene he rarely had sex himself, and increasingly he felt empty and alone.

He maintained good relationships with his family, attending family functions with varying regularity but keeping that life quite separate from his gay life.

The turning point happened when his ex-wife reappeared suddenly with a demand that forced his worlds to collide: She wanted to remarry in the Catholic Church and therefore wanted him to cooperate with seeking an annulment on the basis that he had entered the marriage fraudulently because he was a homosexual.

Jean-Paul plunged into a deep depression on receiving this request. He brought himself to the hospital when he started to seriously consider jumping from the Jacques Cartier Bridge. On the inpatient unit, he was started on lithium carbonate, and over a 3-week admission he showed significant improvement. He found the psychotherapy he engaged in while admitted helpful and asked to be referred on discharge to someone who could do both psychotherapy and medication treatment.

The Catch-22 of Medication Adherence

This leads us back to Jean-Paul's second meeting with me, where I was confronted with his medication nonadherence and hypomanic presentation.

"What can I tell you, doctor, I feel better when I'm this way. Stronger, more confident," he cocked his head to the side flirtatiously, "more attractive."

Having read about the recent depths of his despair from his inpatient discharge summary, it seemed miserly indeed to begrudge him feeling better. We both knew what would come afterwards if the episode continued unchecked, but at that point I was the only one interested in reflecting on that possibility.

Still, Jean-Paul was far from stupid, so as we began our weekly meetings with me insisting on ongoing reflection on his not taking medication, he eventually came around. His mood stabilized as he took medication more regularly, with a brief depressive overcorrection one week. He missed that week's session and left me a semiserious "see-what-you've-done-to-me" voice mail, but he showed up the next week, ready to work.

Identity and Sexual Orientation

We began by looking at the chief complaint, which appears to be an identity statement: "I am a 35-year-old divorced, French-Canadian, Catholic, alcoholic homosexual."

The statement also has the quality of an admission, as in Step 1 of Alcoholics Anonymous (Alcoholics Anonymous 2001), a self-help organization Jean-Paul had joined since his discharge from hospital. It could also be a confession or, alternatively, a self-diagnosis—though, if the latter, it is interesting that Jean-Paul did not include "bipolar" but did include "homosexual."

In the study of sexual orientation, it is common to distinguish among its three components: sexual attraction and fantasy, sexual behavior, and sexual identity (see the Glossary at the end of this book). Jean-Paul's use of the term *homosexual* to describe his sexual identity should be noted with interest, as men with a positive sense of their sexual orientation would be more likely to use the term *gay*.

The word *homosexual* is not necessarily an offensive term to the gay community, but it does come with baggage due to the past use of the term as a clinical diagnosis when homosexuality was considered a mental illness. Jean-Paul's use of the term as a self-descriptor indicated unexamined internalized homophobia (see Glossary). Given the stigmatization associated with both homosexual people and people with chronic mental illness, it is understandable how Jean-Paul might wish to deny seeing himself as a member of these groups.

Identity and Mental Illness

The pharmacotherapy complemented the insight-oriented psychotherapy by reducing the intensity of Jean-Paul's mood episodes, which opened up greater mental "space" for reflecting on the two diametrically opposed ways in which he dealt with strong emotional states. Depressive Jean-Paul expanded and catastrophized life stressors so that they became all-enveloping and unmanageable, his only recourse being to retreat from the world to his bed and hide under the blanket. Manic Jean-Paul, by contrast, denied or dissociated the anxieties of life, allowing for furious bursts of productivity and euphoria but no substantive mental engagement with the core concerns.

As psychotherapy progressed, Jean-Paul was able to see how his anxieties about having a mental illness and being gay had previously been managed rather than addressed.

The idea of a need for consistent mood-stabilizing medication had been kept at bay by rationalizing manic and depressive states as "natural" states. Paradoxically, including manic highs and depressive lows as part of Jean-Paul's identity ("This is just who I am") resulted in him disidentifying with the group of people categorized as chronically mentally ill. By contrast, the acceptance of his mental illness he attained through reflection in therapy reversed that identification, so he could consider the possibility that the manic and depressive episodes were "unnatural" states that could be treated with medication to allow him a more functional range of emotionality.

Similarly, Jean-Paul's dawning awareness of his same-sex attractions as a youth did not lead to an identification with the group of people known as homosexuals. Instead, he compartmentalized those feelings and countered them by rigidly pursuing an idealized heterosexual lifestyle that would be consistent with his religious views and the anticipated expectations of his parents. When that life fell apart, it appeared outwardly that Jean-Paul took some steps toward self-acceptance by coming out. But inwardly, this acceptance was superficial at best and resulted in the equally rigid pursuit of an idealized "A-list" gay lifestyle that eventually came to feel just as false.

In insight-oriented psychotherapy, Jean-Paul was finally able to address the anxieties he had about being gay, rather than manage them:

> I can't be either gay *or* Catholic; I'm both. It's not an easy combination, but it's not made any easier by me pretending otherwise.

In the same way, as he gained more and more experience with reflecting on his feeling states rather than managing them with depressive catastrophizing or manic denial, those states began to feel less explosive. He found, to his surprise, that he could tolerate talking about his anxieties and vulnerabilities not only with me, but also with close friends from both his gay and his Catholic circles. This led to greater intimacy in his relationships and the beginnings of efforts to find a more balanced and genuine way of being in the world.

Key Points

- Identity issues are of considerable importance in psychotherapy for LGBT people, and they are just as important in the treatment of people with bipolar disorder, whose disidentification with "the mentally ill" may lead to medication nonadherence. Treatment with medication and psychotherapy should be strongly considered.

- Rates of substance abuse are elevated in the LGBT community and are also important considerations in bipolar disorder.

- Self-acceptance is an important goal in psychotherapeutic work with these patients, and the process of acceptance of sexual orientation may parallel the process of acceptance of having a mental illness requiring long-term medication management.

References

Alcoholics Anonymous: The Big Book, 4th Edition, 2001. Available at: http://www.aa.org/bbonline/. Accessed November 8, 2011.

American Psychiatric Association: Diagnostic and Statistical Manual of Mental Disorders, 4th Edition, Text Revision. Washington, DC, American Psychiatric Association, 2000

Chauncey G: Gay New York: Gender, Urban Culture, and the Making of the Gay Male World, 1890–1940. New York, Basic Books, 1994

World Professional Association for Transgender Health: Standards of Care for the Health of Transsexual, Transgender, and Gender Nonconforming People, 7th Version, 2011. Available at: http://www.wpath.org/documents/Standards%20of%20 Care%20V7%20-%202011%20WPATH.pdf. Accessed February 27, 2012.

Questions

11.1   Mac, a 22-year-old female-to-male transgender person, is admitted to your inpatient unit in a euphoric manic state. He has a strong family history of bipolar disorder. He recently started presenting full-time in the male role at his university. When you discuss mood-stabilizing medication with him, he asks instead for you to prescribe testosterone injections, stating he believes his mood problems will resolve with proceeding to the next stage of his transition. You do the following:

A. Agree and start testosterone enanthate intramuscular injections every 2 weeks.

B. Diagnose the cross-gender identification as a delusion, prescribe antipsychotics, use female pronouns, and start using the patient's birth name, Tiffany.

C. Provide psychoeducation about bipolar disorder and mood-stabilizing medication, inquire about his social supports, and collaborate with Mac to come up with a treatment plan so that he can be in optimal mental health to proceed with the next stage of transition.

The correct answer is C.

Transition generally improves mental health for transgender people by ameliorating gender dysphoria, but guidelines emphasize that stabilization of mental health concerns and good social and/or therapeutic support are strongly recommended before proceeding (World Professional Association for Transgender Health 2011).

11.2   Marina, a 39-year-old woman in a heterosexual marriage, impulsively visits a lesbian bar during a manic episode and has sex with a woman for the first time ever. In her therapy session with you the next day, she rapidly elaborates her plans to leave her husband and elope to Spain with her new lover. You do the following:

A. Congratulate her on her coming out and give her information about a resort you enjoyed near Barcelona.

B. Tell her frankly that you think her experience was a meaningless fling brought on by the manic episode.

C. Encourage her not to make drastic changes to her life while in the midst of a manic episode and explore more of what this experience might mean to her, while also working with her to optimize mood stabilization.

The correct answer is C.

It is difficult to draw conclusions about the meaning of behavior an actively manic patient engages in, so one should not. Better mood stabilization will bring better self-reflective capacity and thus better understanding.

11.3 Eugene, a 55-year-old gay man whom you treat for bipolar disorder, has begun drinking alcohol heavily at home following a breakup with a long-term boyfriend. You do the following:

A. Advise him of the potentially deleterious effects of alcohol on his mental health and encourage him to explore his feelings about the breakup in therapy rather than numb the feelings with alcohol. You provide him with information about alcohol abuse resources.

B. Encourage him to go out to bars to drink so that he might meet someone new.

C. Start an antidepressant to prevent onset of a depressive episode.

The correct answer is A.

With good mood stabilization in place, and avoiding substances, patients with bipolar disorder are as capable as any others of reflecting on normal sadness in therapy.

Panic Disorder

Seeing Superman

Eric Yarbrough, M.D.

Case Example: Clark

Background: Clark is homosexual. I know because he told me, when he came to me for a psychiatric evaluation to discuss discontinuing the medication he was taking for panic attacks. A psychiatrist had originally prescribed the medication, and Clark had continued it for several years with his primary care physician writing the prescription as part of his regular checkups. Now panic free for some time, he came to me to discuss going off the medication.

In addition to being homosexual, Clark is the oldest son of a Japanese immigrant family. His family moved to the United States just a few years before Clark was born, and most of his childhood was spent in North Carolina with his parents and younger brother. Before moving to New York for medical school, he worked as a waiter in a restaurant and spent his spare time painting landscapes and playing the cello. As he was the eldest son and the first of his family born in this country, his parents expected him to accomplish great things. They were strict with his schooling, painting classes, and music lessons. Clark came into the world with a lot of expectations already placed on him, and he adapted to them with enthusiasm. In fact, he was able to satisfy his parents with almost no disappointments, fulfilling all of their expectations but one.

In addition to being a doctor in training, a cellist, and a painter, Clark is generally a "nice guy." He has a great desire to help people, to avoid confrontation, and to suppress and repress any feelings he thinks might portray him in a negative light. He does a great deal to please his parents. Their approval takes precedence over his own wishes. Most of the decisions Clark makes in his life serve to please them in one way or another, either by being the best at something or by living up to their vision of "the good son."

With all his energy taken up by trying to please his parents, it's unclear to Clark what he wants for himself. When he found himself drawn to an activity that his parents didn't value, he typically let it go. For example, as a child and adolescent growing up near the coast in North Carolina, Clark loved to sail. He was on a racing team in high school and wanted to continue into college. His parents didn't see much use for this pastime. Playing the cello and painting were artistic. These hobbies taught dexterity and attention, which would make their son a better surgeon. What educational use would a man get out of sailing?

Clark knew before college that once he was finished with medical school, he would become a surgeon, run a surgery department, and systematically save the world. For all intents and purposes, his fantasy is to become a modern-day superman.

Every superhero has a weakness, and Clark is no different. When he was a teenager, he would date women and participate in superficial flirtations, but despite his dashing good looks he was largely asexual. School and work were his primary concerns and his excuse for not dating for some time. It was during these teenage years that he started to experience anxiety as well. Most notably, he'd feel anxious at parties in high school and college. He was concerned he would make a fool of himself or be discovered—for what, it wasn't completely clear.

His first panic attack occurred one day while at work. A group of men came into the restaurant where he worked and started to flirt with him. While he waited on them he could feel his pulse quickening, his breathing becoming more rapid, and his palms beginning to sweat. He got dizzy, and just before he felt he would die, he ran out of the restaurant without telling anyone and didn't return to work again for a week.

The panic attack passed, but his anxiety did not. After that experience, Clark became hypervigilant with regard to the men around him in social situations. He started to become aware of his own homosexual thoughts and desires. More panic attacks followed at events where he noticed men and men noticed him. To compensate for his anxiety and panic, he began to drink large amounts of alcohol. The alcohol medicated the panic to a point, but one evening during an episode of severe intoxication, Clark fell and fractured his arm. He decided at that point to stop drinking and seek psychiatric attention.

The psychiatrist diagnosed Clark with panic disorder and started him on a moderate dose of an antidepressant. This helped to control his panic and decrease his anxiety. In therapy, the psychiatrist listened to the significant stressors that had been placed on him and provided general support. Clark talked in therapy about his homosexual desires and his concerns that his parents, should they discover his sexual orientation, would disown him. Although he didn't come out to his parents at that point, he did start to date men. His anxiety symptoms diminished, and he remained panic-free.

Panic attacks are defined in DSM-IV-TR (American Psychiatric Association 2000) as a cluster of physical and psychological symptoms that occur abruptly and usually without warning. They include increased heart rate, difficulty breathing, a choking sensation, paresthesias, depersonalization, derealization, sweating, tremors, and thinking one is about to die (Table 12–1). Clark experienced many of these symptoms during his episodes. When individuals have recurring panic attacks, these symptoms can turn into a disorder, and they change their behavior in the fear the attacks will happen again (Table 12–2). They worry about getting into a situation that might bring on another attack that could escalate to the point of them losing control of their own minds. Social situations created these anxieties for Clark, and he handled the stress mainly through self-medicating with alcohol.

There are several factors in Clark's case that would predispose him to anxiety and panic. Each of them likely contributed, in part, to the clinical picture that emerged.

Clark's personality, likely gained through a combination of genetic and environmental factors, was obsessive in style. He kept rigid schedules, had rules for what his occupation and life's works would be, and tried his best to keep his emotions under control. Feeling anger, sadness, or ambivalence was a frightening experience for him, as it is for many obsessive people. Sometimes emotions, like those people may confront when coming out as gay, become so great that the obsessive defenses can't hold them any longer and they emerge as intense anxiety. During these times some patients can receive a range of diagnoses, from anxiety to personality disorders or even psychosis. It is important to take a good history and evaluate current life stressors that might contribute to the larger clinical picture.

The coming out process is a series of life events and not a single event. The stress and anxiety of coming out to one's parents can be reexperienced when coming out to other family, friends, coworkers, and even strangers. If a coming out experience, including someone coming out to themselves, is stressful and anxiety-provoking to the point of panic symptoms or a panic attack, the same symptoms can reappear with successive coming out events, leading to recurring panic and presenting as a disorder. Without a detailed social history, a clinician may miss this connection.

Having a panic attack while coming to the realization that one is having homosexual feelings is a situation that has been documented since the early twentieth century. Kempf (1920) is most famous for writing about homosexual panic. His writings described a reaction to homosexual advances that led to panic, transient psychosis, and sometimes violent or aggressive behavior. The homosexual panic Clark experienced is instead a reaction to realizing one might be homosexual.

Being homosexual, in and of itself, does not lead one to have anxiety or panic. Being homosexual in a society where it is highly stigmatized, and frequently condemned by many cultural and religious institutions, and where homosexuals are looked on as a group of people with less than equal rights, could lead someone to have such a reaction.

Before Clark became aware of his sexual feelings, his asexual life left him with little to worry about in relationship to his parents, friends, and society as a

---

TABLE 12–1.   Panic attack (DSM-IV-TR)

Note: A panic attack is not a codable disorder. Code the specific diagnosis in which
the panic attack occurs (e.g., 300.21 panic disorder with agoraphobia).

A discrete period of intense fear or discomfort, in which four (or more) of the following
symptoms developed abruptly and reached a peak within 10 minutes:

(1) palpitations, pounding heart, or accelerated heart rate

(2) sweating

(3) trembling or shaking

(4) sensations of shortness of breath or smothering

(5) feeling of choking

(6) chest pain or discomfort

(7) nausea or abdominal distress

(8) feeling dizzy, unsteady, lightheaded, or faint

(9) derealization (feelings of unreality) or depersonalization (being detached from
oneself)

(10) fear of losing control or going crazy

(11) fear of dying

(12) paresthesias (numbness or tingling sensations)

(13) chills or hot flushes

Source.   Reprinted from *Diagnostic and Statistical Manual of Mental Disorders,* 4th Edition, Text
Revision. Washington, DC, American Psychiatric Association, 2000. Used with permission.
Copyright © 2000 American Psychiatric Association.

whole. The rigid and obsessive structure he kept worked in a way that kept him
on schedule, successful, and directed toward his goal of becoming a cello-play-
ing, modern-art-painting trauma surgeon at the command of a hospital. In fact,
it could be hypothesized that his career, hobbies, and personality style were unconsciously chosen to overcompensate for his fear that his parents would discover his homosexuality. This rigid fortress served its purpose for a while, but it
was time-limited. Emotions were building up in Clark, and feelings that he had
ignored for some time started to make their way out in whatever way possible.
For him, it was in the form of panic. He could live only so long in a fortress of
solitude.

Another facet of Clark's personality was the altruistic and giving side. Clark,
like all children, had a desire to please his parents. His intelligence and ability
gave him the chance to make sure they were pleased. Alice Miller (1979/1997)
described in her book *The Drama of a Gifted Child* a person who, from early on
in childhood, develops a false self in taking care of the needs and wants of his
parents. It is not unusual for an emotionally gifted child or teenager to hide a
homosexual orientation from his or her parents in order to protect the relation-

---

TABLE 12–2.   DSM-IV-TR diagnostic criteria for panic disorder without agoraphobia

---

A.   Both (1) and (2):

    (1)   recurrent unexpected panic attacks

    (2)   at least one of the attacks has been followed by 1 month (or more) of one (or more) of the following:

        (a)   persistent concern about having additional attacks

        (b)   worry about the implications of the attack or its consequences (e.g., losing control, having a heart attack, "going crazy")

        (c)   a significant change in behavior related to the attacks

B.   Absence of agoraphobia

C.   The panic attacks are not due to the direct physiological effects of a substance (e.g., a drug of abuse, a medication) or a general medical condition (e.g., hyperthyroidism).

D.   The panic attacks are not better accounted for by another mental disorder, such as social phobia (e.g., occurring on exposure to feared social situations), specific phobia (e.g., on exposure to a specific phobic situation), obsessive-compulsive disorder (e.g., on exposure to dirt in someone with an obsession about contamination), posttraumatic stress disorder (e.g., in response to stimuli associated with a severe stressor), or separation anxiety disorder (e.g., in response to being away from home or close relatives).

Source.   Reprinted from *Diagnostic and Statistical Manual of Mental Disorders,* 4th Edition, Text Revision. Washington, DC, American Psychiatric Association, 2000. Used with permission. Copyright © 2000 American Psychiatric Association.

ship with them. Many gay and lesbian youths grow up in homes where their sexual orientation may not have been accepted by their family, religion, or culture. Clark was no different. Not only did he spend a considerable amount of energy keeping his family unaware of his homosexuality, but he likely spent the majority of his life planning activities to please his parents. This is the creation of a false self, an identity aligned with who his parents and the world want him to be. The true self is the person Clark really is. His true identity in regard to his sexual orientation was buried in his psyche for many years. Only when he was confronted through flirtation did the pieces of his true self start to emerge, but due to his suppression of it, it came out, literally, in the form of panic.

    Panic disorder can be treated with medication or psychotherapy. Medication is usually in the form of antidepressants at higher dosages. Psychotherapy can be cognitive-behavioral or psychodynamic. A defining characteristic of panic disorder is that the attacks come out of nowhere. They seem to be unprovoked. This is a distinction that is not agreed upon by all, and there have been studies to show that with enough history, a stimulus to the panic can usually be identified (Bush et al. 1999). Clark is an example of this.

A general psychiatric evaluation done in a clinic setting would hardly yield time for an extensive psychological and social history. An in-depth interview on more than one occasion would be needed to distinguish the source, should be there one, of panic.

From a dynamic perspective, it would be assumed that there are preceding thoughts that lead to increased anxiety and ultimately panic. Meeting a patient with panic symptoms on a regular basis for support and exploration would likely yield better results than medication alone. If a patient's assessment indicates exploratory work is appropriate, dynamic therapy could be a treatment modality. Allowing emotions to emerge and become conscious is a hallmark of dynamic treatments and would benefit those who may not know their true self by identifying those thoughts through interpretation, uncovering, and processing in a supportive way.

Gay and lesbian patients dealing with the anxiety of coming out, or of accepting their sexual orientation generally, might have other psychiatric symptoms. These could range from substance abuse to severe anxiety, and even paranoia and psychosis under large amounts of stress. Psychodynamic therapy is meant for patients who are more stable and functioning. Unless carefully managed, the uncovering process that takes place can add to a patient's level of anxiety and worsen symptoms.

Treatment course: As mentioned, once Clark arrived at my door, he had been stable on medication for several years. He continued to experience mild social anxiety but was without any episodes of panic. He hoped to stop his medication but was afraid that his panic symptoms would reemerge. I started to see Clark weekly in supportive psychotherapy. This slowly progressed to a more dynamic form of therapy as Clark became aware of his true identity and self. The hallmark of my treatment with Clark was allowing him to show that self. Allowing him to identify and discuss his true interests, ideas, and desires helped him visualize the authentic Clark.

He started to progress in therapy, as demonstrated by changes in his behavior. He was able to choose activities he enjoyed that did not necessarily lead to furthering his career. He started to openly disagree with me about topics and label his beliefs as just as valuable as my own. Clark resumed his old hobby of sailing, and he disclosed his sexual orientation to his parents.

Clark's self-esteem had been underdeveloped, and his anxiety arose out of interactions with others. Exploration helped us identify that he was most anxious when he was in a room of others who might be judging him. One day during our session, he was discussing this anxiety and stated, "It's getting really old talking about this, ya know?" After that, he cried. The anxiety, rather than being a pervasive feeling outside his own awareness, was turning more into a topic of conversation. It was becoming ego-dystonic, and he was starting to improve.

Clark went on to become the surgeon his parents had hoped he would be. He also went on to identify as an out gay man. One who sails, just for fun.

Superman is a fictional character. Clark is a real person. The real person's public alter-ego as a superhero can be thought of as a false self. There are many views about how psychotherapy works, but it is clear that the effects of a supportive and understanding relationship can help heal a patient's anxiety. Successful and highly motivated people like Clark are typically more critical of themselves than others. They can have a strong sense of guilt and anxiety should they venture off the preplanned path that their parents, culture, and society has made for them. As clinicians, we can offer them treatment for that harsh superego. Positive regard and empathy with a patient such as Clark can help to soften the biggest critic he has: himself.

Key Points

- Panic attacks are defined in DSM-IV-TR as a cluster of physical symptoms that occur abruptly and usually without warning. They include increased heart rate, difficulty breathing, a choking sensation, paresthesias, depersonalization, derealization, sweating, tremors, and thinking one is about to die.

- Panic attacks become panic disorder when the person has recurring panic attacks and they change the person's behavior out of fear the attacks will happen again.

- Coming out as gay can be a stressful life event fraught with many emotions. It is during these times that many people can receive a range of diagnoses, from anxiety to personality disorders and even psychosis. It is important to take a thorough history and evaluate current life stressors that might be contributing to the patient's symptoms.

References

American Psychiatric Association: Diagnostic and Statistical Manual of Mental Disorders, 4th Edition, Text Revision. Washington, DC, American Psychiatric Association, 2000

Bush FN, Milrod BL, Singer MB: Theory and technique in psychodynamic treatment of panic disorder. J Psychother Pract Res 8:234–242, 1999

Kempf EJ: Psychopathology. St. Louis, MO, Mosby, 1920

Miller A: Drama of a Gifted Child: The Search for the True Self [1979], 3rd Edition, Revised. New York, Basic Books, 1997

Questions

12.1   Lois is a 19-year-old female with no psychiatric history who presents to an outpatient psychiatry clinic with symptoms of anxiety, depressed mood, and transient moments of rage. Yesterday she had her first panic attack after breaking up with the young man she was dating. Although he was seen as an ideal boyfriend by her parents, Lois found herself more attracted to a classmate named Diana. What would be the best line of treatment initially?

   A. Start Lois on a low dose of a selective serotonin reuptake inhibitor and follow up in 1 month.
   B. Provide supportive and gay-affirmative therapy for several sessions weekly. Evaluate the need for medication on an ongoing basis.
   C. Refer to a specialized dialectical behavioral therapy clinic.
   D. Call in Lois's parents for a private session to discuss their daughter's sexual orientation.

   The correct answer is B.

   Giving Lois the freedom to explore her feelings and sexuality is the more supportive and less invasive initial treatment. Her anxiety symptoms may be due to family stressors or fears that she might be gay.

12.2   Jimmy is a 24-year-old gay man with a prior history of panic disorder without agoraphobia whom you have been seeing in weekly psychotherapy and medication management. He has been working on coming out and has slowly built a support network and started to date other men. He is anxious about telling his parents and fears they will be very upset because of their religious views. What stance should you take?

   A. Jimmy should tell his parents he is gay as soon as possible. The longer he waits, the worse it will be.
   B. Jimmy should never tell his parents, out of respect for their culture and religion.
   C. Coming out is an ongoing process. It is difficult to know when would be the right time for Jimmy to tell his parents. Explore Jimmy's anxiety about telling his parents and advise him to approach them when he feels ready.
   D. Increase Jimmy's medication dosage. It is clearly not high enough to control his anxiety.

The correct answer is C.

There are no definite answers about when and to whom people should out themselves. Providing a supportive environment in which Jimmy can reach these milestones in his own time would be the best treatment.

12.3 Perry is an 18-year-old male referred to you from inpatient psychiatry. He has received a diagnosis of schizophrenia, paranoid type, and was stabilized on intramuscular medications. Perry also reported to the inpatient doctors that he has recently discovered he is homosexual because of looks he's been receiving from men on the street. A panic attack actually brought him in to the emergency room after he says one of these men tried to seduce him. What treatment is best indicated for Perry?

A. Continue the intramuscular medication and start supportive psychotherapy with Perry. His sexual orientation is unclear and may or may not be related to his paranoid symptoms. Further exploration is needed once he stabilizes.
B. Start twice-weekly psychodynamic psychotherapy to uncover what unconscious processes may be causing his panic attacks.
C. The homosexual thoughts are clearly psychotic symptoms. Perry needs more medication treatment to relieve him of these symptoms.
D. Stop Perry's medication. He's been given the wrong diagnosis and is having trouble accepting his homosexuality. He needs gay affirmative therapy, not antipsychotics.

The correct answer is A.

During a psychotic state is no time to do intense exploratory work. Before an individual can delve into his or her sexual feelings, it is important to be relatively stable and well supported.

Obsessive-Compulsive Disorder

Homosexual and Pedophilic Obsessions in a 25-Year-Old Male

Stephan Carlson, M.D.

THIS IS THE CASE of a 25-year-old male who began experiencing symptoms of obsessive-compulsive disorder (OCD) that focused primarily on homosexual, pedophilic, and aggressive obsessions. This case illustrates the clinical nuances of the psychotherapy and medication management with a young man with OCD. Without a clear understanding of the phenomenology of OCD, the case may easily be confused with some lesbian, gay, bisexual, and transgender (LGBT) people's normal developmental struggle during the "coming out" process. This patient's intrusive aggressive thoughts and sexual thoughts of children also must be carefully differentiated from those of violent and sexual offenders. The differential diagnosis, etiology, prevalence, risk assessment, and treatment are explored. The DSM-IV-TR criteria for OCD (American Psychiatric Association 2000) are shown in Table 13–1.

Case Example: Chris

Chris was a 25-year-old white male who presented to my outpatient private practice in Manhattan (accompanied by his mother, who remained in the waiting room) with the chief complaint of depressed mood, anxiety, and insomnia. He was concerned because he was beginning to have trouble at work due to missed days. He reported that he was socially isolated on the weekends, refusing to go out with

TABLE 13–1.   DSM-IV-TR diagnostic criteria for obsessive-compulsive disorder

A.   Either obsessions or compulsions:

Obsessions as defined by (1), (2), (3), and (4):

   (1)   recurrent and persistent thoughts, impulses, or images that are experienced, at some time during the disturbance, as intrusive and inappropriate and that cause marked anxiety or distress

   (2)   the thoughts, impulses, or images are not simply excessive worries about real-life problems

   (3)   the person attempts to ignore or suppress such thoughts, impulses, or images, or to neutralize them with some other thought or action

   (4)   the person recognizes that the obsessional thoughts, impulses, or images are a product of his or her own mind (not imposed from without as in thought insertion)

Compulsions as defined by (1) and (2):

   (1)   repetitive behaviors (e.g., hand washing, ordering, checking) or mental acts (e.g., praying, counting, repeating words silently) that the person feels driven to perform in response to an obsession, or according to rules that must be applied rigidly

   (2)   the behaviors or mental acts are aimed at preventing or reducing distress or preventing some dreaded event or situation; however, these behaviors or mental acts either are not connected in a realistic way with what they are designed to neutralize or prevent or are clearly excessive

B.   At some point during the course of the disorder, the person has recognized that the obsessions or compulsions are excessive or unreasonable.   **Note:** This does not apply to children.

C.   The obsessions or compulsions cause marked distress, are time consuming (take more than 1 hour a day), or significantly interfere with the person's normal routine, occupational (or academic) functioning, or usual social activities or relationships.

D.   If another Axis I disorder is present, the content of the obsessions or compulsions is not restricted to it (e.g., preoccupation with food in the presence of an eating disorder; hair pulling in the presence of trichotillomania; concern with appearance in the presence of body dysmorphic disorder; preoccupation with drugs in the presence of a substance use disorder; preoccupation with having a serious illness in the presence of hypochondriasis; preoccupation with sexual urges or fantasies in the presence of a paraphilia; or guilty ruminations in the presence of major depressive disorder).

E.   The disturbance is not due to the direct physiological effects of a substance (e.g., a drug of abuse, a medication) or a general medical condition.

Specify if:

   With poor insight: if, for most of the time during the current episode, the person does not recognize that the obsessions and compulsions are excessive or unreasonable

Source.   Reprinted from *Diagnostic and Statistical Manual of Mental Disorders,* 4th Edition, Text Revision. Washington, DC, American Psychiatric Association, 2000. Used with permission. Copyright © 2000 American Psychiatric Association.

friends or family. Most troublesome to him were difficulty in sleeping through the night and early-morning awakening. He lost interest in life, and over the last 6 months he became withdrawn, his appetite decreased, and he became more dependent on his parents. He reported no perceptual disturbances or suicidal thoughts. He displayed no manic symptoms. He denied a sexual abuse history. His psychiatric family history was significant for anxiety on his mother's side.

After Chris became more at ease, he reported that he believed the cause of his anxiety, insomnia, and depressive symptoms was his increasingly recurrent, disturbing, and undesired thoughts of wanting to have sex with other men and to sexually touch children. He was concerned that he was "going crazy" and feared he was homosexual. Generally and even irrespective of the sexual thoughts, he feared that he was immoral and "not right with God." His corresponding compulsions included frequent requests for reassurance and avoidance of social contact. He also reported that he was disturbed by unacceptable thoughts of harming his mother and sister with a knife. This he could not understand because he loved them both. He said that he had told his mother about his violent thoughts but could not bear to tell her about his sexual thoughts. He denied ever having acted on these sexual or violent thoughts or ever wanting them to become reality.

Chris denied thoughts of being contaminated or needing to have orderliness and the corresponding compulsions of excessive washing and arranging. He denied any tendencies to hoard.

He had a past medical history of a hidden penis and obesity. He denied a history of traumatic brain injury.

A detailed sexual history was conducted. He denied ever having had sex with women. He attributed this to the embarrassment of his hidden penis. He saw a urologist once who recommended surgery, but he did not follow through because of expense of the elective procedure. He reported occasionally having sexual fantasies of women and becoming sexually aroused by them but said he was usually not very sexual. He denied sexual fantasies for men or children and denied becoming sexually aroused by them. He said that he had attempted to reassure himself that he was not gay and struggled daily with stopping the "homosexual" and "pedophile" thoughts and images.

After conducting the interview, I administered the Yale-Brown Obsessive Compulsive Scale (Y-BOCS) Symptom Checklist (Y-BOCS-SC) to gather information on specific current OCD symptoms. Using the 10-item Y-BOCS rating scale, I then obtained his baseline severity score and subsequently administered this scale at each appointment to measure response to treatment over time. I recommended fluoxetine 20 mg/day initially and titrated this to 80 mg/day over 12 weeks to target his depressed mood and obsessions. Risperidone 0.5 mg at bedtime was added to provide more immediate relief of his anxiety and to aid with sleep. I also recommended cognitive-behavioral therapy with graded exposure and response therapy, which he initially refused but later consented to when he had not received the response he was hoping to achieve.

Over the next 3 months he reported slow improvement in his mood to near baseline. After 3 months also, he agreed to cognitive-behavioral therapy. Within 5 months of commencing the treatment, his repetitive, unwanted thoughts that he was homosexual, a pedophile, and inflicting harm on his sister and mother decreased significantly.

Discussion

Establishing Rapport

The first goal of the treatment was to establish rapport in order to reduce Chris's distress and provide an accurate diagnosis. Chris had fears that he may be homosexual, a pedophile, and a violent person, and he sought reassurance from the treatment. His daily life had become severely impaired. The first step in the assessment phase was to be nonjudgmental so that he would be open about his symptoms and experience. I also was careful not to provide false reassurance—an important consideration in any therapy, but especially so in suspected cases of OCD. For Chris, for example, seeking reassurance was part and parcel of his ritualistic compulsions with his family.

Gay or OCD?

Obsessions about sexual orientation or homosexual obsessions are probably the most misunderstood symptoms for OCD patients, family members, and clinicians alike. Of course, some patients who are homosexual may present to therapy with ambivalence about their sexual orientation, and likewise, homosexual persons may have OCD. In Chris's case, he seemed motivated to seek help to stop the homosexual thoughts rather than to become comfortable with the thoughts. In a study of 485 adults seeking treatment for OCD, 9.9% endorsed past or present obsessions related to homosexuality (Pinto et al. 2008). Chris reported that these homosexual thoughts were inconsistent with his lifestyle, his family's values, and his own desires. This left us in a gray area, as internalized homophobia from societal experience can lower acceptance of one's feelings and thoughts and has been associated with depression and suicide. It was also somewhat confusing because he had only dated a few women for brief periods, but he stated that he hoped one day to be married and have children. His fantasy life had been filled with thoughts of sexual acts with women until the past 2 years, when he began having these intrusive homosexual thoughts. He admitted to a possible form of checking compulsion—watching gay pornography to test the validity of these thoughts. This was not pleasant to him and did not result in the same level of sexual excitement as he had with heterosexual pornography; however, he did not find it entirely repulsive either.

He reported that over the past 2 years he had begun having homosexual thoughts that engendered shame and guilt in addition to anxiety and depression. The obsessions in OCD may have the same content as thoughts of an LGBT person struggling with his or her sexuality; however, in the case of OCD there is usually more sense of the thoughts being unacceptable or ego-dystonic, as was the case with Chris. Some therapists might have the misguided impulse to dismiss the fears by reassuring the patient that the thoughts may be evidence of gay tendencies and that perhaps he should explore this side of himself or, on the opposite end of the spectrum, that this is a form of "latent homosexuality" that can be corrected by reparative therapy. Chris gained some insight into his obsessions from the evaluation, although he continued to have doubts and to think that he may be homosexual.

Sexual obsessions such as those exhibited by Chris are different in quality from other forms of sexual ideation. This will be more clearly illustrated in the section regarding his sexual thoughts of children. Both Chris's homosexual and his child-related obsessions are unwanted thoughts, images, or impulses that make him anxious or distressed when they enter his mind. They are also usually accompanied by other nonsexual OCD symptoms, such as his thoughts of wanting to harm his mother and sister.

Pedophile or OCD?

Much more intrusive and perverse to Chris than his thoughts about homosexuality were his thoughts of having sex with children. A paraphilia such as pedophilia is in the differential diagnosis and should be taken into consideration in the risk assessment. A key initial difference in the assessment is that pedophiles would rarely voluntarily seek treatment to stop the thoughts. Chris reported that he lived with his mother, his sister, and his sister's 6-year-old daughter. His anxiety came from the fear that he might harm his niece. Although he had previously loved to play with her and enjoyed her company, he now avoided her. Together we explored why it was unlikely he is a pedophile. While no single fact could differentiate pedophilia from OCD, he wanted to suppress these thoughts and he avoided being near his niece or any other children. A pedophile would more commonly look for places where children congregate and attempt to be alone with them. Further, these thoughts were not pleasurable to him and he did not want to act on them. Finally, he had other types of obsessions, which helped differentiate the diagnosis as OCD. Any confusion of these symptoms in the treatment with pedophilia would be potentially harmful and counterproductive. I advised Chris to not avoid his niece, as this would only strengthen his OCD symptoms.

Potentially Violent Offender or OCD and Loving Son?

Similar to the sexual obsessions, which were differentiated from other forms of sexual ideation, Chris's intrusive violent images of stabbing his mother and sister needed to be assessed and differentiated from homicidal ideation. Having explored the homosexual and pedophilic obsessions, we now explored the same factors—namely, the absence of past episodes of violence, the ego-dystonicity of the thoughts, his avoidance of handling sharp objects, the high distress, and the sincere motivation to stop these thoughts and get help.

Making the Diagnosis and Initiating Treatment

Chris was 23 when the onset of these reported symptoms began—slightly older than the average 19.5 years age estimate according to The National Comorbidity Survey Replication (Ruscio et al. 2010). The Y-BOCS-SC is an easy way to determine the presence of all major OCD symptoms (Goodman et al. 1989). It can be used clinically also in diagnosing the sexual obsessions that Chris was experiencing. Chris was highly reluctant to discuss these symptoms as well as the aggressive thoughts of wanting to stab his mother and sister. Chris displayed a well-known association of the so-called taboo obsessions (religious, aggressive, and sexual) that cluster together in OCD patients. Often sexual obsessions are less likely to be disclosed to clinicians than other types. Consequently, the prevalence of sexual obsessions found among subjects with OCD has ranged from 6% to 24.9% (Foa et al. 1995; Grant et al. 2006).

After our initial evaluation, I met with Chris's mother to assist in the diagnostic evaluation, round out the risk assessment, and educate the family about the diagnosis of OCD. Chris agreed to discuss all of his symptoms with his mother, which I viewed as favoring a good prognosis. Chris's mother reported that Chris was a gentle, loving person who had never had a significant romantic relationship. I explained to her that there were effective treatments for these disturbing thoughts that were robbing Chris of his young adulthood. I also assured her that a person with OCD is at no greater risk of acting on these repugnant thoughts than anyone else. I informed them both that Chris meets the DSM-IV-TR (American Psychiatric Association 2000) criteria for the Axis I diagnoses of obsessive-compulsive disorder (see Table 13–1) and major depressive disorder (see Table 9–1 in Chapter 9, "Major Depressive Disorder"). Unlike other OCD variants, there is a statistically higher correlation of depressive symptoms in OCD with sexual obsessions, as represented in this case by his comorbid major depressive disorder.

The U.S. Food and Drug Administration (FDA) has approved several selective serotonin reuptake inhibitors (SSRIs), such as fluoxetine, fluvoxamine, paroxetine, and sertraline, as well as the tricyclic antidepressant clomipramine, for treatment of OCD. I recommended fluoxetine because of my personal comfort level with this medication and the patient's reference. The dose was titrated to 80 mg/day, as higher dosages even above the manufacturer's recommendations are sometimes necessary in OCD (Tollefson et al. 1994). Risperidone was chosen as an augmentation agent to attempt to decrease the time to resolution (McDougle et al. 2000).

Unfortunately, sexual obsessions are more resistant to treatment than non-sexual obsessions (Alonso et al. 2001). Unwanted homosexual or pedophilic images and impulses such as those seen in Chris are two subsets of sexual obsessions that can be particularly disturbing because of the stigma and potential consequences of these thoughts becoming reality. The treatment remains similar, beginning with an assessment of the frequency, duration, and intrusiveness of the obsessions. It is best to avoid examining the meaning of the obsessions and just label them as unwanted and part of the OCD. The next step, paradoxically, is not to attempt to suppress them but rather curiously notice them when they arise.

Psychotherapy

Exposure and ritual prevention (ERP), a form of cognitive-behavioral therapy, is the psychotherapy treatment of choice in OCD (Abramowitz 1998). During ERP, the patient is repeatedly exposed to a disturbing obsession, initially by speaking about it in therapy and later by being exposed to actual triggers, while being prevented from engaging in any compulsions to reduce the anxiety. In Chris's case, I met with him weekly to monitor his medication and to implement ERP. After a few months, I encouraged him to view gay magazines and movies and walk in gay neighborhoods to expose him to homosexual cues. In terms of the pedophilic obsessions, I encouraged him to frequently engage in play with his niece. He was asked to notice that both types of sexual obsessions occur much like a wave—that after peaking initially, the obsession and the ensuing anxiety eventually subside. Chris's task was to accept any sensations from these experiences and discuss them in therapy. The habituation decreased his anxiety on its own and led him not to rely on compulsions to manage the obsession. Interestingly, the frequency of the obsession generally decreases in response to the reduced distress. This was Chris's experience, especially for the unacceptable thoughts of touching children sexually.

ERP in combination with the fluoxetine led to a marked reduction in the frequency and intensity of anxiety of the sexual and aggressive obsessions. The aggressive obsessions, surprisingly, extinguished first. The sexual obsessions were never completely extinguished, but Chris learned to manage them much better. His work performance improved, and he was able to function more normally around his niece and other children. Chris's lack of sexual experiences and his struggles with his hidden penis contributed to his continuing doubts about his sexual orientation.

Key Points

- Sexual obsessions in OCD have common themes that must be differentiated from other lifestyle choices and deviant behaviors. These themes include homosexuality/

sexual identity, sexual abuse, sexual thoughts about friends, incest, infidelity, sexual perversions, sex with animals, violent sexual behavior, and blasphemous thoughts combining religion and sex.

- Sexually intrusive thoughts are very common in OCD. As many as 25% of OCD patients have a history of sexual obsessions. These numbers may be underestimated because the stigma associated with sexual obsessions may cause individuals to avoid reporting them.

- Sexual obsessions are treated in the same way as other obsessions: with SSRIs, cognitive-behavioral psychotherapy, or some combination of these. Exposure and response prevention therapy may be particularly important for treating sexual obsessions.

References

Abramowitz JS: Does cognitive-behavioral therapy cure obsessive-compulsive disorder? A meta-analytic evaluation of clinical significance. Behav Ther 29:339–355, 1998

Alonso P, Menchon JM, Pifarre J, et al: Long-term follow-up and predictors of clinical outcome in obsessive-compulsive patients treated with serotonin reuptake inhibitors and behavioral therapy. J Clin Psychiatry 62:535–540, 2001

American Psychiatric Association: Diagnostic and Statistical Manual of Mental Disorders, 4th Edition, Text Revision. Washington, DC, American Psychiatric Association, 2000

Foa EB, Kozak MJ, Goodman WK, et al: DSM-IV field trial: obsessive-compulsive disorder. Am J Psychiatry 152:90–96, 1995

Goodman WK, Price LH, Rasmussen SA, et al: The Yale-Brown Obsessive-Compulsive Scale. Arch Gen Psychiatry 46:1006–1016, 1989

Grant JE, Pinto A, Gunnip M, et al: Sexual obsessions and clinical correlates in adults with obsessive-compulsive disorder. Compr Psychiatry 47:325–329, 2006

McDougle CJ, Epperson CN, Pelton GH, et al: A double-blind, placebo-controlled study of risperidone addition in serotonin reuptake inhibitor refractory obsessive-compulsive disorder. Arch Gen Psychiatry 57:794–801, 2000

Pinto A, Greenberg BD, Grados MA, et al: Further development of YBOCS dimensions in the OCD Collaborative Genetics study: symptoms vs. categories. Psychiatry Res 160:83–93, 2008

Ruscio AM, Chiu WT, Stein DJ, et al: The epidemiology of obsessive-compulsive disorder in the National Comorbidity Survey Replication. Mol Psychiatry 15:53–63, 2010

Tollefson GD, Rampey AH Jr, Potvin JH, et al: A multicenter investigation of fixed-dose fluoxetine in the treatment of obsessive-compulsive disorder. Arch Gen Psychiatry 51:559–567, 1994

Questions

13.1 What factors suggest OCD with pedophilic obsessions over a primary diagnosis of pedophilia?

A. The presence of ego-dystonic thoughts.
B. Motivation to seek treatment.
C. No past behavior consistent with the sexual thoughts.
D. All of the above.

The correct answer is D.

All of the above factors differentiate pedophilic obsessions in OCD from a pedophile. Unlike pedophiles, patients with OCD find their obsessions to be outside themselves or unwanted, not mere sexual fantasies. Patients with OCD also desperately want help. Pedophiles, in contrast, are sexually aroused by their sexual thoughts and usually do not seek help unless forced into treatment. Patients with OCD experiencing a sexual obsession do not want to experience these thoughts, find these thoughts extremely distressing, and do not want to act on them.

13.2 All of the following are *not* a part the treatment of sexual orientation obsessions in OCD except

A. Psychoanalysis.
B. Reparative therapy.
C. Existential therapy.
D. Exposure and ritual prevention therapy.

The correct answer is D.

ERP is the treatment of choice for all types of obsessions and compulsions in OCD. Although often intuitively appealing, psychoanalytic theories of OCD lost favor in the latter part of the twentieth century. Psychoanalytic concepts do little to improve understanding of the underlying processes of OCD and have not led to reliably effective treatments. Reparative therapy is repudiated by the American Psychiatric Association and is aimed at changing sexual orientation, not altering obsessions. Existential therapy deals with an individual's confrontation with the givens of existence, such as death, freedom, responsibility, and isolation.

Posttraumatic Stress Disorder

Handle With Care

CHRISTOPHER A. MCINTOSH, M.D.

MANY, BUT NOT ALL, studies of self-identified lesbian, gay, bisexual, and transgender (LGBT) people identify higher rates of reported childhood physical or sexual abuse compared with heterosexual control subjects (Wilson and Widom 2010). Not all individuals who experience these types of abuse will go on to develop posttraumatic stress disorder (PTSD). Many will have no diagnosable mental disorder, whereas others may develop another anxiety disorder, a mood disorder, or a dissociative disorder. A great number that are seen in clinical situations will have addictions, personality disorders, or clinically significant personality traits (Allen 2001). Not infrequently, patients seen for PTSD from trauma in adulthood have had a history of childhood physical or sexual abuse.

The following case, which describes a patient with a history of physical and sexual abuse as a child, illustrates some of the issues commonly encountered when working with LGBT patients with PTSD.

Case Example: Blake

Blake is a 32-year-old single gay man who was referred for outpatient psychiatric treatment following a "nervous breakdown," consisting mainly of panic attacks, for which he sought help at a hospital emergency department. A bebop jazz musician, Blake had gone to school and had had some early career success in Germany, but a series of relationships with mentors and professional colleagues went sour and led him to abandon his adopted country and return to Canada, although not to a city in which he had lived before.

Blake knew few people in his new home city. He had, through some contacts, made a connection with a talent agent who specialized in jazz musicians and had met some of the other musicians this agent represented. Otherwise, he was rather socially isolated. At presentation, he acknowledged drinking three bottles of wine per week, down from his highest level of drinking of a bottle of vodka per day, but still significant. He left his apartment mostly for necessary errands, otherwise staying in, working on his music in his home studio, and caring for his cat. His parents grudgingly provided financial assistance when he was not making sufficient funds from his career, which was frequently. Although they never failed to eventually provide this support, it was often accompanied by guilt-trips and suggestions that he should leave music to get a "real job."

Personality factors: Blake presented as a bit of a touchy character. His descriptions of his early career success seemed both grandiose and insecure. He implored me to look at the stellar critical reviews of his performances that he had scanned to his website, so that I could verify "that I am who I say I am." He was hypersensitive to the possibility of being slighted, and I wondered privately how this had played out in previous relationships, whether personal, professional, or therapeutic. When asked about his tendency to be wary of close relationships, he offered the following explanation:

> BLAKE: I've spent my whole life building things up from the inside out. Why would I want to threaten that?
> THERAPIST: When you say that, do you mean you've built up your sense of self from the inside out?
> BLAKE: That's exactly what I mean.

Kohut (1971) observed that narcissistic personality disorder is frequently the result of parental empathic failure in childhood. As I later found out, Blake's childhood included not just empathic failure, but also outright denial by his parents of traumatic experiences. It makes sense that this background would lead him to be intensely desirous of close relationships for the validation that was lacking in early life, while simultaneously suspicious that intimacy would torpedo the fragile sense of self he had managed to pull together entirely on his own.

Blake's initial symptom presentation suggested panic disorder, alcohol abuse, and narcissistic personality traits as diagnoses. He was evaluated and thought to be suitable for long-term open-ended psychodynamic psychotherapy, starting at once per week. Medication interventions were deferred initially, as Blake took to heart my psychoeducation about the exacerbating effects of alcohol and wished to reduce his consumption before considering medication. In this early phase of treatment, we would focus on building the therapeutic relationship and assessing whether the alcohol issues could be managed with individual therapy alone or would require other interventions. When I asked Blake on intake about physical or sexual abuse, he initially denied any such history but then modified his answer to vaguely suggest that there had been abuse. It would take Blake another 6 months of therapy before he felt comfortable enough to disclose any more detail.

Safety and the Therapeutic Relationship

Safety and trust in the therapeutic relationship are essential elements of work with any patient with PTSD or, for that matter, any patient with a trauma history. The establishment of sufficient trust is an evolving process and may involve many factors. For some patients, the basic professional frame of therapy (the certified expertise of the therapist, the assurances of confidentiality) is sufficient. Many patients may require more, and usually this involves some version of "getting to know" the therapist. LGBT patients may be particularly interested in knowing the sexual orientation of the therapist.

> Blake had been referred to me with the understanding that I was a gay psychiatrist, but we had not explicitly discussed this until a few weeks into treatment, following a chance meeting with Blake on the street in the "gay neighborhood" in our city. Blake correctly perceived that I seemed awkward in our brief and superficial interaction, and on returning to his apartment he found himself wondering if the awkwardness was because I was a "closet case" caught hanging about the gay neighborhood. (The real source of the awkwardness was simply my own inexperience at that time with how to handle chance public meetings with patients.)

The issue of therapist self-disclosure in therapy has evolved since the original psychoanalytic notion of the "blank slate" analyst (which even Dr. Freud did not often follow in practice) (Cole and Drescher 2006). We reveal a lot about ourselves to observant patients before we say anything by our style of dress, how tidy our office is, and other cues. Most LGBT patients will attempt to discern their therapist's sexual orientation, with varying degrees of success. Many patients indicate that they feel it is important to have something in common with the therapist, whether this is sexual orientation, ethnocultural background, or hobbies and interests.

Two cautionary notes are necessary about self-disclosure. The first is the issue of boundaries. It is the therapist's responsibility to ensure that boundary crossings, such as occasional self-disclosure in the service of the development of a trusting therapeutic relationship, do not develop into boundary violations (Gabbard and Lester 1995).

A second caution about self-disclosure is that the patient's wish for a connection or sameness with the therapist might include a wish to bypass difficult conversations. With gay therapist–gay patient treatment dyads, this is something to keep in mind. It may be important for an LGBT patient to verbalize and properly process the experience of being a member of a sexual minority in an oppressive society and not gloss over this simply because "you must know what I mean."

Medication and Its Meaning

One day, about 6 months into the treatment phase of therapy, Blake was discussing how he had felt betrayed by his agent when a newspaper review of a group recital lauded a younger musician and gave Blake only a brief mention. He irrationally felt physically threatened by this agent, and when we explored why this might be, he disclosed that 15 years ago he had been severely assaulted by three thugs, who had put him in hospital with a skull fracture. He very nearly died from his injuries. He had always felt that his previous agent, an intensely jealous individual with whom Blake had had a relationship, had hired these thugs to punish Blake for leaving him.

"I think about it [the assault] all the time." He displayed significant psychomotor agitation as he talked about this. He also disclosed that this was not the only assault he had experienced. At this point the diagnosis was reevaluated, and he clearly met sufficient DSM-IV-TR criteria for PTSD, with prominent symptoms in each of the three clusters of reexperiencing, avoidance/numbing, and hyperarousal (Table 14–1) (American Psychiatric Association 2000).

Despite ongoing psychotherapy and significantly reduced alcohol use, Blake continued to experience symptoms of panic and PTSD. We therefore explored medication options. It is important to explore the meaning of medication with all patients, but particularly those with PTSD. Blake revealed two incidents that suggested medication management might be problematic. One was that he had been drugged by the assailant in his first adult trauma, a sexual assault by a bartender in a gay bar when he was 19. Second, when Blake had presented acutely distraught for psychiatric care following this incident, he had been misdiagnosed with schizophrenia and had been placed on a high dose of a typical antipsychotic. Because antidepressants are considered standard supportive psychopharmacology for PTSD, I prescribed the selective serotonin reuptake inhibitor (SSRI) sertraline, along with a short-term course of low-dose clonazepam. Blake tolerated the initial side effects of the SSRI, but when the usual antidepressant effects came in at 4 weeks, he wanted to discontinue the medication. While he did acknowledge feeling happier, it seemed somehow "false," and he felt "on edge" and agitated at the same time. He also experienced paresthesias and had difficulty attaining orgasm. Overall, the medication felt like "an agent of control." Blake was prescribed a single dose of fluoxetine to try to ensure minimal SSRI discontinuation symptoms, and the sertraline was stopped.

We eventually found through the course of the psychotherapy that short courses of either clonazepam or low-dose quetiapine were more helpful and acceptable to Blake than ongoing medication in getting through periods of increased agitation. Blake was amenable to taking these when needed, and he did not overuse them. He clearly felt his autonomy was more preserved by taking these medications, in which there was a more observable association between his swallowing the pill and the reduction of anxiety soon thereafter.

TABLE 14–1.   DSM-IV-TR diagnostic criteria for posttraumatic stress disorder

---

A.   The person has been exposed to a traumatic event in which both of the following were present:

   (1)   the person experienced, witnessed, or was confronted with an event or events that involved actual or threatened death or serious injury, or a threat to the physical integrity of self or others

   (2)   the person's response involved intense fear, helplessness, or horror.   **Note:** In children, this may be expressed instead by disorganized or agitated behavior

B.   The traumatic event is persistently reexperienced in one (or more) of the following ways:

   (1)   recurrent and intrusive distressing recollections of the event, including images, thoughts, or perceptions.   **Note:** In young children, repetitive play may occur in which themes or aspects of the trauma are expressed.

   (2)   recurrent distressing dreams of the event.   **Note:** In children, there may be frightening dreams without recognizable content.

   (3)   acting or feeling as if the traumatic event were recurring (includes a sense of reliving the experience, illusions, hallucinations, and dissociative flashback episodes, including those that occur on awakening or when intoxicated).   **Note:** In young children, trauma-specific reenactment may occur.

   (4)   intense psychological distress at exposure to internal or external cues that symbolize or resemble an aspect of the traumatic event

   (5)   physiological reactivity on exposure to internal or external cues that symbolize or resemble an aspect of the traumatic event

C.   Persistent avoidance of stimuli associated with the trauma and numbing of general responsiveness (not present before the trauma), as indicated by three (or more) of the following:

   (1)   efforts to avoid thoughts, feelings, or conversations associated with the trauma

   (2)   efforts to avoid activities, places, or people that arouse recollections of the trauma

   (3)   inability to recall an important aspect of the trauma

   (4)   markedly diminished interest or participation in significant activities

   (5)   feeling of detachment or estrangement from others

   (6)   restricted range of affect (e.g., unable to have loving feelings)

   (7)   sense of a foreshortened future (e.g., does not expect to have a career, marriage, children, or a normal life span)

D.   Persistent symptoms of increased arousal (not present before the trauma), as indicated by two (or more) of the following:

   (1)   difficulty falling or staying asleep

   (2)   irritability or outbursts of anger

TABLE 14–1. DSM-IV-TR diagnostic criteria for posttraumatic stress disorder *(continued)*

<table>
<tr><td></td><td>(3)</td><td>difficulty concentrating</td></tr>
<tr><td></td><td>(4)</td><td>hypervigilance</td></tr>
<tr><td></td><td>(5)</td><td>exaggerated startle response</td></tr>
<tr><td>E.</td><td colspan="2">Duration of the disturbance (symptoms in Criteria B, C, and D) is more than 1 month.</td></tr>
<tr><td>F.</td><td colspan="2">The disturbance causes clinically significant distress or impairment in social, occupational, or other important areas of functioning.</td></tr>
</table>

Specify if:

    Acute: if duration of symptoms is less than 3 months

    Chronic: if duration of symptoms is 3 months or more

Specify if:

    With delayed onset: if onset of symptoms is at least 6 months after the stressor

Source. Reprinted from *Diagnostic and Statistical Manual of Mental Disorders,* 4th Edition, Text Revision. Washington, DC, American Psychiatric Association, 2000. Used with permission. Copyright © 2000 American Psychiatric Association.

By contrast, the concept of him emerging a changed, happier person after 4 weeks on an SSRI seemed false and anxiety provoking. Who would this shinier, happier person be? Would he be a person Blake recognized as "me," or a compliant false self (Winnicott 1965/1990) that would be society's or his parents' (or his therapist's) idea of who he should be? Blake prided himself on having survived thus far by building himself up from the "inside out."

This idea that antidepressant medications "change your personality" may be of particular concern for LGBT patients who are more queer-identified, that is, those who value their status as people living outside of mainstream life and culture. This group of individuals may experience medication as "an agent of control" as Blake did, or an attempt to tame or subjugate the wildness within them. It is advisable here to listen to patients' concerns and to properly educate patients about what antidepressants do and do not do: that they improve symptoms of anxiety and depression but are unlikely, in and of themselves, to change ingrained personality characteristics.

Substance Abuse

A wish for autonomy in controlling one's psychiatric symptoms may explain why so many people with PTSD self-medicate with drugs and alcohol. This had certainly been the case for Blake earlier in life and earlier in his treatment with me. A clinician needs to determine the severity and stage of treatment of any substance abuse disorder prior to engaging in active psychotherapeutic processing of trauma. The therapist should be able to reasonably expect that the patient will not abuse drugs or alcohol after a particularly difficult session or, if a relapse does occur, that a plan has been made to quickly recover from it. A crisis plan for potential substance relapse or return of psychiatric symptoms may include attending an Alcoholics Anonymous meeting, calling a sponsor, reaching out to supportive friends or family, or coming to the emergency department if suicidal thoughts become prominent.

Proceeding With Therapy

Establishing safety in the therapeutic alliance and stabilization with interventions to address substance abuse and other Axis I comorbid disorders are elements of the first of three phases in treatment of PTSD (Herman 1991). The first, stabilizing, stage also includes developing coping strategies and healthy self-soothing skills. This first phase is necessary because the second phase has the potential to be destabilizing, as traumatic events and their impact are examined and a coherent narrative of the experiences is constructed. The third phase involves reconnecting with the world and with important relationships.

The establishment of a strong therapeutic alliance in the first phase pays off in the second phase when inevitable therapeutic ruptures occur. If the alliance is on solid ground, then recovery is possible from such ruptures and strong feelings can be expressed safely by the patient.

> About one year after starting therapy, Blake felt he had developed enough trust in me and in the process to be able to talk about his experiences of physical and sexual abuse in childhood. One significant challenge in reaching this point was the anger he felt. I wondered if, having made a connection with me, he was worried about the anger damaging our relationship:
>
> > BLAKE: I feel this rage when I come closer to talking about it!
> > THERAPIST: Do you feel at times that your rage might hurt me?
> > BLAKE (*looks quizzical*): No. You mean, like I'll explode or something?
> > (*shakes head dismissively*)
> > THERAPIST: Some people could think that.
> > BLAKE (*looks thoughtful*): Yeah, I could see that.
>
> Whether or not any part of Blake was consciously concerned about this, exploring the issue seemed to help, and Blake was able to open up at the next session.
> The sexual abuse was perpetrated by a male member of his extended family, and when Blake told his parents, the entire incident was hushed up and Blake was simply told that the incident did not happen, that he must have been mistaken.

More denials happened when his father started to abuse Blake physically and verbally while intoxicated on alcohol. The reality of these events was simply denied by his mother and father the next day. As Blake came to realize that he was gay in adolescence, he resolutely refused to engage in their attempts to similarly deny this, and he became openly gay at a much earlier age than he might have otherwise. Although this led, in some respects, to worse verbal abuse from his intoxicated father, who now added "faggot" to his list of insults, his sexual orientation became a core reality that he could cling to in the midst of a reality-denying family environment.

The rocky therapeutic process at this stage of the work can be viewed psychodynamically as a reenactment of this early experience of denial/disbelief: Blake was extraordinarily sensitive to the language I used to clarify what he was saying as he disclosed more events in his trauma history. The process in this regard was exacerbated by Blake's (likely defensive) tendency to be vague in his descriptions. One session, I became confused as to whether an assault he was describing was a real past event or part of a nightmare, as both were being discussed. My poor choice of clarifying words—"Did that really happen?"—very nearly lead to a permanent treatment rupture. We worked through it, but Blake continued to describe feeling "like a performing monkey" whenever I would ask for more detail about events he recounted, even about current interpersonal encounters.

Reconnecting With the World

Blake was eventually able to do significant processing of the childhood and adult physical and sexual trauma in therapy, as well as explore the ways in which these childhood experiences informed how he managed adult relationships. Children who have been abused in childhood often develop what is called a disorganized attachment style (Main and Solomon 1986), a confused way of acting in intimate relationships that comes about because of conflicting impulses. An abused child has the instinct that all children have to seek protection from caregivers when threatened. However, in the case of abused children, these same caregivers were also the source of the danger, and the instinct to run away may be just as strong.

Blake's childhood abuse left him ill prepared to deal with the all-important life challenge of how to identify who is safe and who is a threat. As therapy progressed to the point where he was able to begin thinking about reconnecting with the world in a new way (the third phase of PTSD therapy), he had to learn a new coherent way of assessing threat and safety. His past practice of switching between irrational suspiciousness and blind trust gave way to a more reasonable balance of probabilities. This in turn led to a reduction of avoidance and hypervigilance symptoms.

Blake was able to consult a plastic surgeon about a decades-old scar that resulted from one of his past assaults and to have it surgically revised. He became more comfortable with developing professional relationships again and was then better able to promote his music career. He began dating and being sexually active again, and he found this very satisfying. He was on the way to living a new life, no longer in the shadow of past traumas.

Key Points

- Establishing safety in the therapeutic relationship is an essential part of therapeutic work with LGBT people with PTSD. There may be a role for carefully considered therapist self-disclosure of sexual orientation in this process.

- Medication management in PTSD is frequently a challenge, and it is important to support the patient's autonomy in this process. Queer-identified LGBT patients may be particularly concerned about psychiatric medication altering their personality in an undesirable way. It is important to remember that the primary intervention in PTSD is psychotherapeutic and that medication plays a supportive and stabilizing role.

- Treatment of substance use disorders or self-harm disorders is a high priority prior to engaging in an exploratory or exposure-based therapy for PTSD. LGBT-specific substance abuse treatment programs may increase the likelihood of this being successfully addressed.

References

Allen JG: Traumatic Relationships and Serious Mental Disorders. Chichester, UK, Wiley, 2001

American Psychiatric Association: Diagnostic and Statistical Manual of Mental Disorders, 4th Edition, Text Revision. Washington, DC, American Psychiatric Association, 2000

Cole GW, Drescher J: Do tell: queer perspectives on therapist self disclosure—introduction. Journal of Gay and Lesbian Psychotherapy 10: 1–6, 2006

Gabbard GO, Lester E: Boundaries and Boundary Violations in Psychoanalysis. New York, Basic Books, 1995

Herman JL: Trauma and Recovery. New York, Basic Books, 1991

Kohut H: The Analysis of the Self. Madison, CT, International Universities Press, 1971

Main M, Solomon J: Discovery of an insecure-disorganized/disoriented attachment pattern, in Affective Development in Infancy. Edited by Brazelton TB, Yogman MW. Westport, CT, Ablex Publishing, 1986, pp 95–124

Wilson HW, Widom CS: Does physical abuse, sexual abuse, or neglect in childhood increase the likelihood of same-sex sexual relationships and cohabitation? A prospective 30-year follow-up. Arch Sex Behav 39:63–74, 2010

Winnicott DW: The Maturational Process and the Facilitating Environment (1965). London, Karnac Books, 1990

Questions

14.1   Tomas is a 27-year-old American soldier dishonorably discharged from the military under the Don't Ask, Don't Tell policy of the armed forces. You are assessing him in the emergency department, where he has arrived intoxicated on alcohol and expressing suicidal ideation. In the course of the emergency assessment he discloses that he is having nightmares of a firefight his unit was involved with in Afghanistan, in which his good friend was killed and he feared for his own life. You do this:

   A. Advise him to go to a detoxification center, as nothing can be done for him until he addresses the alcohol issue.
   B. Immediately begin exploring details of his trauma.
   C. Admit him for observation, alcohol withdrawal treatment, and ongoing assessment of his suicidality, and connect him with alcohol treatment resources and an experienced trauma therapist with whom he can begin to make a therapeutic connection while he is addressing comorbid substance abuse.

   The correct answer is C.

   Current standards of treatment of concurrent psychiatric disorders and addictions specify that both should be addressed at the same time. In the above case, this would mean that Tomas can begin work on the first, stabilizing phase of PTSD therapy while he is also addressing the alcohol abuse, but work on the second phase (option B above) should not proceed until the addiction has been satisfactorily addressed.

14.2   Mary Jane is a 22-year-old university student whom you have been seeing for psychotherapy for PTSD secondary to a sexual assault. About 2 months into therapy she mentions that something you said in the last session led her to wonder if you were gay. You say:

   A. "Gay? What do you mean? Something I said last session? Are you saying I sound gay?"
   B. Nothing, and resolve to speak less in sessions so you don't contaminate the transference.

    C. "It sounds like you're wondering about my sexual orientation. Maybe we can talk about what it might mean to you if I was gay, or if I was straight?"

The correct answer is C.

Both A and B are defensive responses that do not contribute to building the therapeutic relationship. Additionally, the rationale behind option B is based on an unsophisticated notion of the concept of transference.

14.3   Kaspar is a 35-year-old bisexual artist with borderline personality disorder and PTSD whom you are assessing with regard to his suitability for trauma-related psychotherapy. When you suggest treatment with an antidepressant to reduce levels of anxiety, he refuses and instead asks for benzodiazepines. Possible reasons for this are:

    A. He is a substance abuser and is malingering symptoms in order to obtain the pills.

    B. His father, who abused him in childhood, was prescribed antidepressants and they didn't seem to work for him.

    C. He is concerned antidepressants will affect his ability to make good art.

    D. All of the above.

The correct answer is D.

There are many possible explanations, and one should not leap to assume option A but should explore with the patient the meaning of medication.

Generalized Anxiety Disorder

Jittery Joanne

KENNETH ASHLEY, M.D.
ANTHONY LUJACK, M.D., J.D., M.S.
AARON PATTERSON, M.D., M.B.A., M.A.

THE DIAGNOSIS OF generalized anxiety disorder (GAD) can be difficult in lesbian, gay, bisexual, and transgender (LGBT) persons, both because of variability in presentation and confounding comorbid psychiatric, substance use, and medical disorders. This chapter details the GAD diagnosis and treatment of Joanne, a transgender woman in her forties. It also serves to highlight some of the anxiety-provoking circumstances faced by persons with gender identity/ expression issues, as well persons with a homosexual orientation. Although the data are lacking in transgender populations, it is estimated that the prevalence of GAD is 10%–12% higher in LGB persons than in the general population (Drescher et al. 2008; Meyer 2003). Social stigmatization and isolation are often at the root of anxiety disorders in LGBT persons. Additionally, the absence of role models, the fact that rights of LGBT persons are often poorly defined within the law, and the discrimination faced by many LGBT persons can be factors that may exacerbate an underlying anxiety disorder. As with all persons diagnosed with GAD, depression is often a comorbid finding in LGBT persons.

Table 15–1 presents the DSM-IV-TR criteria for GAD (American Psychiatric Association 2000).

TABLE 15–1. DSM-IV-TR diagnostic criteria for generalized anxiety disorder

---

A. Excessive anxiety and worry (apprehensive expectation), occurring more days than not for at least 6 months, about a number of events or activities (such as work or school performance).

B. The person finds it difficult to control the worry.

C. The anxiety and worry are associated with three (or more) of the following six symptoms (with at least some symptoms present for more days than not for the past 6 months). **Note:** Only one item is required in children.

 (1) restlessness or feeling keyed up or on edge

 (2) being easily fatigued

 (3) difficulty concentrating or mind going blank

 (4) irritability

 (5) muscle tension

 (6) sleep disturbance (difficulty falling or staying asleep, or restless unsatisfying sleep)

D. The focus of the anxiety and worry is not confined to features of an Axis I disorder, e.g., the anxiety or worry is not about having a panic attack (as in panic disorder), being embarrassed in public (as in social phobia), being contaminated (as in obsessive-compulsive disorder), being away from home or close relatives (as in separation anxiety disorder), gaining weight (as in anorexia nervosa), having multiple physical complaints (as in somatization disorder), or having a serious illness (as in hypochondriasis), and the anxiety and worry do not occur exclusively during posttraumatic stress disorder.

E. The anxiety, worry, or physical symptoms cause clinically significant distress or impairment in social, occupational, or other important areas of functioning.

F. The disturbance is not due to the direct physiological effects of a substance (e.g., a drug of abuse, a medication) or a general medical condition (e.g., hyperthyroidism) and does not occur exclusively during a mood disorder, a psychotic disorder, or a pervasive developmental disorder.

Source. Reprinted from *Diagnostic and Statistical Manual of Mental Disorders,* 4th Edition, Text Revision. Washington, DC, American Psychiatric Association, 2000. Used with permission. Copyright © 2000 American Psychiatric Association.

Case Example: Joanne

Joanne, a 44-year-old attorney, had moved to New York from Los Angeles 1 year after having undergone sexual reassignment surgery (SRS) and transitioning from male to female. Joanne had undergone a dramatic upheaval in her life. Not only was she dealing with physical and hormonal changes in her new gender, but she was also struggling to develop a social network and identity in Los Angeles. Work had always been an area where Joanne felt accomplished and comfortable, but at her new job she felt unsteady, and with recent budget cuts, she was constantly concerned about being laid off. Joanne's presenting complaint was that she wasn't sleeping well. She felt tired at work and struggled to remain awake during meetings. Her boss had commented that she often seemed distracted.

Joanne was referred to me by one of her neighbors, an openly gay man whom one of us been treating for many years. At the first session, Joanne indicated that she still felt embarrassed and uncomfortable speaking about her sexual reassignment, even with health professionals. She said that she had avoided finding a new primary care doctor for that reason and, instead, had been traveling back to Los Angeles every 3 months for routine follow-up and prescriptions. Joanne was also extraordinarily concerned about privacy. She asked if notes would be taken or sessions recorded and who would or could have access to these notes or recordings. She also asked if her treating psychiatrist could reveal whether he had clients working at a number of large law firms that she then named individually. The treating psychiatrist told her that he would take occasional session notes and that while he could not reveal where his other clients worked, anything she said in their sessions would be kept confidential. She seemed only marginally reassured by this and said, "I don't mean to sound paranoid, but the legal community in New York is small, and people talk. I can't afford to lose this job because people think I'm wacko."

Joanne had come simply requesting something to help her sleep, but her anxiety was palpable. During her initial session she could not sit still; she was constantly fidgeting in the chair, checking her watch, and patting her hair to make sure it was in place. Her voice was strained and her laugh was nervous. Her psychomotor agitation was so pronounced that the treating psychiatrist wondered if she was perhaps in benzodiazepine or alcohol withdrawal. When asked about substance use, she denied regular use of anything other than the occasional glass of wine, but the possibility of substance abuse was something to consider during the first several months of treatment. Although Joanne had only intended to see the treating psychiatrist for medication management of her insomnia, he thought she would benefit from therapy sessions to discuss the radical changes going on in her life. With some reluctance, she ultimately agreed to see him biweekly.

History: Joanne described herself as "a worrier" beginning in early childhood. She remembered being acutely depressed at age 7 and praying to God that she would die in her sleep. At age 31, she developed self-described "panic attacks" related to work, and on several occasions she was unable to go into important meetings because she had a profound sense of dread. She also described two occasions when she became stranded in other cities on one-day business trips because on the outbound flight, she had had such a severe panic attack that she was unable to take the return flight until 2–3 days later. Joanne had never sought professional help for these prior episodes, and it was only when she began the process of applying for SRS that she began seeing a psychiatrist and a therapist on a regular basis. However, Joanne described her relationship with these professionals as "superficial" and indicated that she did not want to reveal the extent of her underlying anxiety because she did not want to say anything that would jeopardize her chances of having the reassignment surgery. One psychiatrist, with whom she had worked just prior to her surgery, indicated that he felt that Joanne had an underlying anxiety disorder. He prescribed sertraline, which

Joanne took for 1 week and then discontinued without informing him. "The Zoloft shot my anxiety level through the roof, I couldn't sleep, and I couldn't concentrate, so I stopped taking it."

Development of Joanne's gender identity/expression: Joanne (formerly Joe) had gender identity issues beginning in early childhood. She stated that she had known she was a female by the time she was 4 years old. In one of the first sessions, she showed a picture of herself as a little boy dressed up in her sister's cowgirl outfit at a birthday party. There were relatives in the picture smiling and obviously enjoying the spectacle of this little boy dressed up in his sister's clothes. Joanne describes this as the happy period of her childhood. This period came to an abrupt end at age 5 when Joe's father found him dressed in his older sister's First Communion dress, sitting in a wading pool in the front yard and blowing soap bubbles in front of neighborhood children. Sobbing, Joanne recalled how her father had grabbed her by the arm and dragged her into the house with all the neighbors watching. Once inside, he tore the dress off, bent him over his knee, and spanked him. After that, he marched Joe to his bedroom and forced him to put on boy clothes. He said, "You're too old to be acting like a sissy! You need to start acting like a boy! Now, you go back out and start playing with the other boys! If I see you crying anymore, I'll give you something to cry about!" With that, he opened the front door and pushed Joe outside, red-faced and humiliated in front of all of the neighborhood children. Joanne described this as the first of many times in her life when she felt physically and emotionally violated.

In that same session, Joanne recalled that after the beating by her father, she always felt nervous in his presence. She also had ongoing distrust of her mother and spoke of feeling "sold out" by her. That autumn she entered first grade in Catholic school and felt her skin crawl beneath the boy's uniform that she had to wear daily. She recalled feelings of rage when, the week before school began, her mother took her to a barber and her long sun-bleached hair was shaved into a crew cut. She remembers feeling so repelled by how she appeared physically that she was unable to concentrate in school. As a result, her grades dropped and the teacher requested a meeting with her parents to discuss Joe's being "slow." She remembered the disapproving looks from her parents and the shame she felt. For a few weeks, she was placed in a special class with other "slow" children until an astute young teacher recognized that her reading and math skills were actually advanced for her age.

While Catholic school was an awkward experience for Joanne, summers were equally disturbing because her parents forced her to join Little League and the Boy Scouts. Although Joanne never dared to put on her sister's clothes again, she remembers taking her sister's Brownie uniform into the bathroom sometimes as a child and holding it up against her body in the mirror. Joanne recounts living with the constant worry of her parents finding out that she was really a girl mistakenly placed in the body of a boy.

Joanne's first exposure to the mental health community came when one of the nuns at the school found Joanne, and her very effeminate friend Steven, listening to their Walkmans with their neckties wrapped around their foreheads, dancing and lip-syncing the words to "Xanadu," pretending to be Olivia Newton-John. After that, Joanne had several meetings with the school counselor, a priest, who had a degree in social work. Another meeting was held with her parents, and for several weeks there was discussion of sending Joanne to Texas the following summer to attend what she described as "a reprogramming camp for gay kids."

This was a major turning point for Joanne. "This was the episode that broke my spirit. After that, I just gave in and pretended to be the man everyone expected me to be. I went to college, went on to law school, landed a job at a great firm, and never let on to anyone that I was really a woman." During this time, Joanne developed friendships but describes them as mostly superficial. She also had casual sexual relationships with men, but stated that in bed she felt "turned off" by her own male genitalia. The only way she was capable of having sex was in the role of the receptive bottom with all of the lights turned off. For the most part, she denied her gender and sexuality, and the main focus of her life became her work as a highly paid corporate attorney. It was not until her mid-thirties that she started to seriously consider gender reassignment surgery.

Early treatment: Joanne fulfilled all the DSM-IV-TR criteria for GAD (American Psychiatric Association 2000). Patients with GAD have more than 6 months of symptoms present most days that impair social and occupational functioning and that consist of excessive and poorly controlled anxiety or worry paired with somatic symptoms such as insomnia, muscle tension, restlessness, fatigue, and poor concentration.

In her first session, Joanne described how 3 years earlier she lay on a stretcher in the preoperative waiting area with butterflies in her stomach. It was her 41st birthday, and she was about to undergo the SRS that would be the beginning of her new life—her real life as the woman she always knew she was. Yet 3 years later, Joanne found herself sitting in her psychiatrist's office feeling like she had knots in her stomach and complaining of insomnia and poor concentration at work. She looked miserable and anxious, a woman whose reality did not even approach the dreams and expectations she had held 3 years earlier while lying on that stretcher.

Joanne related that the surgery and rehabilitation had been painful, and she was still experiencing recurrent urinary tract infections. Her friends and family had been supportive in the beginning, but the interactions were always strained. Her mother had a hard time not crying when she saw Joanne, and sometimes she still called her Joe. She saw her college roommate a few weeks ago, and he admitted to her that while he was glad she was happy, "it freaked him out" to see and hear her "acting" like a woman. The transition was harder than she expected, and she felt ill prepared for what life was handing her now.

Joanne's anxiety created social impairment because she was now preoccupied with thoughts of how others perceived her. She didn't feel that she "passed" effectively as a woman, and she often found herself worrying about what other people might be saying about her. She was reluctant to enter a women's restroom if female coworkers were in there. Although no one had said anything to her directly, she perceived that some coworkers were staring at her disapprovingly. Her constant worry about how others perceived her prevented her from engaging others and making new friends. She had not been sexually active since her reassignment surgery, and she reported frequently worrying about what might happen if she would have sex with someone. Physically, she was now the woman she had always dreamed she would be, but emotionally, she was a woman at her wit's end. She worried about growing older and being alone, but she worried more about the negative reactions and rejection she might face in the social arena.

Joanne's occupational function was severely affected by her anxiety. After taking a 6-month leave from work, she decided to make a clean start and moved to New York. That too proved difficult. After years of earning six-figure salaries as a corporate attorney, she found herself making a fraction of that working for a small local firm. She had interviewed with a few large national firms, but their reactions to her were not inviting. They looked at her strangely, and she was not ready to explain the "blip" in her career that occurred when she took leave to have her SRS. She was often distracted at work, and she stated that she felt she was always "walking on eggshells" to keep her job.

In Joanne's first therapy session, she made it clear that she was not a "pill person" and was noted to perseverate about the potential side effects of medications she had never tried before. In this first session, trazodone was suggested to help her sleep, and it was only with considerable hesitation that she agreed to take it. On her next visit a week later, she said that it had worked wonderfully and that she had slept through the night for the first time that she could remember. However, she stopped taking it after the initial dose because she had spent hours reading about the potential side effects and had become focused on priapism and how that might somehow derange her sexual reassignment. No amount of medication education by her psychiatrist could resolve this concern for her.

Joanne openly admitted that her worry was excessive. Like many with GAD, she described a family history of anxiety. Her mother had always been a worrier and was fretting about something all the time. It bothered Joanne that she now found herself doing the same thing. She found it ironic that she now spent time worrying about worrying too much. Because of Joanne's reluctance to start medication, her sessions over the first 6 months were dedicated initially to supportive psychotherapy and later to more psychoanalytic therapy. Joanne had a lifetime of trauma to process, and until she was able to identify a few seminal events in her life, she was unable to move forward in any area of her life.

Long-term treatment: In months of psychodynamic sessions, Joanne revealed a pattern of psychological and physical traumas occurring in almost every period of her life. Joanne was typical in that, like many LGBT persons who were gender nonconforming in childhood, she experienced emotional, physical, and sexual abuse early in life. The literature is replete with reports that early childhood trauma, rejection, and poor attachment can lead to lifelong cognitive distortion. These abusive experiences can contribute to the individual perceiving ordinary stimuli as negative or menacing. It can also lead the individual to give heightened conscious and unconscious attention to negative events, circumstances, and interactions, as well as to maintain a heightened vigilance for the occurrence of threatening situations.

Joanne, like many LGBT persons, had been conditioned in early life to catastrophize the world and grew into an adult who experienced ordinary interactions, as well as the world in general, as negative, threatening, and anxiety provoking. In Joanne's case these feelings and perceptions are often based in reality and serve as a self-protective adaptation against the very real threat of violence and discrimination that many LGBT persons face. In addition to the abuse and humiliation her father inflicted on her, she spent her high school years labeled as a "fag" and would find tampons taped to her locker. She reported that the "jock" boys would come up behind her and run their hands down her shirt and ask her if she needed a bra yet. Joanne faced the social stigmatization that many LGBT persons face, and, in addition, she felt at arm's length from her own true identity/expression because of her inability to present herself as the woman she knew she was. Every day of Joanne's adolescent and adult life had reinforced in her the fact that she was different and defective.

In the early months of treatment Joanne often had panic attacks, which she attributed to reliving painful life events in therapy. At one point, she felt her work was so severely compromised by her generalized anxiety and panic attacks that she stated, "I came to you for help, and I feel like things are just getting worse as a result of our therapy sessions." At that time clonazepam was prescribed to relieve the acute anxiety and panic symptoms. At her next visit, Joanne said she had taken a few doses and experienced relief from her anxiety, but ultimately she stopped taking the medication after reading about the side effects—a case of both seeking help and rejecting it. Years earlier, she had bought alprazolam online and had used it briefly. However, after reading on the Internet that alprazolam could be "addictive," she stopped taking it. She didn't want to take the clonazepam because it was in the same class as alprazolam. Joanne laughed nervously and said, "See, I even get anxious about taking the medications that are supposed to help my anxiety." Her psychiatrist educated Joanne about the low probability of becoming dependent on clonazepam when occasionally used over a short course and also told her it was unwise to self-medicate by buying medications on the Internet. He again reviewed her substance use, which consisted of only a couple of glasses of wine a week. However, given the revelation about the illicit alprazolam purchase, her psychiatrist had concerns that she might be minimizing her substance use.

A trial of buspirone was attempted next. However, it made her dizzy and nauseous. The possibility of starting serotonin reuptake inhibitors (SRIs) was discussed, but Joanne was reluctant to try them because her previous trial of sertraline had caused her anxiety to become unbearable. It was explained to her that while some may experience increased anxiety in the first weeks of SRI use, ultimately this anxiety typically resolves, and that SRIs are a first-line treatment for anxiety disorders. Joanne agreed to start escitalopram. The results have been very positive. She did not have the initial spike in anxiety that she had experienced with sertraline, and she found that the escitalopram gave her more energy, improved her mood, and ultimately caused significant remission of her anxiety symptoms. She continued to experience panic attacks occasionally, and we found that gabapentin was an effective medication that she could take as needed for acute panic attacks.

As her psychotherapy sessions continued, a psychodynamic approach was abandoned and a more cognitive-behavioral therapy approach adopted. Joanne and her psychiatrist identified her automatic thoughts that people were judging her negatively for her decision to undergo sexual reassignment and that no one would be interested in knowing her more because she was a "freak." Her negative schemas revolved around not feeling adequate as a woman and not feeling like a normal woman. Her "homework" included assignments that resulted in Joanne speaking to her boss about being transgender. In her session after telling her boss, she was exuberant and indicated that he was very supportive. She reported that he and most of the office staff already knew that she was transgender. While Joanne had always perceived that she was an outcast in the office, she learned that many of her office-mates wanted to express their support but felt unsure how to do so. After coming "out" at the office about being transgender, Joanne developed more meaningful relationships with her coworkers and felt more comfortable in her work environment. Her work performance also improved, and she was promoted.

Another homework assignment included an attempt to be more involved socially. Volunteering at a local homeless shelter was decided upon as a means of making new social connections in a nonthreatening environment. Joanne liked her volunteer work and found that the people at the shelter, many of whom had substance and psychiatric issues, did not judge her for being transgender. She felt accepted there, and she enjoyed being in an environment where the focus was not about her. She also met a chiropractor who was volunteering his services at the shelter. They started dating, and Joanne began an intimate sexual relationship with him. This was the first sexual relationship Joanne had ever had as a woman, and she felt grateful that her first time was with a man who would ultimately become very important in her life. They have since moved in together, and Joanne reported feeling that she is well on her way to creating her new life as a woman that she had been struggling to achieve.

Key Points

- When treating LGBT persons, it is important to factor in ordinary life stressors, which may be extraordinarily anxiety provoking among this population.

- The decision to be "in" or "out" of the closet, as well as the dynamics of being homosexual, bisexual, or transgender within the context of work, relationship, and parenting roles, can be daunting in a world overwhelmingly geared to heterosexuality and cisgenderism.

- A diagnosis of GAD in the LGBT population can be easily obscured by comorbid psychiatric disorders such as depression or substance abuse. Likewise, a GAD diagnosis can be complicated by comorbid medical factors, such as HIV/AIDS, sexual reassignment surgery, and hormone replacement.

- Because many LGBT persons face early social stigmatization and abuse, they may be predisposed to develop negativistic thoughts and behaviors. When available, cognitive-behavioral therapy can play an important role in reversing deeply ingrained negative automatic thought processes and transforming them into more realistic perceptions, which ultimately leads to positive changes in behavior and mood (Gould et al. 1997).

- SRIs are the standard first choice when it comes to the pharmacological treatment of GAD, especially because GAD is often comorbid with depression. Although benzodiazepines are often used in the acute treatment of anxiety disorders, long-term use has been associated with worsening of anxiety. Gabapentin and pregabalin show efficacy in both the acute and the long-term control of anxiety symptoms, without the cognitive, motor, and sleep disturbances seen with benzodiazepine use (Cohen 1995).

References

American Psychiatric Association: Diagnostic and Statistical Manual of Mental Disorders, 4th Edition, Text Revision. Washington, DC, American Psychiatric Association, 2000

Cohen SI: Alcohol and benzodiazepines generate anxiety, panic and phobias. J R Soc Med 88:73–77, 1995

Drescher J, McCommon BH, Jones BE: Treatment of lesbian, gay, bisexual, and transgender patients, in The American Psychiatric Publishing Textbook of Psychiatry, 5th Edition. Edited by Hales RE, Yudofsky SC, Gabbard GO. Washington, DC, American Psychiatric Publishing, 2008, p 1477

Gould RA, Otto MW, Pollack MH, et al: Cognitive behavioral and pharmacological treatment of generalized anxiety disorder: a preliminary meta-analysis. Behav Ther 28:285–305, 1997

Meyer IH: Prejudice, social stress, and mental health in lesbian, gay, and bisexual populations: conceptual issues and research evidence. Psychol Bull 129:674–697, 2003

Questions

15.1 Critical to the acute and long-term treatment for GAD in the LGBT community is

    A. Confronting distorted negative beliefs and encouraging thoughts and social interactions that are more appropriate.

    B. Dealing with the comorbid substance abuse that has a higher prevalence in the LGBT population.

    C. Expressive psychotherapy targeted at reliving, reenacting, and reimagining threatening or stressful life events.

    D. All of the above.

The correct answer is A.

Cognitive-behavioral therapy is a form of psychotherapy targeted at improving basic cognitive skills and social functioning. It has been shown to be a mainstay of treatment in the both the acute and the long-term treatment of GAD. Although dealing with comorbid substance abuse disorders (option B) is certainly necessary in all persons with GAD, it cannot be said at this time that the LGBT population has a higher prevalence of substance abuse disorders in general. The data looking at substance abuse in these populations are equivocal. While certain types of substance abuse and dependence seem to have higher prevalence within certain sections of the LGBT community, it has not been clearly demonstrated that substance abuse disorders are more prevalent in LGBT persons in general. Reliving, reenacting, and reimagining threatening or stressful life events (option C) has not been shown to be useful in either the acute or the long-term treatment of GAD. Rather, recognizing and changing distorted patterns of thought and behavior, as in cognitive-behavioral therapy, has been shown to highly effective.

15.2   Which of the following is *not* true of comorbid anxiety disorders in LGBT persons?

   A. The acute and profound physiological manifestations of panic are specific to panic disorder and define its diagnosis.
   B. Negative early experiences (such as emotional, physical, or sexual abuse during childhood) are often found in the etiology of anxiety disorders, and these early traumatic events may predispose LGBT persons to higher rates of GAD.
   C. Negative cognitive biases in attention and processing of threatening stimuli distinguish anxious persons from non-anxious persons.
   D. Medical stressors such as HIV/AIDS can add to the probability of developing GAD in LGBT persons.

The correct answer is A.

The autonomic symptoms of panic do not exist in isolation with the diagnosis of panic disorder; rather, they live along a continuum, and persons with both GAD and phobic disorder may also experience these autonomic symptoms. Many LGBT persons face stigmatization and abuse very early in life and therefore may be programmed early to give selective attention to negative and threatening stimuli. This excessive focus on the negative aspects of life and social interaction can be a factor in the development of GAD (answer B). Negative cognitive biases can arise from early traumatic experience in LGBT persons (answer C) and result in perceptual distortion, which causes these persons to catastrophize ordinary events and social interactions and can lead to persistent and excessive anxiety. Studies of persons experiencing chronic and grave illness, such as HIV/AIDS, have reported significantly higher rates of GAD (answer D).

Adjustment Disorder

Queer Stressors: Adjustment Disorder in a Lesbian Mother

Serena Yuan Volpp, M.D., M.P.H.

THE DIAGNOSIS OF adjustment disorder is unusual in its approach. It is one of only three diagnoses in (DSM-IV-TR (American Psychiatric Association 2000) to link a stressor to symptom development (the other two are posttraumatic stress disorder and bereavement). In fact, the first criterion of the adjustment disorder diagnosis is the presence of a stressful event preceding symptom formation (Table 16–1). The criteria of the diagnosis have been criticized for lack of specificity regarding both the stressful event and the symptom complex. Studies have demonstrated poor reliability of the diagnosis, but better validity (i.e., that the diagnosis is different from major depression and normal reactions to stress) (Katzman and Geppert 2009).

The prevalence of adjustment disorder varies based on the setting being studied. Few studies have measured the prevalence of adjustment disorder in general community settings, likely because very few structured diagnostic instruments include adjustment disorder. The European ODIN study, surveying various European countries, found a prevalence of less than 1% (Katzman and Geppert 2009). Prevalences are higher in specific clinical settings. In primary care settings, the prevalence ranges from 11% to 18%. Studies in consultation-liaison psychiatry settings have found a prevalence range of 10%–35% (Casey 2009). Although adjustment disorder is thought to occur in all cultures and all

---

TABLE 16–1.   DSM-IV-TR diagnostic criteria for adjustment disorders

---

A.   The development of emotional or behavioral symptoms in response to an identifiable stressor(s) occurring within 3 months of the onset of the stressor(s).

B.   These symptoms or behaviors are clinically significant as evidenced by either of the following:

(1)   marked distress that is in excess of what would be expected from exposure to the stressor

(2)   significant impairment in social or occupational (academic) functioning

C.   The stress-related disturbance does not meet the criteria for another specific Axis I disorder and is not merely an exacerbation of a preexisting Axis I or Axis II disorder.

D.   The symptoms do not represent bereavement.

E.   Once the stressor (or its consequences) has terminated, the symptoms do not persist for more than an additional 6 months.

Specify if:

Acute: if the disturbance lasts less than 6 months

Chronic: if the disturbance lasts for 6 months or longer

Adjustment disorders are coded based on the subtype, which is selected according to the predominant symptoms. The specific stressor(s) can be specified on Axis IV.

309.0   With depressed mood

309.24   With anxiety

309.28   With mixed anxiety and depressed mood

309.3   With disturbance of conduct

309.4   With mixed disturbance of emotions and conduct

309.9   Unspecified

Source.   Reprinted from *Diagnostic and Statistical Manual of Mental Disorders,* 4th Edition, Text Revision. Washington, DC, American Psychiatric Association, 2000. Used with permission. Copyright © 2000 American Psychiatric Association.

---

age groups, the prevalence in the lesbian, gay, bisexual, and transgender (LGBT) community is unknown. However, multiple issues and events that are unique to LGBT individuals could precipitate adjustment disorders. These are discussed in this chapter.

Case Example: Jamie

Jamie is a 33-year-old African American woman living with her partner Michelle and their 5-month-old son Jake in an urban area. Michelle gave birth to Jake. Jamie holds a master's degree in chemistry and works as an eighth grade science teacher in the public school system.

Jamie presented for treatment with the chief complaint "I've been having a lot of trouble sleeping." She reported that since Jake was born, both she and

Michelle had been getting little sleep. Initially, her reduction in sleep was due to the fact that she was trying to feed Jake at least once during the night with a bottle so that Michelle could have an uninterrupted stretch of sleep. After a month or so, however, even though Jamie felt exhausted, she could not fall asleep easily after doing her feeding shift. She estimated that for at least the 3 weeks prior to presentation, she had been getting a total of 5 hours of sleep per night. She felt tired during the day and found it quite difficult to teach until 2:30 P.M.

She was still interested in her job and denied any significant problems with her focus or concentration, although she felt distracted at times. She denied any change in appetite. She denied feeling guilty about working and being away from Jake. She denied feeling like her limbs were heavy. Although she reported some anxiety about getting through her lesson plans, she denied feeling physically restless or fidgety.

When asked if she was depressed, she said, "Of course not—we're so happy to have Jake in our lives." After a pause, she stated, "Well—actually I know that I *shouldn't* feel depressed, but I do feel low, and sometimes I scare myself because I feel irritated with the baby." She denied thoughts of harm toward the baby but had noticed herself feeling overly frustrated a few times when he was crying inconsolably. She stated that although she would "never" kill herself, she had wondered in the past month what Michelle's and Jake's lives would be like if she were "not around" anymore. On further questioning, she stated that a few days prior to coming in, when feeling particularly tired and looking out the window of her classroom, she saw the school buses lined up on the street and briefly visualized herself being hit by a bus. She firmly stated that she did not want to kill herself and denied any intent or plans to do so. She denied any feelings that she was being monitored or followed or that anyone else might wish to harm her. She denied having auditory or visual hallucinations.

She stated that she had been drinking more over the past month, up from one glass of wine at night to two glasses to "try to relax." Michelle was not drinking as she was still breastfeeding, and she had commented on Jamie's increase in alcohol consumption in the past couple weeks. Jamie denied any recent drug use.

Jamie had no history of hospitalizations or of psychotropic medication use. She had seen a therapist in college for a year when she was struggling with the decision about whether to come out to her parents. She reported that at that point she felt quite anxious, but she denied panic attacks and denied significant feelings of depression. She denied a history of manic or hypomanic episodes.

Jamie stated that she thought about suicide toward the end of high school, when she came out to herself as bisexual, but had never made a suicide attempt. She denied a history of physical violence either in her intimate relationships or with strangers.

Jamie started to drink alcohol her junior year in high school at parties. She recalled blacking out a few times her senior year of high school and during college. After college, her drinking pattern evolved to one glass of wine per night during the week and two mixed drinks on weekend nights when she went out with friends. She denied any history of withdrawal tremors. Jamie smoked marijuana about once per month during her sophomore to senior years in college but denied any use since starting her job as a public school teacher 6 years ago. She denied any history of other drug use, and in particular denied any history of injection drug use.

Her medical history was significant only for migraine headaches, for which Jamie occasionally took acetaminophen.

Jamie's father and paternal grandfather both reportedly drank "too much." She reported that while they performed well occupationally, it was well known in the family that they drank excessively and that she thought her grandfather had died of cirrhosis. She reported that her mother was "high strung" and anxious and used alprazolam occasionally.

Jamie was born and raised in the Midwest, the second child of middle-class parents. She has a brother who is 3 years older than she. She was athletic in school and always had a few close friends. She dated her first boyfriend for about 6 months during sophomore year of high school. Although they were physically intimate, they did not have intercourse. Toward the end of high school, she realized that she had developed a serious crush on one of her teammates. She started to think of herself as someone attracted to both men and women. This was quite difficult for her, as she did not know anyone else who was bisexual and wondered whether she was a "freak" or "abnormal."

During college, she played soccer during her freshman year but then stopped after deciding that the team was taking too much time away from her academics. In order to stay active, she started to play intramural rugby. She met her first girlfriend, Anne, on the rugby team. Anne had come out as lesbian in high school and had previously dated a few other women. After becoming involved with Anne, Jamie started to call herself lesbian instead of bisexual. She had a few relationships with women that lasted 1–2 years before meeting Michelle in graduate school. She and Michelle have been together for 9 years.

Discussion

Diagnosis

The diagnosis most consistent with Jamie's presentation is adjustment disorder with depressed mood. The development of her symptoms occurred about 1 month after the birth of her son (Criterion A; see Table 16–1). Criterion B1, "marked distress that is in excess of what would be expected from exposure to the stressor," is designed to help differentiate an adjustment disorder from a normal, nonpathological response to stress. This is subject to clinical judgment; severity of symptoms, cultural norms, and functional impairment should be taken into account (Casey 2009). Although the introduction of a baby into a household is a stressful event, most clinicians would not expect a depressed mood and the level of distress expressed by Jamie (Criterion B1), and her functioning at work is starting to suffer (Criterion B2). In terms of Criterion C, it does not appear that Jamie had a preexisting Axis I disorder. Any Axis II disorder would not account for the constellation of symptoms with which she is presenting.

Next, we need to make sure that she does not meet criteria for another specific Axis I disorder. Although Jamie technically meets criteria for depressive disorder not otherwise specified, that disorder is not any more specific than adjustment disorder. She has the following symptoms: depressed mood, insomnia, decreased energy, and passive suicidal ideation. She does not meet criteria for a major depressive episode now, but it is possible that her presentation represents an evolving major depressive episode. Ongoing monitoring is therefore important. Some students are taught (though this is not specified in DSM) that if a patient presents with suicidal ideation, the diagnosis cannot be adjustment disorder. This is not true. Although not in Jamie's case, it can at times be difficult to differentiate adjustment disorder from posttraumatic stress disorder, when the precipitating event is of a more life-threatening nature.

Moving on to the remainder of the criteria, Jamie's symptoms do not represent bereavement (Criterion D). The stressor has not terminated, and so Criterion E is not relevant. Thus far, the disturbance has lasted about 4 months, so we do not yet know whether the acute or the chronic specifier should be added. Because the baby will be a chronic stressor, if her symptoms last beyond 6 months, she will qualify for the chronic specifier. Although she does not meet the criteria for alcohol abuse, her alcohol consumption has been increasing and should be discussed and monitored, especially given her family history of alcohol abuse. Individuals with adjustment disorder can use, misuse, or abuse alcohol and/or drugs to help mitigate symptoms. In addition, at times a substance-induced mood disorder can be confused with an adjustment disorder.

Treatment Recommendations

The options of pharmacotherapy and psychotherapy were explored with Jamie. There is a very small evidence base for treatment of adjustment disorder, either for psychotherapeutic interventions or for the use of psychotropic medication. The good news is that almost all interventions studied have been found to be helpful, including ego-enhancing therapy, cognitive therapy, supportive psychotherapy, brief dynamic therapy, benzodiazepines, nonbenzodiazepine anxiolytics (etifoxine), herbal remedies (kava-kava, valerian), and antidepressants (tianeptine, mianserin) (Casey 2009). In clinical practice, benzodiazepines are often used to target symptoms of insomnia and anxiety, and antidepressants with sedative side effects are used for the same reasons.

Jamie agreed to try taking a benzodiazepine at night to help with her sleep, but she was more interested in embarking on a trial of psychotherapy to help her understand her reaction to the birth of her son and to help her better adapt to the reality of her new family structure. She agreed to a trial of supportive psychotherapy. The goals of supportive psychotherapy are to ameliorate symptoms, improve ego functions (also known as psychological functions), and increase both self-esteem and adaptive skills.

Treatment Course

Initially, psychotherapy focused on practical measures to help Jamie adapt to the change in her life. Because sleep is so critical to functioning, I helped Jamie with problem solving regarding how to get better sleep. She instituted several changes. First, she was able to cut back from drinking two glasses of wine to one glass of wine at night, as she recognized that the additional glass may have been helping her to fall asleep but ultimately was leading to poorer sleep quality. Second, she was able to persuade Michelle to have the baby sleep in his own room. They had fallen into the habit of keeping Jake in their own bedroom because it seemed easier for middle of the night feeding. However, each time Michelle fed the baby and soothed him back to sleep, Jamie's sleep was disrupted. Third, she was able to negotiate with Michelle, who was still on maternity leave, to give Jamie 2 nights off during the week from feeding duty, in exchange for taking more responsibility on weekend nights.

Jamie was initially resistant to this last change, which precipitated a deeper exploration of Jamie's feelings about the birth of Jake. It turned out that Jamie had been ambivalent about the decision they had made for Michelle to try to get pregnant. Jamie herself wanted to be pregnant, but Michelle was older, and they had agreed for Michelle to try first. Although Jamie was manifestly happy when Michelle was successful, she was able in psychotherapy to express feelings of jealousy and fear. She was envious of the bond that Jake and Michelle had through breastfeeding and worried that Jake would see Michelle as his "primary" mother because she was his birth mother and Jamie was not biologically related to him. She came to understand that this was part of the reason why she stubbornly hung on to doing one of the feedings every night, even though she was working full-time and feeling exhausted. She did not want to be seen as the "lesser" mother.

There are multiple issues around having children that can potentiate feelings of sadness, jealousy, and anger in LGBT individuals. Primary among them is the inability to conceive a child with one's partner (with the exception of some transgender individuals). The lack of traditionally defined gendered parental roles can lead to confusion and feelings of competition and jealousy, especially if one parent is biologically related to the child and the other is not. For lesbians, if both individuals in the couple want to carry the child but they have only one child, one partner must mourn the loss of this experience. Jamie secretly worried that she and Michelle would ultimately decide not to have a second child, even though that had been their plan, and that she would never have the experience of being pregnant and giving birth.

Having a child also precipitates a need for LGBT individuals to negotiate anew how "out" they want to be with family and with colleagues. Although Jamie was not closeted at work, she tended to compartmentalize her home and work life, and she rarely talked about Michelle while at work. She felt very awkward at work asking for short-term maternity leave and telling colleagues and staff that she was going on maternity leave when she clearly had not been pregnant. She needed to come out in multiple other arenas once the baby was born. She felt angry about having to cross out "father" on numerous forms, such as at the pediatrician's office and on day care center applications, and then put her name down as the second parent. This series of small slights or insults brought up hidden shame about being a lesbian for her.

In addition, the birth of the baby created new conflicts between herself and her parents. Her parents had taken years to come to terms with Jamie's identity as a lesbian. They had gotten to the point of inviting Michelle to family events and sending her birthday presents, and Jamie had felt that things were "normal" with her parents. However, the birth of Jake caused unresolved issues to resurface. Although their closest friends were all members of the same church, Jamie's parents did not feel comfortable inviting their friends to Jake's baptism. Jamie was both hurt and angry, as she had witnessed how proud her parents had been at the birth of her brother's daughter, and knew that they had invited ten friends to her niece's baptism even though it was held far from their hometown.

Lee Crespi (1995) aptly describes numerous issues that lesbians need to "mourn" while developing a positive lesbian identity, including heterosexual relationships, as many women in same-sex relationships have had heterosexual sexual experiences and relationships. Even if they come to identify themselves as lesbian, as Jamie has, they often have gone through a period of identifying as bisexual and imagining being in a stable relationship with a man. Jamie had not fully let go of this fantasy, and having a baby with Michelle clearly made the fantasy that much less of a real possibility. In therapy, she was able to recognize that some of the sadness she had been feeling represented emotions related to letting go of the fantasy of being with a man and having a baby with a male partner.

Other Stressors for LGBT Individuals

Becoming a new parent can be a stressor for anyone. As we can see from Jamie's experience, parenthood also raises unique issues for LGBT people. Multiple other events and stressors in the lives of LGBT individuals can serve as precipitating factors for an adjustment disorder, including the process of coming out, relationship breakups, HIV disease, being the victim of antigay violence, and aging (Drescher and Byne 2009). All of these stressors can bring up issues around coming out, just as parenting did in Jamie's case. The developmental process of "coming out" contains multiple points of stress, from becoming aware of one's same-sex attraction to disclosing one's feelings to others. Coming out is not a linear process; people come out in various ways and at various times throughout their lives.

Conclusion

After 2 months of weekly supportive psychotherapy, Jamie was able to start tapering her use of the benzodiazepine at night and was subsequently able to fall asleep after 10–15 minutes. About 3 months later, Jamie noted that she no longer had any of the symptoms with which she had presented, including thoughts of death and depressed mood. She recognized that many of the issues that had been raised in therapy were not fully resolved, but she felt better enough to terminate this round of treatment.

Key Points

- Issues that may precipitate an adjustment disorder in LGBT individuals include coming out, parenting, relationship breakups, antigay violence, HIV disease, and aging.

- Parenthood poses unique stressors to LGBT individuals, including—for some—issues of loss and jealousy around not being biologically related to the child.

- When treating an LGBT individual for an adjustment disorder, pay attention to unresolved issues about coming out that may have resurfaced as a result of the current stressor.

References

American Psychiatric Association: Diagnostic and Statistical Manual of Mental Disorders, 4th Edition, Text Revision. Washington, DC, American Psychiatric Association, 2000

Casey P: Adjustment disorder: epidemiology, diagnosis and treatment. CNS Drugs 23:927–938, 2009

Crespi L: Some thoughts on the role of mourning in the development of a positive lesbian identity, in Psychoanalytic Reappraisals of Sexual Identities. Edited by Domenici T, Lesser RC. London, Routledge, 1995, pp 19–32

Drescher J, Byne W: Homosexuality, gay and lesbian identities, and homosexual behavior, in Kaplan and Sadock's Comprehensive Textbook of Psychiatry, 9th Edition. Edited by Sadock BJ, Sadock VA, Ruiz P. Baltimore, MD, Lippincott Williams & Wilkins, 2009, pp 2060–2090

Katzman JW, Geppert CMA: Adjustment disorders, in Kaplan and Sadock's Comprehensive Textbook of Psychiatry, 9th Edition. Edited by Sadock BJ, Sadock VA, Ruiz P. Baltimore, MD, Lippincott Williams & Wilkins, 2009, pp 2187–2196

Questions

16.1 Which of the following intervention(s) show some evidence of utility in the treatment of adjustment disorder?

    A. Supportive psychotherapy.
    B. Brief dynamic therapy.
    C. Psychotropic medication.
    D. All of the above.

The correct answer is D.

Although the evidence base is small, all of the above interventions have been found to be helpful in treating adjustment disorder.

16.2 A gay male patient comes in for consultation after breaking up with his partner of 8 years. He reports sadness for the past few weeks, poor sleep, poor appetite, low energy, and guilt about abandoning his partner who has HIV. His diagnosis is

    A. Depressive disorder secondary to HIV disease.
    B. Adjustment disorder with depressed mood.
    C. Major depressive episode.
    D. Crystal methamphetamine–induced depressive disorder.

The correct answer is C.

Although it sounds as if the patient's syndrome was precipitated by a stressor, he meets criteria for a major depressive episode, which means that he cannot be diagnosed with adjustment disorder.

Borderline Personality Disorder

Keeping the System Stable: A Systems Approach in Long-Term Treatment of a Patient With Borderline Personality Disorder

Scot G. McAfee, M.D.
David K. Schwing, L.C.S.W.

WORKING WITH PATIENTS who have personality disorders can sometimes be the most exasperating and vexing work encountered by mental health clinicians in any setting (Feinstein 2000). These patients challenge our diagnostic abilities, create doubt about the best ways to help them, and can cause us either to feel rushed to act or to want to avoid treating them altogether.

The following case depicts the treatment of a gay man who displays many of the characteristic features of borderline personality disorder. Through hard work in therapy and drug and alcohol recovery, he has come to see how his personality characteristics and his behaviors have caused him difficulty. By using a therapeutic modality based on the understanding of the interactions between people and the systems around them, he has come to realize that he has an active role in maintaining his stability and continuing to improve his quality of life. Through the use of a variety of modalities including individual therapy, substance abuse treatment, group therapy, and medication management, the patient was able to see himself in a new way, gain insight into the impact he has had on those around him, and enjoy his life. He also gained stability in his jobs, in a new relationship, and with the systems of people around him.

Case Example: Christopher

When Christopher presented for treatment he was a 32-year-old white self-identified gay man who was referred to therapy by an acquaintance. He had no prior mental health treatment. During the assessment sessions with the therapist (D.K.S.), he had difficulty expressing himself or describing his life experiences and it was unclear to him what he wanted out of therapy. He said he was coming to therapy because that was what he saw other people in his circle of friends doing. Indeed, the acquaintance who referred him was in psychotherapy himself and was someone Christopher liked and admittedly wanted to imitate. Christopher was able to work therapy into his schedule and came regularly.

Christopher had a significant history and pattern of recreational use of alcohol and cocaine while partying with friends, while out dancing, or in sex venues to feel more comfortable having sex with other men. He was using cocaine daily at home, either by himself or with a single friend who used as well.

Christopher had been unable to sustain a primary romantic relationship. He initially described his friendships as any other young adult might, but the therapist quickly sensed that Christopher sounded like an adolescent describing friendships. He used the behaviors engaged in to define the friendships instead of describing the benefits the friendships brought to his life. For example, he interacted with his friends by "hanging out," "sneaking cigarettes," gossiping, and all the while wanting to be popular and included in the "in" gay crowd. Christopher observed that other gay men of a certain cohort who were perceived to be affluent, well-connected, body-conscious, and living in New York were open about seeking out psychotherapy. He wanted to both conform to and be part of this rarefied subset of gay subculture.

The therapist felt that Christopher's friendships seemed shallow and fleeting. With time Christopher began to open up about how he was suffering in these relationships and how he wanted them to change. While these relationships were limiting in some ways, he also enjoyed some aspects of them, but he felt lonely.

Christopher had endured significant early life experiences. Most pivotal was the suicide of his father, who also had a history of substance abuse, although Christopher did not think of his father as having major emotional problems. Christopher's mother was conflicted about how to handle the suicide's aftermath, and he remembers her avoiding speaking of it at all. She remarried quickly, which yielded a distant yet tolerant relationship between Christopher and his mother and a strained relationship between Christopher and her new spouse.

Christopher did not do well in school and engaged in social transgressions like abusing his parents' credit cards or stealing directly from them and then lying about it. In the initial therapeutic work, he realized that his emotions were never explained to him by his parents or even considered while growing up. He remembers feeling rageful toward his mother, to whom he later would feel terribly obligated—especially after his father's death. He also felt hurt and sad about his father but had no outlets to express these feelings. He felt quite isolated. In therapy, he enjoyed learning new ways to express his experiences and memories.

Christopher was not sexually active as a teenager, but was aware of having a crush on another boy as well as having fantasies of being a girl in relationships with his other boy friends. His burgeoning sexuality was another way he searched for identification within a peer and social group, finding here a label to explain some part of him. In his twenties, his sexual and intimate life was predominantly lived in sex clubs and in the back rooms of gay bars, where he used cocaine to facilitate seeking sex. However, he felt very little sexual satisfaction with live partners, stating that he was ultimately sexually satisfied in fantasy only. For many years, masturbating to pornography was his primary satisfying erotic outlet.

He admitted creating an idealized image of himself in which he was valued and accomplished. However, while considering this idealized self, he was aware of also facing chronic dissatisfaction with his body and his appearance, which created inner turmoil and continued confusion about who he "really was."

Christopher had a history of significantly unstable employment. He was usually able to interview and secure jobs, but he reported a consistent pattern of interpersonal difficulties within the workplace and with coworkers, and he experienced repeated terminations. His account of these episodes initially discounted his own hostile and provocative behaviors that were obvious factors in his firings. He would be insubordinate to his supervisor by defying requests to stay appropriately silent in meetings, and he would often arrive late to work after having been out partying and taking drugs the night before. He eventually disclosed that he sought employment and positions of status in the workplace mostly for validation among his family and peers, not because work was self-sustaining or fulfilling. It also took him years to admit that his skills and abilities were often not commensurate with the positions he sought.

As the assessment and history-taking sessions led to the beginnings of treatment interventions, Christopher and the therapist agreed that his substance abuse interfered with his ability to fully participate in the therapeutic experience. Having initially gone untreated, the effects of his substance use—irritability, lateness, fatigue—created a barrier to fully seeing or understanding his potential personality issues and his overall psychotherapy treatment goals.

Exploring Christopher's personality issues, he and the therapist worked to discriminate whether his variable outward presentations of frustration and anger were part of his personality, his drug use, or both. They also explored his sexuality further to discriminate any identity disturbance or identity diffusion, core components of borderline personality disorder (DSM-IV-TR; American Psychiatric Association 2000) (Table 17–1). Early in treatment, Christopher would question, "Am I a girl?" "Am I gay?" and would say, "I'm not really enjoying sex with another man." However, the therapist was alert to how someone struggling with sexual identity can raise questions about sexual orientation as an example of identity disturbance, yet that these questions must be viewed in the context of other processes in the individual's life and not automatically seen as an example of the identity diffusion of a person with borderline personality disorder (Meyer and Northridge 2007). Christopher's sociosexual and interpersonal issues of choosing gay friends just because they are gay, wanting to fit in but being unable to, mirroring others in superficial relationships, behaving problematically at work, and engaging in risky drug-taking and sex acts all warranted a consideration of borderline personality disorder (Oldham 2002) regardless of whether he has sexual identity issues or not.

The Treatment: Building a Treatment System

During the early assessment phase Christopher and his therapist agreed this would be a long-term treatment. The approach would be systems-centered

TABLE 17–1. DSM-IV-TR diagnostic criteria for borderline personality disorder

A pervasive pattern of instability of interpersonal relationships, self-image, and affects, and marked impulsivity beginning by early adulthood and present in a variety of contexts, as indicated by five (or more) of the following:

(1) frantic efforts to avoid real or imagined abandonment.   **Note:** Do not include suicidal or self-mutilating behavior covered in Criterion 5.

(2) a pattern of unstable and intense interpersonal relationships characterized by alternating between extremes of idealization and devaluation

(3) identity disturbance: markedly and persistently unstable self-image or sense of self

(4) impulsivity in at least two areas that are potentially self-damaging (e.g., spending, sex, substance abuse, reckless driving, binge eating).   **Note:** Do not include suicidal or self-mutilating behavior covered in Criterion 5.

(5) recurrent suicidal behavior, gestures, or threats, or self-mutilating behavior

(6) affective instability due to a marked reactivity of mood (e.g., intense episodic dysphoria, irritability, or anxiety usually lasting a few hours and only rarely more than a few days)

(7) chronic feelings of emptiness

(8) inappropriate, intense anger or difficulty controlling anger (e.g., frequent displays of temper, constant anger, recurrent physical fights)

(9) transient, stress-related paranoid ideation or severe dissociative symptoms

Source.   Reprinted from *Diagnostic and Statistical Manual of Mental Disorders,* 4th Edition, Text Revision. Washington, DC, American Psychiatric Association, 2000. Used with permission. Copyright © 2000 American Psychiatric Association.

rather than patient-centered, therapist-centered, or diagnosis-centered (Gantt and Agazarian 2006).

The stated therapeutic goals were for Christopher to 1) become more functional in his interpersonal relationships and in the workplace; 2) become more integrated and less split off from parts of himself, especially his sexuality and aggression; 3) become knowledgeable about the dangers and perpetuating effects of his substance use; 4) develop choices; 5) be open to feedback; 6) develop self reflection; 7) develop impulse control; and 8) use all of these goals and techniques, finally, to create a context and framework within which his feelings and impulses could be understood and explored. This represented a great deal of work for Christopher, but he was curious and found this focused attention on himself new and intriguing. He agreed to the plan.

The early part of treatment focused and refocused on engaging in a long-term process of developing the patient and therapist's partnership, bringing them into their different roles with different responsibilities as they worked on their goals together (Gantt and Agazarian 2006). Here, by testing expectations over time, they began to develop trust in the therapeutic alliance and worked on the skills of listening, understanding, supporting, encouraging, learning to see "forks in the road," and identifying driving and restraining forces in relation to the stated goals (Gantt and Agazarian 2006). For example, in many sessions Christopher would appear to be emotionally charged and frustrated and sometimes quite angry, convinced that he was being seen as "a mess." The therapist consistently would have Christopher check out his "mindreads" or cognitive distortions, undo his negative predictions and find out how he felt in the moment, and provide a fork-in-the-road perception that if Christopher didn't just see himself as "a mess" he would discover that he had another fork and had strengths and abilities to organize himself when needed (Gantt and Agazarian 2006). This work helped Christopher see that he has choices and improve his energy toward reaching his goals.

Christopher was referred to and attended Alcoholics Anonymous (AA) meetings and in the beginning really liked them because "there are cute boys there." The therapist encouraged him both to get a sponsor in AA and to participate in fellowship as a part of his recovery program. AA introduced structure into his life, and his therapy system was beginning to stabilize, both in the therapist's office and outside of it. What began as just "showing up" to AA meetings to see "cute boys" became a part of a routine that eventually led Christopher to realize that he was getting treatment by being and staying sober—an insightful and new experience for him.

Another new occurrence within the individual work was Christopher's ability to relate to the therapist in new ways by coming to sessions regularly and on time, allowing himself to tolerate both making and holding eye contact with the therapist, and learning to do breathing exercises together with the therapist when frustrated—all of which he found helpful in containing his impulses and stabilizing his behaviors (Gantt and Agazarian 2006).

Referral to Systems-Centered Therapy Group Treatment

Systems-Centered Therapy (SCT)—enables one to shift from self-centered relationships to an increased awareness of the self in a systems context through learning and practicing with others. With systems-centered awareness comes an increasing ability to make transitions in relationships that are required in the multiple contexts of everyday life, both at home and at work. The goal of all of the steps in SCT work is to keep taking the "fork in the road of choice" away from personal wishes and fears and to enter everyday reality with common sense, curiosity, and a sense of humor (Gantt and Agazarian 2006). Christopher was oriented to the group process and trained in the terminology that would be used, and he became a participant in weekly 90-minute group sessions.

The Psychiatrist as Part of the System

In addition to individual therapy, group therapy, and AA, part of Christopher's treatment system included his referral for a psychiatric evaluation after approximately two and a half years in individual therapy. Christopher was experiencing symptoms of anxiety and difficulty sleeping—not uncommon at his stage of sobriety—and the therapist felt that medications might stabilize some of the intense and unstable affects that were brought up in therapy. One concern in making this referral and connection to a psychiatrist (S.G.M.) was that Christopher would be creating another relationship in the treatment framework, something that until this time would have been difficult for a patient like him. Christopher could see the therapist and psychiatrist as another set of "parents." The two clinicians spoke to each other about how group treatment would be used to normalize this model for him, as many of the group members were working in split treatments, and in multiple instances with the *same* psychiatrist and therapist. Christopher and the therapist were open in their discussions that the psychiatric referral was increasing Christopher's structure and that it would serve as another treatment resource to help stabilize his system.

One week prior to the initial psychiatric evaluation, Christopher went to a local emergency room for symptoms of incapacitating anxiety and insomnia. He was prescribed a low dose of atypical antipsychotic medication and discharged from the emergency room setting to initiate outpatient care with the psychiatrist. At no time during his treatment then or since has he expressed suicidal ideation to the psychiatrist or therapist, although he would express hopelessness and worthlessness during the course of treatment.

As the therapist and psychiatrist had worked together treating many clients, they had become accustomed to each other's styles in practice, and the psychiatrist was quite comfortable offering support for his therapy, AA, and group work. Christopher knew that together, the therapist and psychiatrist would be diagnosing him, providing joint treatment, and tracking his stabilization. He always welcomed the disclosure of clinical material between his therapist and psychiatrist.

Christopher responded well to a low dose of the selective serotonin reuptake inhibitor (SSRI) sertraline, with improvement and eventual resolution of his anxiety, better emotional regulation when overwhelmed, and a slightly more optimistic outlook on life. He requested medication for his insomnia, the choice of which was important to explore with him because of his history of substance abuse and current sobriety. He later complained of developing sexual side effects to the SSRI, including some erectile dysfunction and delayed orgasm. He was ambivalent about dealing with these symptoms because the medication had been so beneficial for his other symptoms, until he entered into a new romantic relationship. For some time before he admitted to the psychiatrist that he was having sexual side effects, he was shopping at naturopathic stores and using herbal preparations in what turned out to be an ineffective attempt to remedy the situation. Christopher and his therapist had discussed that with some of his intimate relationships, Christopher had used sexual symptoms as a way to control the relationships while never being able to openly discuss with his partner what he found sexually satisfying. The addition of a medication that could impair his sexual functioning was something that took a great deal of work in his sessions with the psychiatrist, as well as prolonged discussion in therapy and consultation sessions between the therapist and the psychiatrist.

Over the course of nearly 10 years, we (therapist, psychiatrist, and Christopher) have agreed that we have enjoyed working together. We all have come to realize and accept that when Christopher is having difficulties, he experiences them and "owns" them to the best of his abilities, which have grown considerably. Although the treatment has been exasperating at times, Christopher has shown a consistent interest in getting to know himself, he has been doggedly protective of his sobriety, and he has restructured his life to incorporate his system of care whenever needed. The psychiatrist and therapist feel fortunate that they share similar approaches and understandings when working with patients, and that when working with people with personality disorders, they have gotten used to more frequent consultations and "catch-up" phone calls or supervision meetings, which have been roundly accepted as helpful interactions in the co-treatment of these patients (Linehan 1993). Both feel they can accept these clients and patients into their practice with less anxiety, more hope, and a comfort with the stabilizing forces of the system when it is needed. The psychiatrist does not see medications as the only intervention for the treatment of mood symptoms, and the therapist agrees that medications can be very helpful in many situations. The psychiatrist, while believing that Christopher's work in therapy was helped by ameliorating some of his anxiety and depression with medications, has worked over the years to stop them at times as Christopher attempts to "get to know himself" off medication. Christopher feels that the "best" regimen has continued to be a low-dose SSRI and a sleeping pill, despite the psychiatrist's constant reminders that he could probably sleep without the medications, especially if he were to use more cognitive and behavioral techniques to address his insomnia. Christopher has not taken the view that some in AA take, that a hypnotic agent is just another "addiction," and the psychiatrist has supported him.

Tracking Progress and Outcomes With the Client's Own Observations

As part of the ongoing individual and group work, Christopher and his therapist have had a routine of observing together what has happened within the work. The following are some of Christopher's observations:

> "I think I've developed a bigger sense of compassion for those around me. A genuine feeling and emotion for others, whether it's joy, sadness, or anger for what-

ever someone is experiencing. I can still be jealous and project…this is progress, not perfection!"

"I have really been able to decrease judging others and going one-up. I can just be a person among people. My experience in group is that we all have our stuff and details may be different, but we all experience the same emotions. I think this has really brought out a niceness and sincerity about me. I also get to have conversations on a deeper level with those around me. I think people sense my compassion and ability to listen and give meaningful feedback to friends and family."

"My denial as a defense has been greatly reduced. I may choose not to address an issue or problem, but it doesn't mean I don't have acute awareness. That is a *huge* difference to me…a greater sense of awareness about myself, both good and bad."

"I think also I have a better ability to see people for who they are and always were...both good and bad. I seek out a different type of friend than I did ten or fifteen years ago. I have a keener sense of who and where my friends and family fit in my life."

"My expectations of people and their abilities are more in line and realistic in a healthy way."

Closing Thoughts

Through the use of a combination of therapeutic modalities, namely individual therapy, AA, group therapy, and psychopharmacological treatment, Christopher has learned about himself and how he experiences and understands very complex and powerful feeling states and interpersonal interactions. His growth and understanding were possible because he was intellectually and emotionally challenged to look at the forces in his life that were hindering many of the things he wanted to achieve. Further, he was invited to create a positive relationship with his therapist and psychiatrist in order to jointly embark on this journey. The techniques used by Systems-Centered Therapy, especially being in the "here and now" and developing a way to see oneself and one's choices, were incredibly helpful for this client, as he felt safe to experience himself and to be in control of his own change. The authors posit that using modalities such as an SCT approach to individual and group work along with 12-step programs like AA, and medications when necessary, may benefit many people with personality disorders, especially borderline personality disorder.

Key Points

- Patients with borderline personality disorder present with some of the most difficult challenges in all of mental health work.

- Patients presenting with personality disorders can best be treated by clinicians who avail themselves of work in collaboration and are open to a variety of resources, such as AA, group therapy, and psychiatric co-treatment. *Keep the system stable, and the patient will have a better chance of stability.*

- When a therapeutic treatment system is established, the addition of medications to treat specific symptoms such as depression and anxiety can be an effective way for the overall treatment to move forward and for the client to feel supported and understood.

References

American Psychiatric Association: Diagnostic and Statistical Manual of Mental Disorders, 4th Edition, Text Revision. Washington, DC, American Psychiatric Association, 2000

Feinstein RE: Personality disorders in the primary care setting: diagnosis, management and intervention. Resid Staff Physician 46:47–56, 2000

Gantt SP, Agazarian YM (eds): SCT in Clinical Practice. Livermore, CA, Wingspan, 2006

Linehan MM: Cognitive-Behavioral Treatment of Borderline Personality Disorder. New York, Guilford, 1993

Meyer IH, Northridge ME (eds): The Health of Sexual Minorities: Public Health Perspectives on Lesbian, Gay, Bisexual and Transgender Populations. New York, Springer, 2007, p 22

Oldham JM: A 44-year-old woman with borderline personality disorder. JAMA 287:1029–1036, 2002

Questions

17.1 What is the most useful approach for treatment providers providing "split treatment?"

    A. Wait until the client has a crisis before discussing the case together.

    B. Use open and permitted communication throughout the course of treatment.

    C. Never share information, as it would affect the transference.

    D. Have periodic group meetings.

The correct answer is B.

Open communication between treatment providers, when the patient provides explicit permission for it, is the most effective manner of conducting split treatment.

17.2   A gay, lesbian, or bisexual orientation can be confused for what core feature of patients with borderline personality disorder?

        A. Frantic efforts to avoid abandonment.
        B. Chronic suicidal ideation.
        C. Identity disturbance.
        D. Unstable interpersonal relationships.

The correct answer is C.

All people may react frantically to the loss of a relationship, and being gay or lesbian does not predict more unstable relationships. The inner confusion and coming out process of someone who may be LGBT, during which the person may self-represent as heterosexual in one setting and more stereotypically gay in another, is not to be confused with the identity disturbance of the person with borderline personality disorder, who may never develop an integrated and stable identity.

Parent-Child Relational Problem

When the Kids Are All Right, But the Parents Are Not: Coparenting in Planned LGBT Families

NANETTE GARTRELL, M.D.

IN PLANNED LESBIAN- OR GAY-PARENT families, a decision to rear children precedes the arrival of children through donor insemination, surrogacy, adoption, or foster care (Bos and Gartrell 2011). Family constellations may consist of single lesbian- or gay-parent households, two-lesbian-parent households, two-gay-parent households, and shared custody arrangements between lesbian moms and gay dads (Bos 2010). The case presented here involves a family consisting of two lesbian mothers and two gay fathers who produced two children through donor insemination (illustrated, Figure 18–1). The presenting complaint was that the mothers were increasingly irritable about allowing the fathers equal time with the children, despite their preinsemination agreement to share parenting.

The description of parent-child relational problem from DSM-IV-TR (American Psychiatric Association 2000) is shown in Table 18–1.

Case Example: Four Parents

Bob, the donor (biological) dad, initiated the family consultation. He explained by telephone that the two couples agreed to seek my assistance, since the interactions between the moms and the dads had become quite tense. I first met all four parents for a 90-minute consultation. The parents ranged in age from early

---

TABLE 18–1.   Parent-child relational problem (DSM-IV-TR, V61.20)

This category should be used when the focus of clinical attention is a pattern of
interaction between parent and child (e.g., impaired communication, overprotection,
inadequate discipline) that is associated with clinically significant impairment in
individual or family functioning or the development of clinically significant
symptoms in parent or child.

Source.   Reprinted from *Diagnostic and Statistical Manual of Mental Disorders,* 4th Edition, Text
Revision. Washington, DC, American Psychiatric Association, 2000. Used with permission.
Copyright © 2000 American Psychiatric Association.

---

thirties to mid-forties. All were successful professionals. Alice, the birth mom,
had delivered both children—a 3-year-old daughter and a 7-month-old son. On
their birth certificates, Alice and Bob were listed and the children had the same
last name as Alice. The 3-year-old daughter referred to her parents as Mommy-
Alice, Mommy-Carol (co-mom), Daddy-Bob, and Daddy-Ted (co-dad).

First session: At our initial meeting, I asked each parent to describe her or his
process in choosing to form a family (Gartrell et al. 1999). I also asked each to
specify the current areas of conflict.

Alice said that she had always wanted to have children. She came from a
large Catholic family that had been critical of her lesbianism prior to the birth of
her first child. Her father was alcoholic, with a long history of verbally abusing
her mother. Although her siblings were supportive of her choice to have children, and her parents had come around, Alice rarely visited her parents because
her father's behavior was unacceptable to her. She did not want her children to
witness it. She and Carol had been together 10 years, and Alice described their
first meeting as "love at first sight." Because Carol did not want children, Alice
spent the first 5 years of their relationship convincing her of the benefits of
motherhood. Eventually they reached an agreement to have two children
through insemination, using a known donor. Carol had chosen Bob, one of her
closest friends, as donor; Alice hoped this choice might lessen any residual ambivalence Carol had about parenting. According to Alice, once the children were
born, Carol became very attached to them. As Alice saw it, the conflict that
brought them into treatment was the result of having four parents who loved the
children very much but had "insufficient time for each [parent] to one-on-one
with the kids" (Gartrell et al. 2000).

Carol, the co-mom, came from a Mormon family that had not spoken to her
since she came out as lesbian. She described herself as "fairly OCD," by which she
meant that she was "super orderly, bordering on controlling." She felt this was a
useful trait in setting up the complex child care schedule and keeping track of everyone's needs. She corroborated Alice's report about her initial reluctance to
parent and that she had been thrilled when her best friend, Bob, agreed to be the
sperm donor. What she hadn't anticipated was her own attachment to the children and the distress she felt when the children were with the dads. It also hadn't
occurred to her that she might resent Bob's biological connection to the children
or the presence of his name on the birth certificates.

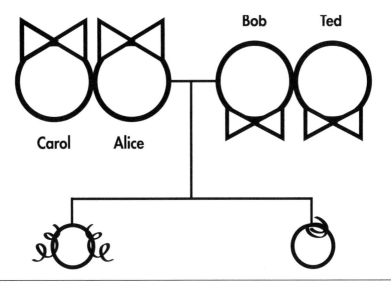

FIGURE 18–1. The family tree.

Bob, the biological dad, grew up in a nonreligious Jewish family that had adjusted relatively easily to the announcement of his sexual orientation when he came out during college. He had always hoped to be a dad. Before Carol had asked him to coparent, he had been saving for adoption or surrogacy. He was pleased that his husband, the co-dad Ted, was supportive of the proposed coparenting arrangement. Bob first experienced tension with the two moms after the delivery of their daughter. His parents were there; the moms' parents were not. Since then, Carol seemed irritable whenever any of the dads' relatives visited. Bob found it stressful to accommodate everyone's wishes to hold, play with, and spend time with the children; he described this conflict as a recurrent theme. Whenever he or Ted raised the possibility of taking the children to visit their respective families, all sorts of obstacles were erected by the moms.

Ted, the co-dad, was raised in a nonreligious family that was accepting of his sexual orientation and nontraditional family structure. His parents and siblings lived nearby, visited frequently, and enjoyed spending time with the grandchildren. Ted's family vacationed at their summer home each July, and he looked forward to taking his daughter and son to these gatherings. He understood the moms' reluctance to be away from the children for days at a time, as he and Bob experienced the same difficulty. From Ted's perspective, the best way for the children to feel secure and happy with all parents was for the children to spend equal time with each of them.

Second and third sessions: I set up a second and a third 90-minute consultation, meeting with each couple separately. During my meeting with the moms, Alice, the birth mom, made it clear that even though she was still breastfeeding their son she hoped to work out a schedule so that all parents could spend equal time with the children, even if it meant doing a lot of pumping so that Carol or the dads could care for their son when she wasn't around. To her, having four loving parents rear the kids felt like a happier version of the large family in which she grew up. She was thrilled that her co-mom loved the children so much—especially after her initial reluctance to parent—but worried that Carol resented the dads' intrusiveness. Because the dads often showed up unannounced, Carol felt that the moms rarely had privacy. Since the dads also took the children home with them, Carol said, "we have no privacy, and less time with the kids in a given week than they do."

I asked Carol, the co-mom, if it was true, as Alice had remarked, that she resented Bob's legal status as a parent. She said she wished they had used an anonymous donor so she could have been the legal coparent. I asked about Bob's observation that the she was often irritable when the dads' parents visited. Carol said she felt that these grandparents were overinvolved. When Alice delivered their second child, Bob's parents brought his baby pictures to the hospital, "pointing out over and over how much he looked like the baby." Carol felt marginalized, since she had neither a biological nor a legal connection with her children. I asked if she thought Bob had similar feelings. She thought not, stating that he wasn't as close to the children as she was.

During my separate meeting with the dads, Bob, the biological dad, said he felt hurt that Carol no longer seemed to value him as a friend. He felt that he had become a source of irritation to her. He said that they had signed a contract before their daughter was born that explicitly stipulated a four-way shared parenting agreement, with equal time allotments, participation in decision making, and financial responsibility for each child. He had envisioned spending holidays with all parents and children together, but because there was so much tension of late, he was beginning to wonder if the dads and moms would celebrate separately.

Ted, the co-dad, felt that Carol was the source of the family tension, describing her as "incredibly uptight." He said that the dads understood the moms' reluctance to have their son overnight with the dads while he was still breastfeeding. He said that the dads tried to accommodate the moms' wishes by visiting the children at the moms' home rather than taking them to the dads' house. Ted resented feeling unwelcome when they stopped in to spend time with the children.

Fourth session: I set up a fourth 90-minute meeting with all four parents together. I began the session by explaining that I would ask each parent to share feelings that been expressed in the separate sessions but not stated in our initial meeting when all four were present. For example, I asked Alice, the birth mom, to describe her hopes for family cohesiveness. I asked if she felt reluctant to stick to the preinsemination coparenting contract. I asked Ted, the co-dad, to explain his desire to accommodate the moms' wish to have the children nearby while the son was still breastfeeding. I asked if he felt that the moms appreciated the dads' efforts to be helpful this way. I asked Carol, the co-mom, to discuss her feelings about not having a biological or legal connection to the children. I asked Ted if he had any similar feelings and, when he replied affirmatively, to discuss them. I asked Bob, the biological dad, to describe how his relationship with Carol had changed. He first spoke of his anger, but on further questioning said he felt sad about the loss of closeness. Carol seemed surprised about this and said that she would give more thought to her own feelings. I asked each parent how their relationship with their own parents might be contributing to the current conflict.

Once the issues that had been brought up in the couples' private sessions had been restated to the entire group, I asked the parents to draw up a list of the top five areas of conflict. They produced the following list:

1. Conflict over time with the children
2. Conflict over the dads visiting the children at the moms' home
3. Conflict over biological/legal connections to the children
4. Loss of closeness between the Carol, the co-mom, and Bob, the biological dad
5. Grandparent involvement in day-to-day life and vacation planning

The parents agreed to meet for six more sessions to tackle these areas of conflict. Because competitiveness was a major theme for this family, I assigned one area of conflict to each parent, with the specific task of developing three or four strategies to resolve it. The assignments were allocated in such a way that none of the parents would be paired with an issue that was most challenging to her or him. I assigned conflict over time with the children to the co-dad Ted; conflict over the dads spending time at the moms' home to the birth mom Alice; conflict regarding biological/legal connections to children to the biological dad Bob; loss of closeness between Bob and Carol to the latter; and grandparent involvement to myself.

Later sessions: In subsequent sessions, we addressed each area of conflict and discussed possible solutions. Regarding the first two items—time with the children and location of visits—Ted said that the dads hadn't previously understood the moms' privacy issues. The dads had assumed that planned or spontaneous visits to the children at the moms' home would be welcome in the interest of accommodating the breastfeeding schedule. In response to inquiries by me, the dads acknowledged that if the situation were reversed, they wouldn't want the moms to pop in unannounced. Ted proposed a new child care schedule, aiming for as much equality as possible. The moms agreed to prepare plenty of frozen breast milk for the times that their son would be with his dads. Both sets of parents promised to call before stopping by the others' home, to inquire whether a visit would be welcome, and to abide by the response. All parents renewed their long-standing promise to contact the others immediately if a family emergency occurred.

Bob had two proposals for equalizing the parents' legal connections to the children. The first was to use Carol's and Ted's last names as their children's two middle names. This idea was vetoed by the other parents as too cumbersome for the children. Bob's second proposal was to investigate the possibility of having both nonbiological parents legally adopt the children. In coparent adoption, the original parent retains legal guardianship of the children, and the other parent gains the same legal status. The other three parents were open to this idea, and Bob said that he would call their attorney to see if it was possible. I mentioned that in my own research, parent-child bonding was more strongly influenced by time spent with the child than by biological connections: egalitarian scheduling offered the best opportunity for multiple parents to feel as though they had a chance to develop meaningful connections with children (Gartrell and Bos 2010). Also, I explained that as they grow up, children go through phases of being closer to one parent than another, that the bonds shift periodically, and that this is a normal part of child development.

Regarding the distance that had grown between Bob and Carol, she proposed that the two of them resume spending time together on a regular basis, without their spouses. An addendum to that proposal was to include the children in some of these outings. Bob was very enthusiastic about this proposal, and the other parents supported it as well. Since the child care schedule was already complicated, I recommended that these outings be officially added to the calendar to ensure that they would take place.

Finally, we discussed the issue of grandparent involvement in the family unit. I pointed out the difference in the dads' and moms' attachments to their families of origin, noting that extended family involvement in their children's lives was a happy prospect for the dads but an unhappy one for the moms. I explained that contact with loving grandparents is generally a positive experience for children, but given the discrepancy between the dads' and moms' feelings about their own parents, it was important to fit the dads' parents' visits within the time already allocated to the dads. I suggested that both couples consider their vacation wishes at the beginning of each year and, if each couple wanted separate travel time with the children, to divide the number of days allocated to such trips equally between the couples. Within the dads' time, vacations with extended family could take place. The moms were more enthusiastic about this proposal than the dads, but all agreed that it was fair.

Last session: At our final session, we reviewed the new child care schedule (including outings for Bob and Carol) and vacation plans for the subsequent year. The moms and dads agreed that if any parent felt that tension had recurred, they would see me again. I reminded them that sticking to a fairly rigid schedule reduced the chances of renewed conflict. I urged them to be as up front as possible about their feelings and choices, to ensure that intended acts of generosity (such as the dads' spending more time at the moms' home while the son was still breastfeeding) are experienced as such.

Key Points

- In shared parenting arrangements between lesbian moms and gay dads, greater family harmony is achieved when child care is equally distributed among all parents.

- Coparenting contracts and coparent adoption enhance feelings of legitimacy for nonbiological parents.

References

American Psychiatric Association: Diagnostic and Statistical Manual of Mental Disorders, 4th Edition, Text Revision. Washington, DC, American Psychiatric Association, 2000

Bos HM: Planned gay father families in kinship arrangements. Australian and New Zealand Journal of Family Therapy 31:356–371, 2010

Bos HM, Gartrell NK: Adolescents of the US National Longitudinal Lesbian Family Study: the impact of having a known or an unknown donor on the stability of psychological adjustment. Hum Reprod 26:630–637, 2011

Gartrell N, Bos HM: US National Longitudinal Lesbian Family Study: psychological adjustment of 17-year-old adolescents. Pediatrics 126:28–36, 2010

Gartrell N, Banks A, Hamilton J, et al: The National Lesbian Family Study: 2. Interviews with mothers of toddlers. Am J Orthopsychiatry 69:362–369, 1999

Gartrell N, Banks A, Reed N, et al: The National Lesbian Family Study: 3. Interviews with mothers of five-year-olds. Am J Orthopsychiatry 70:542–548, 2000

Questions

18.1   Planned lesbian- and gay-parent families are formed through

    A. Surrogacy.
    B. Donor insemination.
    C. Adoption.
    D. All of the above.

The correct answer is D.

The word *planned* in reference to lesbian and gay family formation refers to the decision to become a parent *before* conceiving or adopting children.

18.2   Coparent adoption refers to

    A. The biological parent adopting the nonbiological parent so that all family members can have the same last name.
    B. Coparents adopting a child who is not yet a member of the family.
    C. The biological parent relinquishing legal jurisdiction over a child so that the nonbiological parent can become the child's guardian.
    D. The coparent gaining legal jurisdiction over the child without changes to the original parent's guardianship of the child.

The correct answer is D.

Regardless of whether the original parent's guardianship came through biological connection or adoption, she or he does not relinquish parental rights when the coparent acquires legal status as the child's co-guardian.

Partner Relational Problem

Listening Beyond Homo-Ignorance and Homo-Prejudice

VITTORIO LINGIARDI, M.D.
NICOLA NARDELLI, PSY.D.

THIS CHAPTER ILLUSTRATES a case of a partner relational problem (PRP) as described in DSM-IV-TR (American Psychiatric Association 2000). PRP involves patterns of negative interaction and communication problems between partners or spouses, associated with impaired functioning of the individual or symptom development in one or both partners (American Psychiatric Association 2000) (Table 19–1).[1] In this chapter, we provide clinical examples of coming out, internalized homonegativity, and sexual compulsivity. We also alert clinicians to some of the difficulties that arise when clinical listening is affected by "homo-ignorance" or "homo-prejudice" (Lingiardi and Drescher 2003).

Case Example: Antonio

First session: Antonio is a 32-year-old Italian bank clerk who is a nonpracticing Catholic. He has consulted a psychiatrist in the public mental health services for his growing difficulty in handling feelings of anxiety and irritability, thinking "a bunch of pills" could be the right solution. When the psychiatrist asks for

---

[1]The PRP is part of the wider diagnostic group of "relational problems," syndromes associated with more or less severe distress levels. There are no criteria provided in DSM-IV-TR for these codes, included as "other conditions that may be a focus of clinical attention" (V-codes).

TABLE 19–1. Partner relational problem (DSM-IV-TR, V61.10)

This category should be used when the focus of clinical attention is a pattern of
interaction between spouses or partners characterized by negative communication
(e.g., criticisms), distorted communication (e.g., unrealistic expectations), or
noncommunication (e.g., withdrawal) that is associated with clinically significant
impairment in individual or family functioning or the development of symptoms in
one or both partners.

Source.   Reprinted from *Diagnostic and Statistical Manual of Mental Disorders,* 4th Edition, Text
Revision. Washington, DC, American Psychiatric Association, 2000. Used with permission.
Copyright © 2000 American Psychiatric Association.

---

more details about the origin of Antonio's anxiety, the patient reluctantly says it
probably has to do with his "private life." At this point, the psychiatrist—we will
call him Dr. Ricciardi—awkwardly hazards a guess: "Problems with your wife?"
Antonio, becoming more and more anxious and irritated, turns his eyes away
and does not answer. "What do you mean by 'private life'?" continues the doctor. "I have a boyfriend," Antonio mutters.

Dr. Ricciardi, realizing the inappropriateness of his question, tries to start
over: "Oh…I see. Well, that is not a problem. Go ahead." However, this second
try is even more awkward and reveals his uneasiness with gay or lesbian clients.
Dr. Ricciardi has had very little professional experience with gay clients and even
less personal experience with gay people. Both Antonio and his psychiatrist live
in a provincial, somewhat small-minded town, characterized by a "don't ask,
don't tell" culture toward gay people. However, Dr. Ricciardi's problem has more
to do with knowledge and experience than it does with either prejudice or hostility; he ordinarily would not think about homosexuality as something having
to do with relational or family problems. For him, homosexuality has meant,
above all, solitude and shame. In a second, the many things he *does not* know
about the lives of gay people pass through his mind. He feels professionally inadequate, but at the same time, challenged. He courageously asks, "What's your
boyfriend's name, and how long have you been together?"

After a few seconds of silence, Antonio says: "His name is Paolo. He is thirty.
He teaches art at a secondary school. We met four years ago. Ever since last year,
things started going wrong." Antonio's face turns sad, and Dr. Ricciardi catches
a glimpse of some concern about the relationship.

"I dislike labels," Antonio goes on to say. "And I would not say I am gay. I've
had some women in my life. If I must label myself, then let's say I am bisexual."

"And what about Paolo?" says Dr. Ricciardi.

"Jesus, he is gay. Definitely. He told me he knew since he was ten."

"Why don't you tell me something about your relationship?"

Antonio says their first year went pretty smoothly. Paolo lived in another
town about 500 km away. During the weekends, they would meet at Paolo's
house, where they spent beautiful Sundays together. "Mostly sleeping, fixing the
garden, and having sex." Silence. "I'm the active one," Antonio wants to specify,
by which he wishes to let the doctor know he is the "top" or insertive partner in
anal intercourse. Then, 2 years ago, Paolo decided to move to Antonio's town.
Since that moment, "we started fighting for pointless reasons."

Although some moments of reciprocal uneasiness and discomfort are still present, the atmosphere of the consultation now seems more relaxed on both sides. The session is reaching its conclusion, and Dr. Ricciardi asks Antonio if, besides the aforementioned "pointless reasons," he and Paolo are able to talk about and deal with the relational problems underlying their disputes.

Antonio answers, "Generally, I don't talk at all, and I withdraw. Mostly, I leave home." Then, clearly stressed, Antonio adds that on those occasions, he goes to a cruising place, picks up a hustler, and penetrates and abuses him verbally. Initially, these "escapes" did not worry Antonio. On the contrary, he was convinced that this was a good way to loosen up and to "save" his relationship with Paolo. Then, when he returned with Paolo, he "forgot" everything. During the last year, however, these episodes would happen more frequently, until Antonio realized that they had become completely compulsive. At the same time, he realized that his relationship was deteriorating.

The session time has finished. The psychiatrist, still surprised and confused, is able to conclude the visit in a positive way. "Antonio, you have given me a clear picture of the situation, but I think that in order to understand how I can be of any help, we will need to meet a couple more times. Then I can get to know you better, and I will be able to choose the best solution for you and consequently, for you and Paolo." Antonio seems relieved.

Internally, Dr. Ricciardi had morally judged Antonio's compulsive behaviors. Sometimes, personal ideology can influence clinical practice (Lingiardi and Capozzi 2004). To his credit, after this first session, Dr. Ricciardi consulted a senior and more expert colleague. Acting as a supervisor, the senior psychiatrist helped Dr. Ricciardi understand how his own prejudices (e.g., "all homosexuals are sexually promiscuous") might obstruct fuller comprehension of the psychological and relational meaning of certain behaviors and can, paradoxically, strengthen a patient's dissociative defenses.

The supervisor turned out to be very useful, and with his help, Dr. Ricciardi started to think that some of Antonio and Paolo's problems might have to do with internal conflicts about disclosure of their homosexuality. In different ways and probably without being aware of it, both men seem to present this problem. However, this problem is at the same time the origin of their interpersonal conflicts and a shared factor that indirectly keeps them together.

Second session: Antonio arrives early to his second appointment. He immediately begins to talk, saying that the day before he had a fight with Paolo, who again and again insisted on being introduced to Antonio's parents. Dr. Ricciardi asks Antonio if his relationship with Paolo is kept a secret from Antonio's parents. "Of course, it's none of their business," he answers. He adds that once, by chance, his parents saw him with Paolo.

"So, now Paolo already knows my parents! What more does he want?" asks Antonio. "Why does he want them to pry into my personal matters? What's the point of telling my parents what I do in my bed? Friends or lovers, what does it matter? Yet for Paolo it matters. It matters more for him than for me. But they are *my* parents, and I am the one who has to decide what to do with them. There is nothing to do. Paolo doesn't understand; he does not want to understand. Yesterday, he crossed the line, and…(coughing) he made me beat him."

Antonio explains that Paolo is too insistent. For example, they recently met at a party of Antonio's old friend. Antonio presented Paolo just as "a friend," and Paolo "started with his usual protest." Once again, the discussion turned into a violent quarrel, with Paolo accusing Antonio of being ashamed of kissing or cuddling in public. Antonio told him that he neither wants to kiss nor to cuddle in public because it doesn't seem "polite" to him. He also reminded Paolo that Paolo hadn't come out to his own parents. "'I would not have problems in doing that,' says Paolo, 'if you were able to do it with yours.'"

"At times," Antonio says, "Paolo talks with me about his intention to reveal his homosexuality to his parents, but then he never does! What does he want from me?" Antonio believes that someone has to do "certain things" only in private. After these wrangles, Paolo often feels the need to reconstruct the serenity of their "happy days," becoming more agreeable and giving little gifts to Antonio. "I really don't understand these behaviors of Paolo!" Antonio goes on. "I have even thought that there is someone else! Otherwise, I have to conclude that after so many years, he still does not know me." Then he adds, "When he is acting so childish and insistent, I hate him. I get dreadfully angry, and I can calm myself only by…well, what I told you about last time."

The session is about to end, and the psychiatrist feels the need to offer his perspective of the situation to Antonio: this is a multifaceted but often confusing situation, in which Antonio is torn between alternating feelings: on one side, anger, dissatisfaction, and a desire to give up this relationship but, on the other, guilt and concern for his sexual compulsivity and a fear of his inability to handle it. Antonio nods and sighs.

Third session: During the third session, Dr. Ricciardi asks Antonio to tell him more about the way he has lived and now lives with regard to his attraction toward men and asks him if he feels affected by particularly painful memories and/ or experiences. Suddenly, Antonio bursts into tears. With some hesitation, he begins to tell how homosexuality has always been mocked and stigmatized by his family—by his father, in particular. His adolescence was affected by feelings of shame and inferiority. He remembers having been bullied at school, something he has hardly ever spoken about, trying to "forget" it. He never disclosed his feelings to his parents, nor did he have the courage to tell them the stress he suffered from being bullied at school. "One of the reasons I 'chose' the silence is because I heard my father defining a TV character as a 'pathetic fag.'"

Dr. Ricciardi realizes how, in order to cope with these "microaggressions in everyday life" (Sue 2010), Antonio learned to act defensively in a dissociative way, putting his being a "faggot" in a sort of "mental drawer," at the edge of his consciousness (Drescher 1998; also see Chapter 1 of this volume). Every time he finds himself in a situation in which his homosexuality becomes detectable, it is as if the episodic memory implicitly linked to his traumatic experiences is reactivated. Even if he is not completely aware of it, Antonio expects that "coming out" necessarily implies a negative reaction from somebody. On these occasions, feelings of anxiety, guilt, and inferiority emerge, and Antonio tries to cope with them by identifying with the aggressor. In this way, he is "turning the tide" and externalizing his distress. When problematic painful and dissociated mental memories are reactivated (for example, when Paolo wants Antonio to introduce him to his parents), the burden of anxiety becomes too heavy and cannot be managed in a functional way anymore. Antonio either withdraws or acts compulsively.

Although Antonio's compulsive sexual behaviors had initially led Dr. Ricciardi to misjudge him, he has now arrived at nonjudgmental listening to Antonio and exploring with him some of the possible underlying meanings of his behaviors. In other words, listening and attunement have enhanced the possibility of focusing on some previously unacceptable mental contents that Antonio could only tolerate and manage through dissociation and sexually compulsive behavior.

Again, our psychiatrist consults with his supervisor. Both of them believe some aspects of Antonio's sexual actions could be linked to the reactivation of internalized experiences of stigmatization. They reflect on a particular detail of Antonio's narrative: when he penetrates and insults a hustler, he enters a state of fantasied hyperarousal in which Antonio plays the role of a policeman raping a prisoner of war. It seems that Antonio's self-contempt, rage, and anxiety are enacted as dissociated and exciting fantasies that give him the possibility of attributing those intolerable feelings to another person and, at the same time, creating an illusion of actively controlling them.

The supervisor also notes that instead of recognizing his distress about his own sexual orientation and the possibility of coming out, Antonio criticizes Paolo's incoherence: "Sometimes, Paolo says he would like to come out to his parents, but he never does it! What the hell does he want from me?" Paolo is probably troubled about his homosexuality as well, and this puts the couple in a "funhouse mirrors" situation. The supervisor presents this as just a working hypothesis, the most important aspect of which is that Paolo, on one side, and the hustler, on the other, represent for Antonio "containers" for his unacceptable and painful thoughts and feelings.

Final session: During their fourth and last meeting, Dr. Ricciardi decides to directly convey to Antonio something of what has emerged from their brief consultation. In particular, he explains that Antonio's current emotional state and all his past sufferings connected to same-sex attraction can affect his present life, undermining his relationship with Paolo.

Instead of "a bunch of pills," Dr. Ricciardi suggests psychotherapy. Antonio realizes how their four meetings have made him feel better. Moreover, he understands how helpful it has been to share his memories and experiences of having to hide his homosexuality. Further, he realizes how his family and personal history have adversely affected his relationships. He willingly accepts the proposal, and Dr. Ricciardi refers Antonio to a psychotherapist.

Conclusion

Partner relational problems are a "human heritage" that pertain to all sexual orientations and to every kind of romantic relationship. However, as anticipated, minority stress (Meyer 1995) can complicate these relationships and obstruct their resolution. Psychiatrists and mental health professionals need to understand the role of minority stress in gay and lesbian psychological and relational development.

As is widely known, the process through which gay men and lesbians acknowledge their homosexuality and feel comfortable without hiding their identity is called coming out (see Chapters 1 and 2). Coming out "stages" or "stops" always constitute an important dimension to be explored with a patient experiencing difficulties with his or her homosexuality. It is also important to pay attention to how a patient experiences a partner's coming out.

In seeking out a psychiatric consultation, Antonio had begun his coming out process; but his presentation was as someone frightened, ashamed, and insecure. Saying, "I would not say I am gay...let's say I am bisexual," can be considered, in his case, a defense mechanism to cope with anxiety, shame, and self-contempt connected with "being gay" (Isay 1989).

Antonio grew up in environments (family, school, town) where homosexuality was characterized negatively. He suffered from internalizing the homonegativity around him. The range of attacks against his identity and sense of self ranged from the psychological to the openly verbal and even to the violently physical. Those real-life experiences led him to expect, fear, and imagine future attacks. These experiences, both in a focal and a cumulative way, affected his cognitive and psychological development (for example, considering homosexuality to equal weakness and submission, or masculinity to equal power and success). Or as Corbett (2001) puts it, "faggot=loser."

Like many young victims of bullying, particularly those being bullied for effeminacy or being perceived as being gay, Antonio felt he could not ask his parents for help. He wanted to avoid further humiliation. Having no other way to cope with these difficulties, Antonio developed heightened dissociative defenses that ended up in compartmentalizing his homosexuality and reinforcing its associated stereotypes (Drescher 1998; also see Chapter 1 in this volume).

At the end of the consultation, the psychiatrist decided not to prescribe drugs. Instead, he presented to Antonio the usefulness of psychotherapy aimed at understanding the relational and psychological meaning of his anxiety, rage, and irritability as well as his compulsory and increasingly ego-dystonic sexual behaviors. Following his psychiatric consultation, Antonio began to interact with his dissociated and previously unprocessed mental contents. This led him to gradually understand that engaging in psychotherapy could be a good idea. Previously compulsive behaviors gradually became less "necessary." At the same time, he began more open communication with his friends and parents. Even the bickering with Paolo decreased, and their relationship became more communicative and intimate. Antonio continued to be sexually dominant with Paolo, but this became more consistent and integrated into his psychological and relational life. Sometimes, Antonio and Paolo were even able to see a little humor in that.

Paolo began his own psychotherapy a year after Antonio. But this is a different (and also a similar) story.

Key Points

- Minority stress can affect a gay couple's well-being.

- Past stigmatizing traumas can negatively influence a gay couple's intimacy in the present.

- "Homo-ignorance" and "homo-prejudice" can bias clinical listening.

References

American Psychiatric Association: Diagnostic and Statistical Manual of Mental Disorders, 4th Edition, Text Revision. Washington, DC, American Psychiatric Association, 2000

Corbett K: Faggot=loser. Studies in Gender and Sexuality 2:3–28, 2001

Drescher J: Psychoanalytic Therapy and the Gay Man. Hillsdale, NJ, Analytic Press, 1998

Isay R: Being Homosexual: Gay Men and Their Development. New York, Farrar, Straus, & Giroux, 1989

Lingiardi V, Capozzi P: Psychoanalytic attitudes towards homosexuality: an empirical research. Int J Psychoanal 85:137–158, 2004

Lingiardi V, Drescher J (eds): The Mental Health Professions and Homosexuality: International Perspectives. New York, Haworth Medical Press, 2003

Meyer IH: Minority stress and mental health in gay men. J Health Soc Behav 36:38–56, 1995

Sue DW: Microaggressions in Everyday Life: Race, Gender, and Sexual Orientation. New York, Wiley, 2010

Questions

19.1 When seeing a gay patient and judging gay sexuality to be immoral, the psychiatrist should

    A. Appeal to the patient's religious and moral values and explore the risk of contracting sexually transmitted diseases.

    B. Inform the patient that the psychiatrist is not an expert on sexual problems and prescribe antidepressants.

    C. Explain to the patient that promiscuity is a consequence of homosexuality and, according to this notion, declare that homosexuality must be "cured.".

    D. Ask oneself why one judges the patient's sexual behaviors as immoral.

The correct answer is D.

A clinician's prejudices can heavily obstruct the understanding of the patient. If clinicians think they are influenced by prejudice, it is useful to consult a supervisor or to discuss the case with colleagues.

19.2   A young gay man requests a psychiatric consultation because he has problems in handling his partner's being in the closet. The psychiatrist

     A. Infers that the patient is talking about himself because he does not accept his own homosexuality anymore and asks the patient if he has ever thought of undergoing "reparative" therapy.

     B. Tries to understand whether the partner's "closetedness" could be somehow related to the patient's "outness" and starts to explore how they live with this disparity and how they talk at home about this aspect of their relationship.

     C. Suggests that the patient should respect his partner's choice.

     D. Condemns the patient's need to disclose his homosexuality in public.

The correct answer is B.

It is often important to consider how the patient experiences his or her partner's being "out" or "closeted." With a gay couple, it is important to address the (different) ways they came to terms with their homosexuality and the specific ways in which they have or have not come out.

Bereavement

Bereaved, Bothered, and Bewildered

KENNETH ASHLEY, M.D.
DICKSON JEAN, M.D.
DANIEL SAFIN, M.D.

Bereavement or Depression?

In this chapter we present the features and discuss the appropriate diagnosis and treatment of a case in which grief after a partner's death was accompanied by worsening mood symptoms.

Case Example: Louise

Background: Louise is a 58-year-old lesbian living in a rural community in central Pennsylvania. She has been coping with the death of her partner, Rachel, 6 months ago. The loss has proved difficult for Louise in many ways. She has not found the support and compassion she had anticipated from family and friends. In her grief, Louise did not anticipate all the things with which she would have to deal, including various financial issues and unexpected concerns about housing that came up following Rachel's death. In the midst of all this, Louise found her mood deteriorating. She told her primary care physician how difficult it was to fall asleep following Rachel's death. The physician gave her a prescription for a hypnotic sleep agent and made a referral to a nearby counseling center to further explore her mood symptoms.

When Louise met Rachel: Louise had grown up in rural Pennsylvania, raised by two Italian American parents who had moved there from Brooklyn, New York, in the early 1950s to open a small grocery store. She and her three sisters spent most of their childhood helping out around the store when not at school. In their strict Catholic home, the girls were raised to value hard work, perseverance, and sacrifice. As a teen, Louise had begun to have sexual feelings toward other women but did not know what to do with them. In her early twenties Louise had her first sexual encounter, with a woman she met at a state fair. She struggled with her sexual identity, experiencing various sexual encounters with both women and men, before accepting her homosexuality in her late thirties. She avoided telling her family about her sexuality until she was in her forties, and then did so only after much questioning from her sisters as to when she would start seriously dating and get married as they had all done. Following that disclosure, her parents were not at all supportive and refused to have a relationship with her. Her sisters were supportive, although they said they did not fully understand her feelings.

At age 40, Louise was working in a small business as a night cashier when she met Rachel at a local bar. They began dating 3 months later and moved into Rachel's home the following year. Rachel, who was the same age as Louise, had been previously married to a man and had two adult children who lived in the area. Louise found a new calm and happiness in this life. Her sisters met Rachel and often invited them both to barbeques and social functions. Rachel had a civil service job, and together they were able to maintain their home and take small road trips each year. Louise found it difficult to save any money for retirement on her salary. Both believed that Rachel's savings and pension from her job would support them in their retirement.

As they both approached age 55, Louise noticed Rachel becoming significantly more fatigued. At Rachel's yearly physical, her primary care physician found a lump in her left breast. Although devastated by Rachel's diagnosis of breast cancer, Louise assisted Rachel through a double mastectomy, chemotherapy, and radiation therapy. When it was discovered that Rachel's cancer had metastasized, Louise was supportive but often had a hard time expressing her own feelings related to Rachel's deterioration. Louise kept her sadness and fear to herself.

Rachel's last months of life involved more chemotherapy and radiation therapy, followed by a hospice admission for pain control. During this time, Rachel's children were often at odds with Louise over medical decision making and communications with hospital staff, even if ultimately they agreed. Louise's sisters and many of her friends encouraged her to defer to Rachel's children in these matters. Louise felt unimportant and unsupported. Rachel died of a pulmonary embolism 16 months after her initial diagnosis.

Starting treatment: Rachel's children had only minimally involved Louise in the planning of the funeral. She also felt that while the children received an outpouring of support for their loss, she received only terse condolences from others, including her sisters. Louise felt that people minimized the relationship that she and Rachel had shared. Rachel was often on her mind, and Louise had trouble envisioning a happy future without her. Louise accepted that Rachel was gone but still yearned for her. She at times felt guilty over not being able to save Rachel from her illness.

At the counseling appointment arranged for Louise by her physician, she met Becky, a social worker. In reporting the loss of her partner of 17 years, Louise said that in the 6 months since Rachel's death she found herself crying frequently without provocation. Although Louise was not comfortable telling strangers about her relationship with Rachel, she felt it important that Becky know the truth. She told Becky that whenever she attempted to share her feelings of loss and disclose the nature of her relationship she felt as if she was coming out again. She spoke of her religious conflict with her own sexuality and how this made it difficult to turn to her church for support. She remembered how she had been rejected by her congregation for being in a lesbian relationship. Rachel's death seemed to be a confirmation that her love for Rachel was a sin. Louise wondered if she should also die as a result of these feelings.

Louise reported that her work performance, while satisfactory, was not at her usual level. She felt people at work did not think of her loss as a big deal and told her to "just go out find someone else." She did not reach out to the few friends who did check on her, and she did not respond to messages her sisters left on her voice-mail. She had lost 15 pounds and had given up her exercise routine. She found it hard to fall asleep and often woke in the night with thoughts of Rachel.

Louise shared with Becky the emotional challenges she endured during Rachel's illness and death. She remembered being excluded by Rachel's children from medical decisions and feeling marginalized. She was shocked when the physicians tended to defer to the children during treatment discussions. She felt particularly hurt when she was not consulted on the funeral arrangements. She reported that Rachel's children were contesting all her claims to Rachel's estate. In the state where they resided, domestic partner legislation or marriage for same-sex couples did not exist (see Chapter 3 in this volume, "From Outlaws to In-Laws: Legal Standing of LGBT Americans' Family Relationships"). Louise said that she and Rachel never sought legal advice, fearing that they would not find a lawyer who would be understanding of their relationship. Without formalized legal arrangements Louise was left with no recourse for survivor benefits in regard to the savings that Rachel had built up for them.

Louise's case was presented at the Counseling Center's team meeting. It was decided that she should attend the bereavement support group led by Becky and have an evaluation with Dr. Smith, the staff psychiatrist. At their follow-up meeting, Becky explained that the process of grieving can touch on family, housing, financial, and spiritual issues as the living try to find a way forward without a loved one present. Louise agreed to attend the bereavement support group, although she feared that others would not be understanding of her loss. Dr. Smith and Louise met later that week to further evaluate her condition and decide if other treatment was needed in addition to the sleep agent provided by her physician.

Becky and Dr. Smith tried to determine how far beyond the boundary of normal bereavement Louise's symptoms had progressed. Attention focused on the extent of Louise's feelings of worthlessness or guilt, and her thoughts about death and suicide were assessed. She had difficulty with functional impairment, but it was not yet marked enough for others to notice. Dr. Smith felt that Louise exhibited symptoms that raised suspicion for complicated grief and warranted close, continued monitoring. The length of time of bereavement, her yearning for Rachel, and her preoccupation with death were particularly concerning.

Discussion

In the face of loss, clinicians are confronted with myriad signs and symptoms. Sadness, relief, and happiness can all be a part of normal bereavement, as can tearfulness, isolation, trouble with concentration, hearing the deceased's voice, or even seeing the deceased briefly. Some of these overlap with symptoms that clinicians associate with major depressive disorder (MDD). It is therefore critical to determine a patient's baseline level of mental health along with past history and family history of psychiatric illness. Louise told Becky and Dr. Smith that she had no known history of psychiatric illness but that she suspected her mother had mild depression. If the focus of psychological symptoms is not restricted solely to the grieved and includes other domains of a patient's life, then greater clinical suspicion of a major depressive episode should be entertained (see Table 20–1). Somatic symptoms that can be associated with MDD, such as changes in appetite, weight, sleep, and energy level, are also common in bereavement. Patients may seek assistance for these somatic symptoms, as Louise did when she spoke with her primary care physician about her sleep disturbance. If these symptoms are found to be related to bereavement, not to another mood disorder, the patient may nonetheless benefit from intervention. Increased frequency of visits with the clinician, support groups, grief counseling, individual therapy, and family therapy can all be considered. Antidepressants are not recommended in cases of normal bereavement. Hypnotics may be considered for brief periods to aid with insomnia.

Many of the signs of acute grief and bereavement are part of the natural process of healing and resolve with the passage of time. If they persist and impair functioning, as happened with Louise, clinical focus should be directed to evaluating for MDD and complicated grief. These two disorders carry significant morbidity and may require different treatment. Generally, if criteria for an MDD episode exist 2 months following the death, a depressive episode can be diagnosed and treated. This differs from what some have called complicated grief, in which the patient exhibits more severe and debilitating bereavement symptoms.

Complicated grief, known alternatively as prolonged grief reaction, is a disorder in which diagnostic criteria and best treatment practices are evolving. It is not included in DSM-IV-TR (American Psychiatric Association 2000) but may be considered for inclusion in DSM-5 (American Psychiatric Association 2010). Clinical criteria for complicated grief vary between research groups. Diagnostic screens such as the International Complicated Grief (ICG) tool and the Texas Revised Inventory of Grief can be helpful to assess for the presence and severity of symptoms. In general, criteria sets include a constellation of symptoms lasting more than 6 months that include a sense of disbelief regarding the death; anger and bitterness over the death; recurrent pangs of painful emotions, with intense yearning and longing for the deceased; and preoccupation with thoughts of the loved one, often including distressing intrusive thoughts related to the death (Shear et al. 2005). The incidence of complicated grief seen in study samples ranges from 10% to 20%. High comorbidity is also seen with major depressive disorder (21%–54%) and posttraumatic stress disorder (30%–50%); some groups consider complicated grief to have symp-

---

TABLE 20–1. Bereavement (DSM-IV-TR, V62.82)

This category should be used when the focus of clinical attention is reaction to the death of a loved one. As part of their reaction to the loss, some grieving individuals present with symptoms characteristic of a major depressive episode (e.g., feelings of sadness and associated symptoms such as insomnia, poor appetite, and weight loss). The bereaved individual typically regards the depressed mood as "normal," although the person may seek professional help for relief of associated symptoms such as insomnia or anorexia. The duration and expression of "normal" bereavement vary considerably among different cultural groups. The diagnosis of major depressive disorder is generally not given unless the symptoms are still present 2 months after the loss. However, the presence of certain symptoms that are not characteristic of a "normal" grief reaction may be helpful in differentiating bereavement from a major depressive episode. These include 1) guilt about things other than actions taken or not taken by the survivor at the time of the death; 2) thoughts of death other than the survivor feeling that he or she would be better off dead or should have died with the deceased person; 3) morbid preoccupation with worthlessness; 4) marked psychomotor retardation; 5) prolonged and marked functional impairment; and 6) hallucinatory experiences other than thinking that he or she hears the voice of, or transiently sees the image of, the deceased person.

Source. Reprinted from *Diagnostic and Statistical Manual of Mental Disorders,* 4th Edition, Text Revision. Washington, DC, American Psychiatric Association, 2000. Used with permission. Copyright © 2000 American Psychiatric Association.

tom clusters from each of these two disorders and propose then that it is a distinct clinical entity (Shear et al. 2011).

Standard treatments for depression have been evaluated for complicated grief (Shear et al. 2011). Nortriptyline and bupropion have not demonstrated efficacy in open-label studies, whereas there is evidence of potential benefit from serotonergic agents. Interpersonal psychotherapy (IPT) and a cognitive-behavioral-model psychotherapy for complicated grief (CGT) have been studied head to head in a randomized clinical trial. The CGT treatment group showed better response than the IPT group, although both groups showed improvement. Notably, 45% of the study subjects were also taking antidepressant medication, and patients in the CGT arm and taking antidepressants showed the best response (Shear et al. 2005).

Treatment and recovery: Louise fit well into the bereavement support group. She found a kinship with those undergoing similar significant losses. Although Louise found her participation in the support group a way to remain connected and to address her issues of loss, she continued to experience significant feelings of depression and otherwise felt isolated. Dr. Smith continued to note Louise's chronic feelings of depression and episodes of tearfulness. Louise reported that it remained a struggle to get out of bed to go to work, or to do much of anything, as nothing was very pleasurable. She also said that she still felt her work performance remained below her previous levels, noting difficulty with focus. Dr.

Smith suggested a combination of therapy and medication to address her continuing feelings of depression. It was agreed that starting weekly individual cognitive therapy and escitalopram 10 mg daily were warranted. In the following 4 months, Louise noticed a marked improvement in her mood, she gradually found it easier to go to work, and she began accepting invitations from friends to go to dinner and the movies. Though she still missed Rachel every day, it was refreshing that she could think of her and the happy times that they had shared.

Louise wound up having to move out of the home she had shared with Rachel as a result of further conflicts with Rachel's children. The children gave Louise a small amount of money that allowed her to rent a small home near one of her friends. Louise reported that she was starting to reconnect with other friends and her sisters. She had also begun to do some reading related to her religious beliefs that allowed her to explore her feelings in the context of those beliefs. Louise felt grateful for the care she had received at the counseling center but knew that the years ahead still would present struggles. Louise said she now felt strong enough to face these struggles.

Key Points

- The existence of "chosen families" in the lesbian, gay, bisexual, and transgender (LGBT) community means that partners and friends often play the role of primary caregivers to someone dying. Clinician awareness of this will help when key health care decisions need to be made and will facilitate the support and interaction that both the dying individual and the chosen family need (Almack et al. 2010).

- There are unique psychosocial issues that affect both how loss is experienced in the LGBT community and how bereavement progresses.

- Clinicians should evaluate for complicated grief or MDD during the bereavement process and, if these conditions are present, direct patients to appropriate treatment interventions.

References

Almack K, Seymour J, Bellamy G: Exploring the impact of sexual orientation on experiences and concerns about end of life care and on bereavement for lesbian, gay, and bisexual older people. Sociology 44:908–924, 2010

American Psychiatric Association: Diagnostic and Statistical Manual of Mental Disorders, 4th Edition, Text Revision. Washington, DC, American Psychiatric Association, 2000, p 740

American Psychiatric Association: DSM-V: conditions proposed by outside sources. 2010. Available at: http://www.dsm5.org/PROPOSEDREVISIONS/Pages/ConditionsProposedbyOutsideSources.aspx. Accessed November 14, 2011.

Shear K, Frank E, Houck P, et al: Treatment of complicated grief: a randomized controlled trial. JAMA 21:2601–2608, 2005

Shear MK, Simon N, Wall M, et al: Complicated grief and related bereavement issues for DSM-5. Depression and Anxiety 28:103–117, 2011

Questions

20.1   Normal bereavement can include which of the following signs and symptoms?

    A. Sadness.
    B. Tearfulness.
    C. Relief.
    D. Insomnia.
    E. Reduced appetite.
    F. All of the above.

The correct answer is F.

A patient coping with the death of a loved one can present in various ways, and the response can fluctuate over time. Clinicians should remain vigilant for signs that something beyond normal bereavement is occurring.

20.2   Which of the following can affect bereavement in the LGBT community?

    A. Being asked not to attend the funeral.
    B. Eviction from a shared home.
    C. Being included in all end-of-life decisions.
    D. Denial of claims for survivor benefits.
    E. Legal recognition of a partnership or marriage.
    F. All of the above.

The correct answer is F.

Customary spiritual, financial, and legal arrangements, which may be issues during bereavement, can present stronger challenges for the LGBT bereaved. By keeping current on local and national legislative LGBT issues that may affect their patients, clinicians will better understand the relevance and influence of these issues during bereavement.

Occupational Problem

The Case of Iris: Occupational Problems in the LGBT Community

SHANE S. SPICER, M.D.
LAURA ERICKSON-SCHROTH, M.D., M.A.

LESBIAN, GAY, BISEXUAL, AND TRANSGENDER (LGBT) people are often faced with stress in the workplace that can lead to problems with attendance, and performance, as well as depression, anxiety, and other emotional and behavioral difficulties. Workplace stressors faced by the LGBT community are often different from those of the general population. Although many people still experience being terminated from or demoted at work because of their actual or perceived sexual orientation or gender identity, many more people are subject to more subtle, yet often overwhelming, workplace difficulties. These include feeling isolated and fearful of being discovered as a sexual minority in a nontolerant environment, being subjected to homophobic or transphobic comments or jokes, and experiencing internal conflict about if, when, and how to come out in a workplace environment. In this chapter, the case of Iris, a transgender woman, illustrates some of these types of workplace stressors. The relevant description from DSM-IV-TR (American Psychiatric Association 2000) is included in Table 21–1.

It will be helpful to define some terms and concepts used in this chapter. *Gender* is a culturally constrained concept including the combination of social, psychological, and emotional traits associated with masculinity or femininity.

TABLE 21–1.   Occupational problem (DSM-IV-TR, V62.2)

This category can be used when the focus of clinical attention is an occupational
    problem that is not due to a mental disorder or, if it is due to a mental disorder, is
    sufficiently severe to warrant independent clinical attention. Examples include job
    dissatisfaction and uncertainty about career choices.

Source.   Reprinted from *Diagnostic and Statistical Manual of Mental Disorders,* 4th Edition, Text
Revision. Washington, DC, American Psychiatric Association, 2000. Used with permission.
Copyright © 2000 American Psychiatric Association.

Gender identity relates to someone's internal sense of being male, female, or
something else. *Gender expression* refers to how people demonstrate their gender to the outside world through things like clothing, behaviors, and appearance. In contrast to gender, *sex* describes someone's genetic and anatomical expression of being male, female, or something else. *Sexual orientation* describes
whether someone is attracted to same-sex partners, opposite-sex partners, both,
or neither.

   Transgender is often used as an umbrella term to describe those whose gender identity or gender expression falls outside of typical cultural expectations.
Commonly, transgender is used to refer to someone whose gender identity (or
gender expression) and sex are discordant with each other or do not conform to
social norms. For example, if someone is born in a genetically and anatomically
female body but has an internal identity of being male, this person may identify
as transgender. Some transgender people make changes to their bodies using
hormones or sexual reassignment surgeries to *transition* their physical features
to align with their gender identity. Often, terms such as *trans woman* and male-
to-female (MTF) are used to describe someone born anatomically as a man, but
identifying as a woman, whereas *trans man* and female-to-male (FTM) are used
to describe someone born anatomically as a woman, but identifying as a man.
Sometimes people do not identify as *trans,* but feel that they are simply a *man* or
woman, and that they were always this gender. Another term that some people
use to describe their gender-nonconforming identity is *genderqueer,* a word that
conveys more of a sense of being between two genders. It is important to note
that gender identity and sexual orientation are different concepts; transgender
individuals can be heterosexual, homosexual, bisexual, or something else.

Case Example: Iris

Initial presentation: Iris is a 34-year-old single African American trans woman
who entered a court-mandated intensive outpatient addiction treatment program because of cocaine and alcohol use as well as recurrent arrests related to
prostitution.

   During her first visit to the program, Iris was guarded and hostile with the
staff. She created quite a commotion in the waiting area and was quick to point

out that she had been in many jails, psychiatric clinics, and substance use treatment programs throughout her life and had never found any of them useful. "It's always the same thing. Nobody ever knows what it's like to live my life." However, when she noticed that the front desk staff and social worker doing the intake consistently used her preferred female name and pronoun, she became more comfortable. Although Iris was reluctant to disclose her history, during the course of the intake interview she began to appear a bit more relaxed. At one point she looked around the office at the trans-affirmative signs and flyers posted on the walls and commented that this was the first time she had ever been in an LGBT-affirmative treatment program. "I never knew places like this existed."

Mental status examination: When she first arrived, Iris was wearing a short skirt, a tube top, and high-heeled sandals. She was well nourished and appeared older than her stated age. Her hair was well coiffed, she had long, painted fingernails, and she was wearing makeup and gold jewelry. She vacillated from being very flirtatious and engaged to being easily upset and offended. Her speech was loud at times, and she had a pronounced southern accent. She described her mood as "pissed" because she had to come to this treatment program, and her affect was full, irritable, and appropriate to content. Her thinking was goal-directed, and there was no evidence of psychosis, suicidal ideation, or homicidal ideation. Her cognition was not impaired, and she had fair intelligence. Her insight was fair, and her judgment was fair to poor.

Background information: When asked about her reason for seeking treatment at the program, she said, "Honestly, I'm here because the court says I have to be here. I'm not sure I'm even addicted to drugs. I probably use more than I should, but you would, too, if you had to sleep with the men that I sleep with!" Iris went on to describe how closely related her substance use was with her current sex work. She often drank alcohol prior to doing sex work, about 2–3 drinks, 3–4 days per week, and smoked crack cocaine with her clients approximately once weekly. She stated that she used substances only during her work. Although she bought alcohol for herself, she used crack cocaine only when her customers provided it. She had a history of multiple past rehab admissions, incarcerations, and psychiatric hospitalizations—all typically due to either needing shelter or having used substances in the context of sex work. She denied current and past withdrawal symptoms and stated that she had never been in ongoing outpatient psychiatric or substance use treatment.

Iris moved from her hometown in rural Georgia to New York City prior to graduating from high school, with the hope of living in a more tolerant and welcoming environment. Although she stated she had always been feminine and "felt like a woman," she did not begin to live and dress as a woman until she moved to New York City. Her father, who was alcohol dependent, had physically abused her throughout her life "for being a sissy boy." Her mother and younger brother had tried to keep in contact with her after she moved to New York, but they had stopped communicating with her over the past few years after learning about her recurrent incarcerations for prostitution. She was from a very religious family, and although her mother and brother loved her even though she was "different," they could not understand why she worked as a prostitute.

"That was too much for them. They just couldn't accept that I was doing the devil's work."

Once arriving in New York City, Iris was able to transition to living as a woman. She slowly met some other trans women in the city and learned where she could receive hormone injections on the streets. She was eventually invited to "pumping parties" where she could receive injections of silicone, which helped give her the curves and shapely body that she found appealing. Over the years, she found temporary housing either in single-resident occupancies (SROs), with friends, or with older, wealthier men who supported her with food and housing in exchange for sex. She often found herself homeless, and she recalled being unwelcome in both male and female shelters, frequently needing to sleep in parks and on the streets. She quickly realized that it was very difficult to get a "real job" as a trans woman. "Nobody wants a tranny working for them. People get scared about how others are going to react." Although she had been able to assume a more feminine appearance and was able to "pass" for the most part, she still had a prominent Adam's apple, which she had not been able to afford to have surgically altered. In addition, many of her legal documents still had her male name and male gender listed, which was difficult to explain to prospective employers. "Then if I actually was able to get hired somewhere, there would always be talk. Somebody would end up having an issue with me. So I turned to working the streets. It pays well when I get the work, and they *want* me there. It's a hard life…but a few cocktails make it a little less painful."

Participation in treatment: While in the program, Iris slowly integrated into the treatment milieu and used groups and counseling effectively. At first she was quite irritable, anxious, and easily upset in groups and was referred to see the staff psychiatrist. She was found to have an underlying posttraumatic stress disorder (PTSD), which was effectively managed with psychopharmacological interventions and psychotherapy. She adhered to court mandates such as random urine toxicology screenings, which were negative. With motivational interviewing, she began to identify that her substance use was at times causing difficulties in her life, and she became more invested in her recovery and treatment. As she had not seen a medical provider outside of jail settings in more than 15 years, she was referred to an LGBT-affirmative community health clinic where she received testing for HIV, hepatitis, syphilis, and other medical problems. She was relieved to find that she had not contracted any sexually transmitted diseases despite occasionally having barrier-free sex during her sex work. With these results, she felt empowered and more motivated to have safer sex moving forward. She was eventually engaged in primary care and was initiated and monitored on appropriate hormone treatment.

Throughout her treatment, Iris maintained housing in an SRO. She was gaining new skills and engaging in a welcoming community, and she remained optimistic about "getting my life together" until growing frustrated in her job search. Despite applying for work at trans-affirmative organizations and working with a legal aid program to help change her documents to her female name and gender, she continued to have difficulty finding gainful employment. She began to express to her substance use counselor her desires to return to doing sex work until she was able to find other work. She explained her motivation to do this as not wanting to spend all of the money she had been saving for sexual reassignment surgeries. Although she and her counselor identified this as a potential trigger for relapsing on substances of abuse as well as placing her in danger, she decided to move forward using sex work in a "safe, cautious way."

However, just prior to returning to sex work, Iris received a call offering her a job in a temporary firm as a receptionist in a medical clinic. She was very eager to work and attended her job consistently. Although she aimed to please her supervisor, she was written up repeatedly by coworkers over issues such as dressing inappropriately or being unprofessional with patients. Iris felt strongly that these complaints were unfounded and simply a way to get her fired. She was concerned that a nurse at the clinic had suspicions that she was a trans woman. The nurse would frequently make comments about Iris's "large hands" and Adam's apple in front of the other staff. Eventually, the nurse managed to recruit other coworkers to stop speaking to and socializing with Iris at work. After some time the other office staff became quite hostile toward Iris, and to Iris's disappointment, she found that her supervisor was not supportive. Her supervisor encouraged her to quit, stating that she felt that Iris was "not the right kind of person for the job." Iris did eventually resign from her job as a result of discrimination based on her gender identity.

Iris had extreme feelings of hopelessness and was fearful that she might never be capable of successfully working outside of the sex industry. She explained to her counselor that she was going to return to sex work, but agreed to continue attending the program and to remain abstinent from substances of abuse. Iris's attendance in the program became more inconsistent. At first she was not responding to outreach calls and letters, and then it was discovered that her cell phone was disconnected and that she was no longer living at the SRO listed in her chart. On speaking with the case manager who was coordinating her court-mandated treatment, the program staff learned that Iris had been found to have urine toxicology results consistent with alcohol and cocaine use twice over the past week and was incarcerated. Iris has not yet returned for treatment at the program.

Discussion

Transgender Mental Health

This case illustrates many of the common mental health concerns within the transgender community. Trans communities have a long history of interaction with psychiatry, and this contact has frequently involved diagnosis of transgender people with a mental illness due solely to their transgender status. Many mental health care providers currently use the DSM diagnosis of gender identity disorder to describe transgender experience. Because of the stigma of assignment with a mental illness, and also because of the psychiatrist's historical role as gatekeeper to accessing hormone treatment and sexual reassignment surgeries, many transgender people are suspicious of the mental health care system and avoid psychiatric care unless absolutely necessary. Even when motivated to seek care, transgender patients often worry that providers are not properly trained to treat them. Their concerns are valid, as transgender health care is not a required part of medical school curricula and few psychiatry residency programs provide education and training on the needs of this population.

One of the most notable parts of Iris's story is her remarkable change in attitude about being in a program as she engaged in treatment. She progressed from "guarded and hostile" to attending groups regularly, engaging in primary care, and finding a job. When first presenting, she was precontemplative in regard to identifying her substance use as a problem, stating, "I'm here because the court says I have to be here. I'm not sure I'm even addicted to drugs." However, by employing motivational interviewing techniques, Iris was able to identify how her substance use was at times causing problems and getting in the way of her achieving her ultimate goals. She eventually became more invested in discontinuing her alcohol and crack cocaine use with the hope of having a brighter future by doing so. It might have been easy early on for providers to label Iris as "difficult to treat." However, she responded with increasing trust as she was confronted with a respectful, understanding environment. It is important to allow adequate time for engagement and rapport building. As mental health providers learn more about transgender people and begin to develop more positive relationships with trans patients, transgender community members will begin to see psychiatric care as a more positive and helpful option in their lives.

Transgender people can face the same mental health issues as all people and can have any DSM diagnosis. For example, just because someone has a psychotic disorder does not mean that they cannot *also* have a transgender identity. There are, of course, instances in which psychotic disorders can cause patients to have delusions involving gender, but like anyone else, transgender people can have schizophrenia, bipolar disorder, borderline personality disorder, or any other possible diagnosis. In general, there is very little research on transgender mental health. Few studies directly address rates of mental illness in transgender people as compared with the general population, but those that do exist suggest that transgender patients may have increased rates of depression, substance use disorders, body image issues, and eating disorders (Spicer 2010).

Mental health concerns may disproportionately affect transgender people because of their experiences living within a culture that is not tolerant of and is often hostile toward their sense of self. Trans people face *transphobia,* which is discrimination against transgender and transsexual individuals. Like Iris, gender-variant people may experience greater levels of childhood trauma than some other groups, and this can often lead to mental health sequelae as adults. In retrospective studies of transgender people, high levels of childhood abuse, both physical and sexual, were reported (Veale et al. 2009). It is likely that gender-variant children are recognized by others at an early age and targeted for abuse. Iris describes being abused by her father "for being a sissy boy." Transgender people often face rejection, social isolation, and sometimes violence as they continue to develop into youths and then adults.

Our patient, Iris, has experienced incarcerations and involvement in the legal system. Corrections environments can be particularly difficult for transgender people, as they are often targeted for violence and rape. Further, officers may not report or intervene in such activities, whether in the mistaken belief that the person enjoys such behavior or due to frank discrimination. In some cases, police are involved in brutality and sexual violence against transgender people. In addition, sexual minorities may be arrested more often than others for the same crimes, or arrested for crimes they have not committed.

Likewise, our nation's shelter systems often are not equipped to provide safe accommodations for transgender people, and trans people can be exposed to the same sort of perilous situations as in prison. Both transgender women and men are often harassed or not permitted in women's shelters and can be at risk for violence and rape in men's shelters.

A number of studies have shown increased rates of depression and suicidality in transgender individuals (Spicer 2010), and one demonstrated a relationship between abuse and subsequent major depressive episodes and suicidal ideation (Nuttbrock et al. 2010). There is anecdotal evidence that some transgender people diagnosed with depression achieve symptom remission and no longer require medication after they transition, suggesting that for some people, depression is situational. Suicide rates may also decrease after transition (Pfafflin and Junge 1998). Some research demonstrates that transgender individuals experience suicidal ideation and attempts out of proportion with their levels of mental illness, indicating that something other than depression, such as the extenuating social circumstance of living as a transgender person, causes transgender people to commit suicide in increased numbers (Terada et al. 2011).

Problematic drug and alcohol use is also a common issue for transgender people. Substance and alcohol use is a coping strategy for many people, transgender or not, and trans people are often faced with numerous social stressors, social isolation, and lack of trans-affirmative mental health care. In addition, because of increased rates of unemployment and homelessness, transgender people are often in situations where those around them are abusing alcohol and substances. Many times, substance abuse treatment programs lack staff that are sensitive to and knowledgeable about transgender-specific concerns. Substance use treatment programs frequently include group treatment modalities. In order to receive the benefits of this type of intervention, people must be able to be open and honest about their lives and substance use. Often, trans people are not comfortable discussing such details in mainstream programs because of a lack of understanding or support from other treatment program members and/or staff.

Although it might seem quite obvious, an area of mental health that is often overlooked in transgender people is their body image and relationship to their bodies. Transgender individuals may develop eating disorders in an attempt to control bodies that they are unhappy in. Some transgender patients also engage in self-harm behaviors. Some people cut themselves in areas that represent their nonchosen gender. For example, trans men may cut their chests and trans women may cut their genitals. It is important to ask clients about their relationships to their bodies and whether they have engaged in any of these behaviors.

When providing treatment for transgender clients, it is essential to be understanding, open, respectful, and willing to provide thoughtful care. Given the long history of trauma and rejection that many transgender clients have experienced, being shown respect can not only help with engagement and communication, but also be powerfully therapeutic in repairing the damage caused by past traumas they may have experienced within the health care system. When first meeting with someone, ask what that person prefers in terms of gender, name, and pronoun, and record this specifically on the chart for future reference. Respect your clients' wishes regarding using their preferred gender, preferred name, and preferred pronoun in conversation, independent of their anatomical sex or surgical status. As in the case with Iris, simply using the client's appropriate pronouns and name can help the person feel more comfortable and be more apt to engage in treatment.

Whether working as an individual practitioner or as part of a large hospital or organization, it can be useful to take an inventory to assess how *trans-affirmative* your practice is in *relational* and *structural* terms.

Relationally, one can establish a guideline that all practitioners become familiar with the gender, pronoun, and name that their clients prefer. It is important that no one make assumptions about behaviors or bodies based on initial presentations. It can be very helpful to practice using gender-neutral language such as asking about a "partner" or "significant other" instead of boyfriend or wife. It is of great importance to learn from your clients. When appropriate, reflect your patient's terminology for sexual behavior and anatomy and ask for clarification when necessary.

Simple structural changes in an organization or practice can make transgender clients feel much more welcomed. For example, including LGBT information on brochures and educational materials sets a tone that being a sexual minority can be acknowledged and discussed in the program. In addition, it can be helpful to post and enforce a nondiscrimination policy, which includes gender identity/expression. As was helpful in the case with Iris, openly displaying signs of LGBT acceptance clearly identifies that the organization is a safe space for LGBT people and will foster better communication and engagement. Also, forms and paperwork used by staff should at minimum allow "transgender" options when recording gender, as well as a place to record "preferred name" and "legal name." It is important to be open about positive messages towards transgender people in particular, because even within LGBT organizations, transgender individuals may face discrimination from lesbian, gay, and bisexual groups.

In addition, when providing care for transgender clients one must pay attention to issues regarding access to care. It can be helpful to become aware of useful transgender and trans-affirmative resources in your community. Be familiar with insurance and legal issues involved in transgender care and create relationships with other trans-affirmative providers and organizations for support and referral streams. When referring a client to a vocational program or a medical or mental health care provider, be certain that transgender clients will feel safe and receive appropriate care in that setting. Sometimes it is useful to first call or visit an organization to inquire about their ability to provide trans-affirmative services. Help clients with the referral and provide support and follow-up regarding their engagement as indicated.

LGBT Occupational Problems

While this case discusses a transgender patient, occupational problems affect all groups within the LGBT community. The DSM category of "occupational problem" can be used when the focus of clinical attention is an occupational problem that is not due to a mental disorder or, if it is due to a mental disorder, is sufficiently severe to warrant independent clinical attention. As is evident in Iris's case, the formality of a workplace does not necessarily protect people from being harassed by colleagues, and daily abuse at a place where someone spends a good portion of their day can be greatly distressing. People do not always overtly discriminate against LGBT coworkers or employees, but may hide the true reason for not hiring, demoting, not promoting, or firing an LGBT person. Employers may use vague complaints about job performance or personality characteristics to put forward an alternative reason for the action. For example, Iris was told she was "not the right kind of person for the job."

Although much workplace discrimination against LGBT people is covert, people are still openly fired because of their actual or perceived sexual orientation or gender identity. The media has recently been attuned to the multiple elementary school teachers who have been fired for this reason. Current laws in many states allow employers to discriminate on the basis of sexual orientation and gender identity in their hiring and firing processes. The Employment Non-Discrimination Act (ENDA) is a proposed federal bill that would protect against this type of discrimination. Early on, controversy around ENDA involved the fact that the original bill did not include protection based on gender identity. In addition to transgender people, many gay, lesbian, and bisexual people are the objects of discrimination based on their gender presentation (e.g., butch lesbians, effeminate gay men), and an expanded bill could protect them as well.

LGBT people often struggle in the workplace because of issues surrounding coming out. People who work in careers or workplaces that are not tolerant of sexual minorities feel conflicted regarding how to balance being authentically themselves with being successful at work. Sometimes the conflict is more de-rived from the person, the fears and anxieties more related to the internalized homophobia or transphobia held by the individual. However, in other situa-tions, the workplace can actually be overtly or covertly homophobic or trans-phobic, with potential occupational and financial consequences if the person comes out or is outed by others. Frequently, situations are more complicated and the anxiety about coming out at work results from a combination of inter-nal and potential external conflicts, so there must be a careful process of exam-ining the risks and benefits of coming out at work. If someone strongly desires to come out but coming out in a certain workplace could be dangerous or un-manageable, treatment may include linkage to legal and advocacy resources, as well as to other career opportunities.

For transgender people in particular, there are specific concerns related to em-ployment that do not necessarily apply to other LGBT people. The case of Iris highlights some of the unique experiences and challenges for transgender people in the working world. When someone is commonly read by others as transgender, it can sometimes invite ridicule and hostility in our culture and can make one a target of attack. It may also affect trans persons' self-esteem by reminding them that they are not seen as they see themselves. Iris is a transgender woman and may have some residual male physical characteristics due to changes she experienced with male puberty: an Adam's apple, a deeper voice, male-typical height, and male-typical body hair growth. Trans clients will sometimes discuss whether they "pass" or not—meaning, whether they appear as their identified gender to others.

Many transgender people spend years dealing with the internal and external conflicts of coming out in a culture that is not tolerant of gender nonconfor-mity. This can not only lead to mental health issues, as discussed in the previous section, but can also result in leaving school prior to graduation and having un-steady employment, preventing the building of skills and confidence necessary for stable, legal work. When beginning to seek out legal work, many people do not have the appropriate wardrobe (or the funds for this wardrobe) to match their appearance, and also may be unaware of the subtleties of professional dress and mannerisms required of their gender. For example, Iris is written up by co-workers for "dressing inappropriately." Often, in helping clients with these sorts of occupational stressors, linkage to concrete vocational services for guidance and support in building a professional wardrobe can be very important.

For those who have already built careers in their previously assigned gender, one major obstacle is that their degrees and past employment history remain un-der their prior name and gender. Reference providers may be unaware of the tran-sition. Those who wish to keep their transition private may not be able to include significant education or work experience on their resumes without outing them-selves. In addition, many professions require background checks, which would lead to being outed whether a person wanted this or not. In some cases, coming out or being outed can lead to losing one's job in a particular field and not being able to return to that field of work. Frequently, the professional networks that people have cultivated over the years contain people who are not as supportive once someone transitions. When working with trans clients in such situations, it is very useful to help clients locate legal and practical support in navigating name and gender changes on legal and educational documents. One can also work with clients to find trans-affirmative professional contacts, mentors, and community supports to help with career changes and professional growth.

Some trans people seek new lines of work and have to essentially restart their professional lives when they transition. Transgender people seeking employment may also self-select out of certain fields, such as those with environments that hold the possibility of increased harassment or decreased safety. Sales and public service careers can expose people to many consumers per day, and the thought of this can be very frightening. Trans employees may also prioritize jobs that have health care benefits, as their health care needs may be very important to them as they transition.

Because of the challenges outlined in this chapter, transgender people often have difficulty finding and maintaining employment. This can lead to homelessness or marginal housing situations. According to research, one in five transgender people has unstable housing or is at risk or in need of shelter services (Minter and Daley 2003). In addition to employment difficulties, one of the many reasons that some transgender people find themselves struggling with homelessness is that their families often reject them. Studies show that up to 35% of homeless youths are LGBT (Cochran et al. 2002). Iris's childhood was difficult, but she seems to have a family that is willing to go to some lengths for her. While her mother and younger brother reached out to Iris to stay in touch despite her transition to female, they are heavily influenced by their own sense of morality and draw the line at prostitution. For someone like Iris, reestablishing a relationship with her family may be something to work towards, as family support, when possible, can be very powerful. Family acceptance of LGBT youth has been shown to improve self-esteem and general health status and to decrease depression and substance abuse (Ryan et al. 2010).

Employment difficulties can also lead transgender people to seek out illegal means of supporting themselves, such as engaging in sex work, as Iris does. In some cases, transgender women report being gratified by some aspects of sex work, as it can validate the desirability of their body and trans identity. Others, like Iris, would prefer not to do this work but believe it is their only option for making money. Sex work can be dangerous and can put transgender people, who are already at increased risk of violence, in unsafe situations. In addition, some transgender sex workers have a difficult time advocating for, or negotiating, the use of condoms in their work. In this case, because Iris uses substances primarily in the context of sex work, one of the most important interventions in addressing her substance use is to help her engage in alternative modes of work. Unfortunately, Iris is involved in sex work because she sees no other way to survive financially, so in her case it may be difficult for her to stop using substances unless her work situation can be successfully altered.

In addition to being a sexual minority, many LGBT people also face additional workplace stressors and barriers to employment. For example, transgender *women* face both transphobia and traditional sexism. Transition brings about differences in the way trans women are treated by others, including blatant transphobia, but also experiences similar in some ways to those of non-transgender women—being seen as less smart and capable than men. In addition, trans women experience what writer Julia Serano calls "trans-misogyny," which is when transphobia and sexism combine to cause a type of discrimination that is a unique experience for transgender women. Jokes, sexual remarks, and harassment are based on other people's extreme upset at seeing a "man" expressing femininity.

Compared with other transgender people, Latina and African American trans women, like Iris in this case, have increased difficulty accessing health care and have been found to have higher rates of HIV infection. Trans people of color face not only discrimination from the non-transgender world, but also from within the mainstream trans community. Even programs designed specifically for LGBT people do not necessarily take into account the specific needs of LGBT people of color.

Financial difficulties and unemployment also result in lack of insurance coverage, and for transgender people this can lead to the use of street hormones. For trans men, this may mean the use of unsafe needles or unregulated amounts of testosterone, which can result in liver problems. For trans women, using too much estrogen can lead to pulmonary emboli and death. Pumping parties, like the ones Iris attended, where women inject themselves with silicone to produce curves, may expose them to non-medical-grade silicone, problems with silicone migration causing misshapen bodies, contaminated needles carrying risk for infections, and emboli.

When LGBT people present with occupational problems, one should assess and offer treatment using a holistic approach. Clients should be evaluated for underlying psychiatric disorders and be offered individual treatment if indicated. In addition, social, vocational, educational, medical, and legal supports should be provided as necessary.

Conclusion

Like the general population, LGBT people often face challenging stressors in the workplace. However, as the case of Iris demonstrates, the occupational stressors affecting LGBT people are often unique to this population and deserve specific discussion. Iris's case not only illustrates how occupational problems can be quite distressing and problematic, but also portrays some specific needs and issues in the transgender community.

Although Iris was lost to contact at the end of the case, her story is still a hopeful one. While she was engaged in the addiction treatment program, she was able to find support, make significant changes in her behavior, and find relief from her psychiatric symptoms. When the program and providers she met with were respectful and provided holistic trans-affirmative care, Iris was able for the first time in her life to engage in medical care, a substance abuse program, and psychiatric treatment. Although her occupational problem was not fully resolved, she was able to gain some experience working legally. As is clear in this case, people do not live in a vacuum and should be offered individual care as well as linked to appropriate psychosocial, legal, and vocational resources as indicated. This case illustrates that even when addiction and psychiatric issues are addressed, occupational problems can greatly affect mental health.

Key Points

- LGBT people often face internal and external conflicts in the workplace due to overt and covert homophobia and transphobia. These occupational problems can lead to significant difficulties in people's lives, and they may benefit from mental health treatment as well as vocational, psychosocial, and sometimes legal interventions.

- When providing treatment for LGBT clients, it is necessary to use a holistic approach in order to address the many potential medical, psychological, social, legal, and occupational needs of the person in a community context.

- Transgender people face many barriers to accessing well-informed and trans-affirmative mental health care as well as other medical and psychosocial services. When getting to know a client, allow ample time for engagement because of possible past traumas, and make every effort to link the client to appropriate trans-affirmative care.

References

American Psychiatric Association: Diagnostic and Statistical Manual of Mental Disorders, 4th Edition, Text Revision. Washington, DC, American Psychiatric Association, 2000

Cochran BN, Stewart AJ, Ginzler JA, et al: Challenges faced by homeless sexual minorities: comparison of gay, lesbian, bisexual, and transgender homeless adolescents with their heterosexual counterparts. Am J Public Health 92:773–776, 2002

Minter S, Daley C: Trans realities: a legal needs assessment of San Francisco's transgender communities. 2003. Available at: http://www.transgenderlawcenter.org/trans/pdfs/Trans%20Realities%20Final%20Final.pdf . Accessed November 14, 2011.

Nuttbrock L, Hwang S, Bockting W, et al: Psychiatric impact of gender-related abuse across the life course of male-to-female transgender persons. J Sex Res 47:12–23, 2010

Pfafflin F, Jung A: Sex Reassignment: Thirty Years of International Follow-Up Studies SRS. A Comprehensive Review, 1961–1991. Dusseldorf, Germany, Symposium Publishing, 1998

Ryan C, Russell ST, Huebner D, et al: Family acceptance in adolescence and the health of LGBT young adults. J Child Adolesc Psychiatr Nurs 23:205–213, 2010

Serano J: Whipping Girl: A Transsexual Woman on Sexism and the Scapegoating of Femininity. Berkeley, CA, Seal Press, 2007

Spicer S: Healthcare needs of the transgender homeless population. Journal of Gay and Lesbian Mental Health 14:320–339, 2010

Terada S, Matsumoto Y, Sato T, et al: Suicidal ideation among patients with gender identity disorder. Psychiatry Res May 23, 2011 [Epub ahead of print]

Veale JF, Clarke DE, Lomax TC: Biological and psychosocial correlates of adult gender-variant identities: new findings. Pers Individ Diff 49:252–257, 2009

Questions

21.1 All of the following are true *except*

A. Currently there is no federal bill protecting employees against discrimination based on sexual orientation or gender identity.

B. Employers often use vague complaints about job performance to discriminate against LGBT people.

C. The majority of occupational problems faced by LGBT people are due to being fired based on their sexual orientation or gender identity.

D. Transgender people face some similar and some different challenges than other LGBT people in the workplace.

The correct answer is C.

Although many LGBT people do experience frank discrimination and terminations in the workplace, the vast majority are subject to more subtle workplace difficulties such as feeling isolated and fearful of being discovered as a sexual minority in a nontolerant environment, being subjected to anti-gay or anti-trans comments or jokes, and ongoing internal conflict about if, when, and how to come out in a workplace environment.

21.2 Which of the following is *not* a common reason for transgender people to have trouble accessing health care?

> A. Transgender people often feel uncomfortable in offices and clinics when they are unsure about whether the staff will respect their identities.
> B. Many transgender people have occupational problems that prevent them from obtaining health insurance to cover the costs of medical care.
> C. Even providers in LGBT health centers are sometimes not as well-trained in transgender health care as they are in gay, lesbian, and bisexual health care.
> D. Transgender people are not interested in engaging in health care programs and do not like mental health providers.

The correct answer is D.

Transgender people are often interested in maintaining good health, and some seek out mental health care, but there are cultural, personal, financial, and legal barriers to accessing appropriate medical and mental health treatment in the transgender community. All of these barriers are greatly influenced by the core issue of *transphobia*—the discrimination against transgender and transsexual individuals.

21.3 A new patient comes in to see you in your clinic. You have appropriately added a blank line for "gender" on your intake form, and the patient has written "transgender man." When the patient arrives for the first visit, you note that the individual is short, with cropped hair, wearing male-typical clothing, but has breasts. How do you address this patient?

> A. You should address this person as "Mr." or "Sir" since he is obviously indicating that he is male on his intake form.
> B. You should address this person as "Ms." or "Ma'am" since she has not yet had top surgery to remove her breasts.
> C. You should ask the patient to explain what pronouns they use and how they would prefer to be addressed because the patient is the best source for this information.
> D. Don't worry, you can address this person as either male or female because the patient is still in transition.

The correct answer is C.

When it is at all unclear, you should always ask the patient to tell you what pronouns they prefer and how they would like to be addressed. It is never a good idea to make assumptions. Just because someone is still physically transitioning does not mean they do not identify fully with their new gender. Many transgender people do not have surgery, for personal or financial reasons, and this does not necessarily say anything about how they identify. Other people identify as genderqueer and would prefer to be addressed with more gender-neutral language such as "they" rather than male or female pronouns.

Identity Problem

Doctor, Am I Gay? Identity Problems Associated With Homoerotism

Karine J. Igartua, M.D., C.M., F.R.C.P.C.(C)

WHEN INDIVIDUALS SEEK therapy because of conflicts or confusion about their sexual orientation, the DSM-IV-TR code for Identity Problem can be used (American Psychiatric Association 2000) (Table 22–1). Patients often consult our clinic searching for an identity label that fits how they feel (gay, lesbian, bisexual, queer...) but find it difficult to find a term that adequately captures their particular combination of physical and emotional attractions to men and women. When the layers of sexual behavior patterns, group identification, and cultural values are added, it may be impossible to find a satisfactory label. Therapy becomes less about finding or defining a label than about understanding oneself in terms of all these dimensions and feeling comfortable with where one falls within each.

The vignettes that follow are based on the stories of patients who consulted at the McGill University Sexual Identity Centre (MUSIC), a specialized outpatient psychiatric clinic dedicated to providing services to individuals, couples, and families with issues of sexual orientation (see www.mcgill.ca/cosum). The clinic treats people who are questioning their sexual orientation or are unhappy about it, individuals and couples seeking to improve their interpersonal relationships, and couples and families with concerns about a loved one's sexual orientation. The Centre's clientele reflects the multiculturalism of Montreal.

TABLE 22–1.   Identity problem (DSM-IV-TR, 313.82)

This category can be used when the focus of clinical attention is uncertainty about
multiple issues relating to identity such as long-term goals, career choice, friendship
patterns, sexual orientation and behavior, moral values, and group loyalties.

Source.   Reprinted from *Diagnostic and Statistical Manual of Mental Disorders*, 4th Edition, Text
Revision. Washington, DC, American Psychiatric Association, 2000. Used with permission.
Copyright © 2000 American Psychiatric Association.

Occasionally, individuals will present with obsessional doubt about their sexual orientation in the total absence of homoerotism. These individuals should be
investigated for obsessive-compulsive disorder, and most of the work will be standard treatment for OCD. This clinical situation is not the focus of this chapter,
which deals rather with identity problems related to homoerotism. (Obsessions are
discussed in Chapter 13 of this volume, "Obsessive-Compulsive Disorder.")

Case Example: Maria

Maria was a 53-year-old from Argentina who was married and the mother of
three teenagers. Despite discovering her husband's infidelities, she decided to
stay with him as the family was in the process of emigrating to Canada. She arrived in Montreal with her family 2 years prior to consulting at MUSIC. Because
her education was not recognized and her language skills in English were limited, she took a job in a factory. While working there, she developed an emotionally intense relationship with another woman, Katherine. This relationship
eventually became sexual, and Maria presented to the clinic stating: "I need to
figure out if I am a lesbian."

Maria felt a level of intimacy and emotional connection with Katherine that
she had never experienced before. Sex was equally satisfying. Prior to Katherine,
Maria had had one close relationship with another woman during her under-
graduate years, but there had never been any acknowledged sexual attraction on
either part. In general, Maria felt that her relationships with women were more
emotionally satisfying than her relationships with men. She believed that the
distance she felt with men may have come from the macho society in which she
was brought up. She felt angry that women were expected to be subservient to
men and did not accept the way women in general, and herself in particular,
were treated by the men in their lives. However, she had always felt sexually attracted to men, had previously only had sexual experiences with men, and fantasized exclusively about men.

Case Example: Thomas

Thomas was a 24-year-old university student who was in a relationship with Jenny
for 18 months. He had worried about "being gay" for the last 10 years, despite
having many satisfying romantic and sexual relationships with women. "Being
gay" was unacceptable to him because he wanted "a wife and children." He de-

scribed episodes of intense homoerotic fantasies accompanied by anxiety that led him to visit a sauna in order to have anonymous sex, which was strictly genital (no kissing, no talking). These experiences were followed by much self-recrimination and a depressed mood that could last up to 2 weeks, during which he would become convinced he was gay. He had other periods when the homoerotic impulses were not so present and he felt happy to be heterosexual. He had described these mood fluctuations to another psychiatrist and received a bipolar diagnosis. In a moment of emotional intimacy, he expressed his homoerotic impulses to his girl-friend. Jenny was quite open-minded, having grown up with a gay uncle, yet she became perturbed, wondering what this might mean for their future together.

It was in this context that Thomas presented to our clinic. On further exploration, it became clearer that the homoerotic impulses usually occurred in the context of unexpressed anger at his girlfriends. In his current relationship, he would at times feel frustrated but would not express his feelings for fear of losing Jenny. He would then have a homoerotic impulse, which he would act upon, then feel guilty about. This would lead him to want to separate from Jenny because of his "negative" sexuality.

Case Example: Theresa

Theresa was a 36-year-old customer service agent who lived alone but had been in a 10-year relationship with Marc. She presented to the clinic in a state of "crisis" because she had begun a sexual relationship with a woman. She stated that she loved Marc and had a sexually satisfying relationship with him. She was also content with the level of intimacy they shared and felt that he provided her with "stability and structure." She had no intention of leaving Marc, since she felt they were "right for each other." However, she had been aware of her same-sex eroticism since adolescence, had had many previous relationships with women, and described women as "HOT!" Though she had ignored these feelings for most of her relationship with Marc, this new experience with a woman had reignited her libido, and she no longer felt that she could give up this side of herself. Because she felt her greatest emotional connection was with Marc, a man, yet her sexual yearnings were more towards woman, she did not know how to define herself. Was she "gay, straight, or bisexual?"

Case Example: George

George was a 39-year-old second-generation Vietnamese Canadian who worked as a graphic designer for an advertising company. He presented to the clinic complaining of a lack of self-confidence. George identified as gay, although he did not like "the label." He complained that once one is labeled, "that is all people see." He was first aware of same-sex eroticism at age 12, and he dated girls briefly in high school but was never comfortable with physical intimacy with them. He came out to himself at age 18 and had his first same-sex romantic relationship at age 21. Since then, he had had half a dozen relationships, never lasting longer than 2 years. He had not told his parents about his sexual orientation, and his father continued to ask him when he would bring home a nice girl. He did not like being gay and expected rejection. In addition, he did not like being Vietnamese, as he felt this too had subjected him to ridicule. He thus had a negative identification as a "Gay-sian," wishing he were both Caucasian and heterosexual.

Case Example: Nadia

Nadia came to Canada from Lebanon at age 21 years to study engineering. She was financially supported by her family. She had always focused on her studies and excelled in school. She was never really interested in boys, and this gave her the image of the "good Muslim girl." At age 16, she had an intense emotional connection with her best friend, and this relationship became romantic and sexual. The two felt that their sexuality was "wrong," but the attachment was too strong to ignore. They fantasized about how they would find brothers to marry so that they could be a part of each other's families and continue to be together.

Once in Canada, Nadia was exposed to the concept that she could actually create a life for herself with a woman. This went against everything she knew. Not only was it culturally forbidden to be in a same-sex relationship, but also it was unacceptable to go against one's parents' wishes. If she was not to marry the chosen man, then she would at least be expected to return to Lebanon, live in the family home, and care for her parents.

While in university, she again fell in love with her best friend, and the two of them maintained a clandestine sexual relationship for 4 years. Once on the job market, she remained closeted at work, believing that she would lose contracts if her sexual orientation were known. In her thirties, she had three significant relationships with women lasting a couple of years each. She never dated boys.

Nadia was quite uncomfortable with the term *lesbian,* which she was unable to identify with. She associated the word with *man hater, tomboy,* and *sexually promiscuous,* none of which described her. The word was also connected with maternal disapproval, exile, sin, risk of corporal punishment, and even death.

Discussion

Patients often come to MUSIC with notions of gay, straight, and bisexual, as if they were three distinct categories and each human could easily be classified into one of them. The first part of our approach is therefore an exploration of the different dimensions of sexuality, and education about how these dimensions are distinct and not always concordant. Table 22–2 compares the five patients in terms of emotional intimacy, sexual attraction, and sexual behavior. Relevant cultural or religious attributes are also noted.

When sexual attraction, emotional intimacy, and sexual behavior all coincide as for Nadia and George, it is relatively easy to fit into one of the three categories, but for most patients, the overlap is not perfect. A study done in Montreal-area high schools in 2003 showed a lack of concordance between sexual behavior, attraction, and identity (Igartua et al. 2009). An earlier U.S. study found a similar pattern in adults (Laumann et al. 1994). Thus, many patients will have some difficulty recognizing themselves in the constrictive labels of "gay," "bisexual," or "straight." Learning this was quite reassuring for Thomas, Theresa, and Maria.

TABLE 22–2. Comparison of case examples along the different dimensions of sexual orientation

	Emotional intimacy	Sexual attraction/ fantasies	Sexual behavior	Cultural/ religious/ political	Identity
Maria	F	M	F ≥ M	Anger at men's mistreatment of women	?
Thomas	F	F ≥ M	F ≥ M	Expectation of nuclear family	Heterosexual
Theresa	M	F	M ≥ F	—	?
George	M ~ F	M	M	Double minority	"Gay-sian"
Nadia	F	F	F	Culturally nonexistent, religiously unacceptable	Uncomfortable with "lesbian"

Note. F = toward females; M = toward males.

For Thomas, learning this distinction between attraction, behavior, and identity was the most important step of therapy. Once he understood that heterosexually identified people can have same-sex attractions, and that his sexual behaviors were an expression of frustration and a means to free himself from what he felt was a suffocating relationship, he became more comfortable and certain of his heterosexual identity. He and Jenny continued together as a couple.

Theresa was also relieved by distinguishing behavior, attraction, and identity, and by the realization that there were different choices she could make. She had decided that she wanted to be coupled with Marc, whom she truly loved and depended on, but wanted to have sex with women. She identified as a lesbian who was committed to a man. Marc, who was as attached to her as she was to him, accepted Theresa's homoeroticism. He did not mind if she had sex with women, as long as he retained emotional primacy. They reviewed their couple contract and decided on an open relationship, where guidelines were put into place in order to protect the emotional bond between them.

Based on their feelings, behaviors, relationships, and socially taught conceptual frameworks, patients construct their identity. One doesn't just wake up one day with a gay identity. The concept that identity formation is a process is also a useful one for both patients and their family members.

Gay identity is a Western construct. In other cultures, men can have penetrative sex with other men without it meaning they are gay. In some parts of the world, a woman's self-definition is to be a wife and mother. For Nadia, having a life with a woman was not even a conceptual possibility. Contextualizing gay identity as a North American way of categorizing sexuality somehow made it less dogmatic for Maria. It afforded her the freedom to associate with the label or not. It also reduced the urgency of the questions about etiology: Why am I gay? She understood that "being gay" is an identity that is constructed given the right constellation of homoerotic feelings, same-sex intimacy, and sociocultural environment.

> As Maria progressed through therapy, it became clearer to her that her primary emotional and sexual attractions were toward women. She understood her lack of sexual experience with women as a limitation imposed by her culture of origin. She left her husband, and later, because of significant age and stage-of-life differences, she also left Katherine. The two have remained emotionally intimate, though Maria knows they have no future together because Katherine wants children and Maria has already raised her family. She no longer feels pressure to identify as lesbian or heterosexual, understanding that identity formation is a process. She feels that her next relationship is likely to be with a woman but has decided not to talk about her sexuality with her family until there is someone significant in her life.

Even when all dimensions of sexual orientation coincide, as with George and Nadia, there may still be discomfort and difficulty accepting the labels gay, lesbian, or bisexual because of the many negative associations these labels still carry. Using a stage model (Cass 1979), we teach patients about a graduated awareness of same-sex eroticism, understanding the potential implications of their attractions, grieving heterosexual privileges, undoing negative stereotypes about homosexuality (internalized homophobia), working through anger at having been made to feel illegitimate (through heterosexism and societal antigay bias), and finally accepting one's homoerotism and integrating it into a positive identity.

> For George, the components of sexual orientation converged fairly well: he understood himself as "gay." His difficulty lay more with his internalization of negative stereotypes about homosexuality, his erotophobia, and his desire never to make waves. During group work, he became aware of his own stereotypical belief that all gay men are "sluts, interested only in sex." He was able to see how this belief 1) made it difficult for him to develop a positive gay identity, because he did not want to identify as a "slut"; 2) inhibited him from enjoying his own sexuality, because when he had sex, he felt like a "slut"; and 3) kept him from investing emotionally with anyone, because of his belief that all gay men are "sluts" and thus incapable of meaningful relationships.
>
> He also came to understand the price he paid by not sharing his sexual orientation with his family. He longed for more closeness with his father but had kept all conversations superficial. After another group member came out to his parents, George gathered the courage to do the same. The response from his parents was not perfect, but it was far less rejecting than he had anticipated. He was encouraged that in time both he and his parents could develop a positive view of same-sex relationships. George is still in group therapy, where he is learning to be more assertive and to better identify and express his feelings.

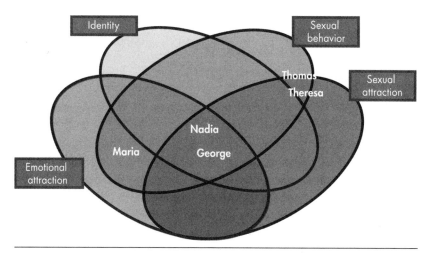

FIGURE 22–1. **Partial overlap of dimensions of sexual orientation.**

The various dimensions of sexual orientation (sexual attraction, emotional attraction, sexual identity, and sexual behavior) are independent and only partially overlapping. To illustrate, the five case examples in this chapter are placed on the diagram according to each one's particular confluence of the dimensions.

Nadia's difficulties, like George's, were not in understanding her sexual orientation, but rather in finding a way to accept it. She had ingrained religious beliefs that marred her self-esteem and relationships with women. Examining her relationship to and understanding of religion was necessary. Distinguishing the central tenets of her spirituality (being kind and generous, not hurting others) from some of the customs associated with her religion helped her. We also acknowledged the very real persecution that gay men and lesbians face in other countries. Ensuring her safe travels to different Arab countries to visit with her family became part of the therapy. Taking steps to protect herself made her feel that she did not deserve the persecution.

When patients present with identity problems related to their homoerotism, therapy progresses through three stages. In the beginning, we explore patients' dimensions of sexuality (emotional attraction, sexual attraction, behaviors, identity), and their familial and cultural restrictions on sexuality. This occurs along with psychoeducation about the dimensions, their nonperfect concordance (Figure 22–1), and the cultural underpinnings of "gay" identity.

During the second part of therapy, patients are made aware that creating one's sexual identity is a process. Part of that process is identifying and addressing the patient's own homophobia. At MUSIC, we have developed a 6-week cognitive-behavioral therapy (CBT)–based group treatment program aimed at reducing the distress from internalized antigay bias. The group format is useful because it increases the sense of normalcy by sharing similar experiences relative to homophobia and heterosexism and to understanding how these two concepts—and not homosexuality—are sources of stress. Recognizing the extra burden of stress underscores the need to enhance protective factors, both psychological and social. Group exercises are designed to bring out all the stereotypes patients have about homosexuality. Using CBT techniques, patients then challenge these beliefs and come to see that most of them are cognitive distortions.

For example, in one exercise, 10 photos of well-known individuals are passed around the group. Participants are asked to identify the sexual orientation of these people. The group leader then asks how participants arrived at their conclusion, what thoughts went through their minds, what evidence they had to support their thinking, what evidence is missing, and whether there is another possible conclusion.

Another way to explore stereotypes is to have patients free-associate to the words *homosexuality, gay,* or *lesbian.* In Nadia's case the associations were all negative and spoke volumes about her fear of isolation and persecution, but also about her beliefs that homosexual women were unfeminine and angry. Thomas's word set was *solitude, difference, marginalization, freedom, sexuality, freed, no family, multiple partners, softness, friendship*—a much more ambivalent set of associations. The word *freedom* hinted at the function and meaning of his sexual escapades: an expression of anger and frustration. For Thomas, homoerotic attraction became less distressing when he was able to differentiate it from the urge to act on a sexual impulse to express anger.

The third part of therapy is aimed at helping patients solidify their identity and increase their resilience to stress by finding community supports. Most minority patients share their minority status with their family of origin, yet for sexual minorities this is usually not the case. The sexual minority patient may need to create a substitute family, a group of people who share this identity and can be supportive. The therapist can help the patient explore different resources, both locally and on the Internet. It is at this point that the previously constraining labels may finally feel useful. The words *lesbian, gay, bisexual,* and *homosexual* become shorthand for any kind of same-sex emotional or sexual attraction, activity, or affiliation. The words become a way of identifying and finding community.

Key Points

- Sexual orientation is multifaceted. Finding a label that adequately captures where one "fits" with regard to emotional connectedness, physical attraction, behavior, group identification, and cultural beliefs may be difficult or impossible.

- The labels *gay, lesbian,* and *bisexual* are oversimplifications and may feel constraining. These same labels are, however, useful for finding community.

- When a patient comes in asking "Am I gay?" the therapist's role is not to answer the question but rather to explore the various facets of sexuality and help relieve any discomfort the person may feel with any aspect of their eroticism. This is accomplished by exploring the origin of the discomfort (both in the personal and family narratives and in the broader sociocultural context) and challenging the dysfunctional beliefs that perpetuate it.

References

American Psychiatric Association: Diagnostic and Statistical Manual of Mental Disorders, 4th Edition, Text Revision. Washington, DC, American Psychiatric Association, 2000

Cass VC: Homosexual identity formation: a theoretical model. J Homosex 4:219–235, 1979

Igartua K, Thombs BD, Burgos G, et al: Concordance and discrepancy in sexual identity, attraction, and behaviour among adolescents. J Adolesc Health 45:602–608, 2009

Laumann E, Gagnon J, Michael R, et al: The Social Organization of Sexuality: Sexual Practices in the United States. Chicago, IL, University of Chicago Press, 1994, p 299

Questions

22.1   Components of sexual orientation include

   A. Sexual attraction and sexual behavior.
   B. Sexual attraction, sexual behavior, and identity.
   C. Sexual attraction, emotional intimacy, and sexual behavior.
   D. Sexual attraction, emotional intimacy, sexual behavior, and identity.

The correct answer is D.

Sexual attraction, emotional intimacy, sexual behavior, and identity are all components of sexual orientation. Examining each of these separately is important because in many patients, gender preference for sexual attraction, emotional intimacy, and sexual behavior will not be exactly the same. Identity is constructed based on these and the sociocultural environment within which the patient is evolving.

22.2 When a patient consults because of confusion about his or her sexual orientation, the therapist should (choose all that apply)

    A. Explore which gender the patient is sexually aroused by.
    B. Take an inventory of the patient's sexual behaviors.
    C. Explore which gender the patient is emotionally attracted to.
    D. Deduce that the patient is "gay" or "straight" based on A, B, C.
    E. Treat the patient's discomfort with his or her homoerotism.
    F. Understand the patient's family, cultural, and religious circumstances as they relate to homosexuality.

The correct answer is A, B, C, E, and F.

Helping patients define who they are attracted to sexually and emotionally, inventorying who they are sexually involved with, determining how religious, cultural, and family beliefs have affected them with regard to their sexuality, and treating any discomfort they may have in relation to their erotism are important steps in helping patients create their sexual identity. Therapists should not attempt to define the patients' identity for them. When patients become aware of their patterns of erotism and comfortable with them, they will be free to choose the identity that fits them best.

Religious or Spiritual Problem

Damage and Repair

UBALDO LELI, M.D.

DSM-IV-TR HAS A V-CODE (V62.89) that can be used when the focus of clinical attention is a religious or spiritual problem such as "distressing experiences that involve loss or questioning of faith" (American Psychiatric Association 2000a) (Table 23–1). What follows is the case of a gay man who, in addition to his Axis I and II diagnoses, had a spiritual problem that was a major focus of his psychotherapeutic treatment.

Case Example: Robert

Robert initially came to treatment referred by his health insurance company, for help with depression and anxiety. A tall, big-boned man in his late twenties with bright red hair, he was soft-spoken and gentle. At the same time, he evinced an internal tension that clouded his clear green eyes and twisted his posture, nearly giving him the appearance of a hunch on his back. His personal story, related with profound sadness from his first session on, was permeated with a pervasive sense of failure and rejection that made him tearful when he spoke.

Robert reported he had been previously diagnosed with type I bipolar disorder, but I had difficulty finding substantial evidence of a credible manic episode in his history. This made me wonder whether, rather than suffering from a

TABLE 23–1.   Religious or spiritual problem (DSM-IV-TR, V62.89)

This category can be used when the focus of clinical attention is a religious or spiritual problem. Examples include distressing experiences that involve loss or questioning of faith, problems associated with conversion to a new faith, or questioning of spiritual values that may not necessarily be related to an organized church or religious institution.

Source.   Reprinted from *Diagnostic and Statistical Manual of Mental Disorders*, 4th Edition, Text Revision. Washington, DC, American Psychiatric Association, 2000. Used with permission. Copyright © 2000 American Psychiatric Association.

bipolar spectrum syndrome, he was instead affected by a personality disorder or by a form of chronic posttraumatic stress disorder. The alternative diagnoses were suggested by the intensity of Robert's mood lability, pervasive impulsivity, and intensely fluctuating anxiety. Because his presenting symptoms were consistent mostly with a major depressive disorder, such alternatives could be only entertained and not immediately confirmed. He had been briefly hospitalized 2 years earlier because he had spoken of suicide in the aftermath of breaking up with his previous partner. At the time of his initial consultation he was taking valproic acid and clonazepam.

A serious problem, which did not surface until after the first few interviews, was Robert's binge drinking. He went bar-hopping nearly every weekend and on every excursion got extremely drunk, often making numerous rambling phone calls to acquaintances both close and removed. Most of these evenings ended with somebody calling Robert's live-in partner, who would come pick him up either passed out on the sidewalk or in the gutter outside a bar from which he had been ejected. The next day Robert would remember nothing of what had happened. This additional piece of history called into consideration a differential diagnosis of substance-induced mood disorder. However, I believed that Robert's traumatic experiences involving his family dynamics and his experience of reparative therapy were aggravating factors superimposed on a primary mood disorder, strongly suggested by a family history positive for psychiatric illness. The history of affective disorders in Robert's family was extensive. His mother and one of his brothers had bipolar disorder, his sister suffered from major depression, and alcoholism could be traced back for as many generations as Robert knew about.

Past history: From 7 through 17 years of age, Robert had been educated in a Roman Catholic seminary in another part of the country, where he had been born to parents of Northern European origin. As a child, his emotionally distant parents treated him rigidly. At the time of his first visit, his younger sister was in the process of leaving a convent just before taking her final vows. Of his two older brothers, one had cut off contact because Robert had come out as gay. He had only sporadic contacts with his other brother, although Robert described their relationship as "good."

A strictly observant Roman Catholic, Robert's mother wanted all her children to become priests and nuns. She had repeatedly told Robert since early childhood that if someone was destined to become a priest but did not do so, he would be responsible for all the lost souls he could have saved through his ministry; they would go to Hell and burn forever, and he would follow them to damnation as soon as God deemed it. Robert entered the seminary while still in grammar school, aware already of his homosexual feelings but convinced that they were natural and not sinful, provided he was chaste and did not engage in any sexual activity. He did, however, discover masturbation at age 9 and practiced it daily as a secret delight.

During his seminary years, Robert did not have sex with anyone. He went to confession daily to be absolved of his private impure acts and thereby take communion at Mass. As part of his priestly formation, Robert revealed to his spiritual director the nature of his same-sex desire. Despite the confidential nature of the relationship between a spiritual director and his acolyte, which is supposed to be as confidential as the Sacrament of Confession, his spiritual director revealed that Robert was gay to the seminary authorities. As a consequence, upon completing high school he was instructed to leave the seminary, return home, and enter into treatment with a sexual conversion therapist. At that juncture, Robert felt that the reason he had been mistreated at the seminary—having to carry out unpleasant duties such as cleaning the toilets and never being given due credit for his skill in various sports, in which he excelled—was because he was gay.

Once back home, he felt hopeless and without a sense of self-direction. His lifelong ambition had been to become a priest, and now this had been thwarted. He still felt his call to the priesthood, but he had to come to terms with the fact that there was no way he could ever be ordained within the Roman Catholic Church, which still defines homosexuality as an innately disordered condition.

Robert was in sexual conversion therapy for one year, during which time he was sent on retreats, was counseled to be "manly," and gave testimony at events of the "evil of the gay lifestyle" and of the possibility that one could become heterosexual if one tried hard enough. His eventual departure from that "treatment" occurred following a series of prayer sessions with Bill, another man who had been "cured" of his homosexuality. Bill, whom Robert met as part of the socialization required by his therapist, locked himself up with Robert in the bathroom and raped him while his wife and two children watched television in the living room. The combination of physical pain, sense of violation, shame, and resentment evoked an unprecedented behavioral change in Robert. He entered a downward spiral of sexual promiscuity and heavy drinking. Gravitating to roughneck clubs, he met in one of them Carl, the leader of a biker gang, who became his lover and with whom he took to the road, eventually ending up in New York City.

Carl kept Robert as a "mascot" for his biker gang. Their pattern was to settle down for short periods of time in various cities, slowly moving across the country. They eventually settled and lived communally in one of New York City's outer boroughs. The biker gang treated Robert relatively well. As the boss's boy, he was respected, fed, and given accommodations. During this period, Robert felt a sense of security despite the group's pervasive heavy drinking and cannabis use. When the relationship with Carl collapsed, Robert moved to Manhattan, met his current partner David—a Protestant priest—and found an office job. This allowed him to obtain health insurance and to enter psychiatric treatment for what he felt was depression.

Initiating treatment: Robert initially sought medication treatment. However, because of his history of abuse, his lack of self-direction, his poor impulse control, and his binge drinking—which affected him the most acutely—I suggested that in addition to medication, he might benefit from psychotherapy. At the time we began weekly psychotherapy, he was already taking citalopram and clonazepam, prescribed by his previous psychiatrist. I discontinued clonazepam because of the possibility of abuse and its potentially lethal interaction with alcohol. His antidepressant was changed to desvenlafaxine because citalopram had been ineffective in improving his mood. Finally, lamotrigine was added to his regimen in an attempt to mitigate his mood swings. Robert was compliant with medications and with psychotherapy. During the first year of his treatment, much history surfaced. His struggle with the pervasive sense of meaninglessness he felt toward work, as well as his lukewarm feelings toward his current partner, David, remained central to his therapeutic discourse. However, the sense that a central piece of his life was missing became progressively clearer.

For many months, the topic of Robert's call to priesthood and the painful events at the seminary did not surface directly in his associations. With time, I realized I was countertransferentially tiptoeing around the issue of his vocation. I felt inhibited by an unspoken wish to remain as neutral as possible that caused me to not offer any suggestions, with the rationalization that doing so would cloud Robert's path to self-discovery. During the first year, an additional factor that kept our exploratory work closer to the surface was the turbulent issue of Robert's alcohol abuse. He was unable to control his binge-drinking episodes, and despite efforts to contain them by using a contract-setting approach, they continued to be serious and frequent. His impulsive drinking was accompanied by frequent episodes of promiscuous sexual behavior: Robert's favorite entertainment outside working hours, when he was not home, was to pay for massages "with release." His wish to be accepted and loved often dulled his judgment, and he became infatuated with several masseurs.

Robert's alcohol abuse often escalated and led to severe fights with David, who strove to maintain some degree of discipline within the household. On two occasions, Robert became so drunk while dining at home that in the midst of the ensuing fights, he threatened to kill himself with a kitchen knife. On both occasions, after being subdued by David, Robert was taken to the hospital by the police.

His first hospital stay was short—72 hours of observation in the emergency room—but on the second occasion he was kept in an inpatient unit for a week for additional stabilization. During this second admission, Robert was placed on quetiapine, which helped to contain his mood swings. About 8 months into his treatment, he also finally agreed to attend Alcoholics Anonymous (AA) and decided to attempt full sobriety.

The spiritual crisis: During Robert's second year of treatment, a deepening of the therapeutic process developed and there was a progressive decrease in his impulsivity. Binge drinking became less frequent as Robert attended AA. He also became more involved with the church where David was the assistant pastor. Transference phenomena emerged and could now be brought to Robert's awareness. From the start, he had treated me with the utmost respect, which, together with his strict compliance with the treatment, betrayed a clear tinge of idealization. Our therapeutic relationship at this time was based on my continuously mirroring Robert's feelings and offering him a deeply empathic presence: I felt myself more like a guide or a witness, perhaps even a little like a father.

At this stage of the treatment Robert comfortably shared the details of his many sexual escapades. These evoked, in my countertransference, feelings toward him of a warm, protective nature. This allowed me to validate his feelings and encourage his ambitions, including his yearning to live with a gay sexual identity and to pursue his goals in life.

In the second year of treatment, it was clear—to me, at least—that the missing piece in Robert's identity was his call to the priesthood. During the hours, hope and disillusionment, desire and guilt, and sin and Divine Grace increasingly became the hot topics of discussion. This led eventually to a more focused inquiry into Robert's life direction, his aspirations, and his future. At first, conversations about Robert's call to the priesthood were tentative and noncommittal, lest he face another terrible disillusionment, one that I would have possibly encouraged. Over time, however, the discussions about his vocation became more concrete, to the point that he started asking himself if he might follow again the path to the ministry. While the treatment was taking this turn, outside the consulting room Robert started to participate more and more actively in David's religious services, functioning as a deacon. At the same time, he was expressing greater dissatisfaction with his job: what he did in the office was meaningless, and he felt trapped there.

In the middle of his third year of treatment, Robert announced that he had been speaking with his partner's congregation and elders and had scheduled an appointment with their bishop to discern his vocation and explore the possibility of entering the seminary.

Robert was eventually accepted into a Lutheran seminary and started classes there. At that time, he was sober, was compliant with medications, and had had no significant mood swings for 18 months.

Discussion

This case reports the history and treatment course of Robert, a 27-year-old Caucasian man with an admission diagnosis of bipolar disorder in partial remission, posttraumatic stress disorder secondary to rape and reparative therapy, and alcohol abuse/dependency. In addition to his Axis I diagnoses, Robert had a personality disorder not otherwise specified, with narcissistic and borderline features.

An important aspect of this case is the role of spirituality in the psyche, and specifically its role in the development and consolidation of human identity. While Robert's irritability, mood swings, labile affect, and impulsive behaviors improved with antidepressants and mood stabilizers, the incorporation of his spiritual dimension into the psychotherapeutic process allowed him ultimately to accept his sexual orientation and follow his call to religious life.

The psychotherapeutic treatment focused on the development and reparation of Robert's sense of self, with the emergence of a mirroring transference met by a stable and consistent empathic stance on the part of the therapist. Although parameters such as contract setting and recommendations for cognitive-behavioral intervention in the form of self-help group treatment were used in the treatment, the process unfolded along the lines of a supportive psychoanalytic psychotherapy, with an eye to holding and validation and with positive affirmative aspects in relation to the patient's spirituality and sexual orientation.

Robert was also a victim of reparative therapy, that is, the attempt to change one's sexual orientation. Since 2000, the American Psychiatric Association (2000b) has viewed these "treatments" as unethical and potentially harmful. In 2009, an American Psychological Association (2009) task force report found no scientific evidence that such treatments were effective. In Robert's case, reparative therapy added a whole new layer of damage to someone who was already traumatized, having seen his erotic, emotional, human, and spiritual aspirations violently assaulted by his church. This trauma compounded the basic damage he had suffered from the emotional neglect he had experienced within his family. Robert was not only genetically susceptible to affective disorder, but also his basic life aspirations and identity attributes had been negated by organized religion and societal prejudice.

The crucial element that contributed to the success of Robert's treatment was the therapy's affirmation and support of his gay sexual orientation and of his faith-based call to religious life, with the biological and behavioral interventions functioning as essential prerequisites for Robert's psychological healing.

Key Points

- The effects of biologically based mental illness can be exacerbated in lesbian, gay, bisexual, and transgender (LGBT) individuals by a hostile social and religious environment, to which attention must be paid if treatment is to be successful.

- For many people, spirituality is a constitutive element of their identity and must be integrated with other structural aspects of the patient's personality for a fully positive outcome.

- A supportive, positively affirmative stance on the part of a therapist is indispensable for the reconstruction of the damaged self in LGBT individuals suffering the effects of abuse and discrimination.

References

American Psychiatric Association: Diagnostic and Statistical Manual of Mental Disorders, 4th Edition, Text Revision. Washington, DC, American Psychiatric Association, 2000a

American Psychiatric Association, Commission on Psychotherapy by Psychiatrists: Position statement on therapies focused on attempts to change sexual orientation (reparative or conversion therapies). Am J Psychiatry 157:1719–1721, 2000b

American Psychological Association: Report of the American Psychological Association Task Force on Appropriate Therapeutic Response to Sexual Orientation. Washington, DC, American Psychological Association, 2009

Questions

23.1   When religious beliefs, faith, and spiritual issues emerge in psychotherapy, the therapist should do this following:

A. Think about religious and spiritual issues as resistances and interpret them as such in order to enhance the patient's psychological freedom.

B. Treat religious beliefs as a respected and immutable part of a patient's psychological makeup to be ignored and kept out of treatment interventions.

C. Regard religious and spiritual issues as basic aspects of a patient's identity to be acknowledged and met with a positive attitude, while keeping an open mind to their potential role as resistance against change.

D. None of the above.

The correct answer is C.

Religious beliefs, spirituality, and faith are constitutive elements of one's identity and, while they tend to be constant, they may also evolve during a person's development and as a consequence of treatment. One treatment goal is to integrate them into a more coherent sense of self through the therapist's attitude of maintaining respect and keeping an open mind.

23.2   For an LGBT patient who presents simultaneously with an affective disorder, substance abuse, and issues of religious and spiritual nature, the treatment priorities should be as follows:

A. First treat substance abuse, then affective disorders, and, when the patient is stable, consider adding individual psychotherapy to address problems caused by religious and spiritual issues.

B. Address substance abuse and affective disorders aggressively, while simultaneously exploring in psychotherapy the implications of the religious and spiritual issues for the patient's LGBT identity.

C. Treat substance abuse and affective disorder with medication and behavioral interventions while discouraging psychodynamic psychotherapy, which may cause a relapse in substance abuse.

D. None of the above.

The correct answer is B.

A complex clinical presentation that includes substance abuse, affective disorders, and spiritual and religious issues in an LGBT patient requires an eclectic approach, with a variety of interventions administered simultaneously. These include cognitive-behavioral, self-help, pharmacological, and psychodynamic treatment.

Acculturation Problem

I Am Fukushima (But You Can Call Me Lady Marmalade, Honey)

Khakasa Wapenyi, M.D.

MENTAL HEALTH CLINICIANS with an interest in culturally competent diagnostic formulation welcomed the addition of the condition Acculturation Problem to the fourth edition of the *Diagnostic and Statistical Manual of Mental Disorders* (DSM-IV; American Psychiatric Association 1994). Acculturation problem (V62.4) falls within the V codes category "Other Conditions That May Be a Focus of Clinical Attention" (Table 24–1) (American Psychiatric Association 2000). Examples: An 8-year-old boy, a first-generation child of Korean descent, is sent to a doctor for disruptive, oppositional, and out-of-control behavior. As a child growing up in the United States, he becomes socialized to his American peers, learning that it is normal to be outspoken and rambunctious. His parents take this to be a psychological problem that must be addressed by the proper authorities. A middle-aged woman from rural Kentucky moves with her husband to a densely populated metropolis when he gets promoted. She becomes a shut-in, and her husband, exasperated and confused, brings her to a therapist for the treatment of depression.

In this chapter, I focus the discussion on acculturation problems as they relate to transgender individuals, illustrated here by the case of a person called "Lady Marmalade."

TABLE 24–1.   Acculturation problem (DSM-IV-TR, V62.4)

This category can be used when the focus of clinical attention is a problem involving adjustment to a different culture (e.g., following migration).

Source.   Reprinted from *Diagnostic and Statistical Manual of Mental Disorders*, 4th Edition, Text Revision. Washington, DC, American Psychiatric Association, 2000. Used with permission. Copyright © 2000 American Psychiatric Association.

Case Example: Mariana

Mariana is a 24-year-old Latina, originally from Belize, a woman of transgender experience (i.e., male-to-female [MTF]) who was referred by her friend, Immaculata. Mariana was distressed and depressed, self-isolated, unable to sleep, and inconsolable. Immaculata thought this might be an *ataque de nervios* (Guarnaccia 1993). As Mariana sat down on the therapist's couch, she cried (invoking the Japanese nuclear power disaster), "Honey, I'm a living Fukushima!"

Mariana was distressed because her childhood nanny, Blanquita, was alone in Belize and dying of terminal cancer. Blanquita had essentially raised Mariana on her own. Mariana was born to wealthy, cosmopolitan parents who traveled extensively during her childhood.

Mariana was unable to travel home to Belize because she was undocumented. After she was born in the United States, she and her parents traveled back home to Belize in the first year of her life. She came back to the United States 6 years ago, using her Belizean passport. If she were to travel to Belize, she feared she could not return to the United States. Her birth certificate issued in the United States listed her as a baby boy. She showed the therapist a manila envelope stuffed with documents for a U.S. passport.

She did not understand why she was having such a hard time with the authorities. At airports, she was accustomed to Homeland Security agents being a little taken aback when she told them she was American. She always thought it was because she was a sassy Latina who wore "Spandex, Lycra, and Spanx" and spoke broken English (i.e., Spanglish). She assured the therapist that she spoke and sang French, German, and Italian fluently, without an accent. She had studied these languages in school because she always knew she would be a performer. Her childhood dream had been to become an opera singer.

She knew her beloved nanny had been taken ill years ago, something they never discussed on the telephone. Mariana had planned to return to Belize 6 months after landing on U.S. soil, but life intervened. She always sent money home to her nanny, and until recently that had sufficed. In the last year, her nanny's health had swiftly declined and she was spending more time in the hospital than not. Mariana's fervent wish was that she could be with her nanny before she died and thank her.

Blanquita had been seminal in Mariana's psychosexual development. Mariana, then Mario, had known he was different since he was 6 years old. Mario always wanted to dress in girl's clothing and liked to wear his hair long. He enjoyed playing house with the girls rather than playing soccer (*futbol*) with the boys. Blanquita recognized early on that Mario was a sensitive boy and never chastised him for being different. The boys, later everyone, ridiculed Mario for being a girl (or effeminate) and a "sissy."

Initially Mario thought he might be gay. When he traveled with his parents to major urban cities, he saw androgynous men and thought he might belong to this alien species. Mario had always thought of himself inside as "Mariana" because this is what Blanquita called him. By the time he was 12 years old, he was introducing himself to well-heeled strangers as Mariana. By 16 years old, after receiving a large gift of money from his mother, he had breast implant surgery.

With much urging from her nanny, Mariana decided to travel to the States after high school. Blanquita told her she should go to New York City, to "the Heights," where there was a little Spanish New York. Mariana would be able to meet people like her and finally meet the man of her dreams while doing the samba down streets paved with gold.

Unfortunately, New York City did not turn out as Mariana expected. She arrived without knowing a soul. She was friendless for months and alienated from the *macho* Dominican culture of Washington Heights. Finally, she found a thriving Latin LGBT (lesbian, gay, bisexual, and transgender) community. She became fast friends with Immaculata, another Latina transgender woman from Panama.

As quickly, Mariana was introduced into local New York City transgender survival culture: drag performance, sugar daddies, recreational drug use, and sex work (sex in exchange for favors, housing, drugs). Most New Yorkers knew her as Lady Marmalade. She did not know when she went from being "a good girl to a bad girl…this was not how I was raised." She was still thick into living *la vida loca* when she heard her nanny had taken to bed.

Medications (dosages unknown): Mariana reported taking "street" premarin, spironolactone purchased from an Internet pharmacy, and, as needed, Ambien obtained "from a friend," street Xanax, and Percocet prescribed by a doctor for lumbago.

Mental status examination: Mariana was colorfully attired in feminine clothing. She had long brown hair with highlights, wore full makeup, and sported nails painted with the flag of Cuba ("I love Cuban men"). She appeared younger than her stated age, was very animated, engaged easily, and maintained good eye contact. Upon arrival, she behaved in a dramatic, entitled manner but slowly became deferential, fawning, and almost obsequious. She was clearly distressed and agitated, but she exhibited no adventitious movements.

She spoke fluently with a slight Spanish accent. Her mood was dysphoric and anxious, with a high level of expressed emotion. Congruent with her mood, she was labile, tense, and tearful throughout the interview. She spoke in a roundabout manner, loquacious and at times overinclusive, but logical. She was mired in grief and guilt regarding her nanny's impending demise and hardly spoke on any other topic. On further exploration, she denied any hallucinatory or paranoid ideation. She adamantly denied any impulse to hurt herself or others, as her sole focus was to travel home to see her nanny.

She was simultaneously hyperalert and internally preoccupied with thoughts and feelings about her nanny. She immediately acknowledged *la doctora* and commented on the tasteful design of the therapist's office. Her recall was excellent, and she appeared to be an intelligent and articulate woman. In spite of talking in highly metaphorical and poetic language, she was able to respond appropriately to direct questions. She knew she was acting *loca* but insisted that all her troubles would be solved if she were able to travel. Her judgment was clearly impaired in multiple domains.

Diagnoses

Mariana's differential diagnosis is as wide as it is challenging to even seasoned clinicians. However, although we find that the patient's life is populated with a variety of possible psychiatric syndromes, medical conditions, social problems, and complex interactions of these forces—most notably the interplay of DSM Axis I with Axis IV—acculturation themes are ubiquitous. Throughout the five axes, we encounter cultural components that appear to be fundamental in determining Mariana's overall mental and physical health (Paniagua 2001; Smart and Smart 1997).

I. Adjustment disorder vs. mood disorder vs. bereavement vs. *ataque de nervios,* acculturation problem, polysubstance use disorder, rule out post-traumatic stress disorder, gender variance/gender incongruence, rule out gender identity disorder

II. Cluster B traits

III. History of breast implants, silicone injections in lips, hips, cheeks, thighs and buttocks, cheek enhancement, tracheal shave, surgical voice augmentation, false rib removal, electrolysis

IV. Immigration, occupational, environmental, and other psychosocial problems

V. Current Global Assessment of Functioning score: 58

Discussion

Berry (2001) sets up four modes demonstrating immigrants' attitudes towards acculturation. *Integration* refers to identifying with and participating in both cultures. *Assimilation* refers to choosing to identify solely with the new culture. *Separation* refers to being involved only in the traditional culture. *Marginalization* is characterized by lack of involvement in and rejection of both cultures.

Berry posits that changes in mental health vary across the four acculturation modes because of different levels of acculturative stress. He writes that integration is the form of adaptation where the best mental health might be expected because of the lowest level of acculturative stress.

Tip One: Mariana would be defined as a person falling within the "Separation" category per Berry's (2001) formulation. In New York City, she remained within the Spanish culture, even when she joined the novel, yet personally familiar, Latin LGBT community.

Tip Two: Mariana had experienced "shell shock" upon arriving in New York City. Shell shock, particularly in recent immigrants, may be conceived as a forme fruste of "cultural" posttraumatic stress disorder (Gaw 2001). For her, the initial acculturation to New York City, specifically to the Washington Heights neighborhood, was a traumatic experience. (This is not to say that moving to Washington Heights is a universally traumatic experience!) Mariana withdrew into herself and became isolative until she found a welcoming Latin LGBT community.

Mariana can be helped clinically in moving from separation to integration. In theory, this process would decrease her acculturative stress and help her cope with and master her emotional distress in a healthier, more adaptive manner. A tried-and-true method would be for the therapist to help Mariana incorporate treasured memories of her indigenous culture and loved ones by memorializing her positive experiences in the here and now. The goal of therapy is to help maintain her past, self-affirmative memories/objects, while developing and sustaining ties to her adopted culture.

Tip Three: Always refer to your transgender patient with his or her stated, preferred gender pronoun. The fastest and easiest way to alienate a transgender person is by using the wrong gender pronoun. For example, Homeland Security officers referring to Mariana as "he," based on her birth certificate, caused Mariana severe anxiety and distress.

Mental health clinicians, respecting patients' autonomy, should strive to align with the patient's self-defined gender identity as one of the primary means of establishing and solidifying the therapeutic alliance.

Moreover, when the therapist evaluates Mariana's presentation, clinical judgment should remain open. Mariana's apparently contradictory and unpredictable changes in gender identity while telling her story may be perceived as "psychotic." For Mariana, this way of narrating her history is entirely natural and perfectly rational.

Tip Four: It is not advisable to ask a transgender MTF person whether they "have a penis" in an attempt to definitively clarify gender. This question is based on a belief in biological determinism, inconsistent with the concept that gender, like "race," is fluid and essentially a social construct. Individuals are shaped by multiple factors that combine to determine gender: genetics, family environment, culture, society, media, and one's self-definition or self-knowledge. (In an effort to determine her identity, Homeland Security officials might ask Mariana to agree to physical examination by an authorized, official government medical doctor.)

Tip Five: Expanding on the concepts of gender fluidity and gender as social construct, clinicians should have the capacity to move beyond the idea of binary gender (either male or female). For example, a transgender MTF person may have undergone multiple feminizing procedures and yet have no interest in undergoing sexual reassignment surgery/gender reassignment surgery. Transgender individuals may choose to identify as female, which is a decision we should respect and strive to understand.

Key Points

- If you don't know, *ask*. This principle applies to all cultural questions, be they related to ethnicity, language, sexuality, gender, or other matters. If the therapist asks clinically relevant questions in a respectful, nonjudgmental way, LGBT individuals probably will not take offense or become defensive.

- The clinician may have a responsibility to do "homework"—that is, to independently research unfamiliar aspects of a patient from a different culture. In this way, the clinician can ease the patient's comfort level in disclosing intimate details of his or her history.

References

American Psychiatric Association: Diagnostic and Statistical Manual of Mental Disorders, 4th Edition. Washington, DC, American Psychiatric Association, 1994

American Psychiatric Association: Diagnostic and Statistical Manual of Mental Disorders, 4th Edition, Text Revision. Washington, DC, American Psychiatric Association, 2000

Berry JW: A psychology of immigration. J Soc Issues 57:615–631, 2001

Gaw AC: Concise Guide to Cross-Cultural Psychiatry. Washington, DC, American Psychiatric Publishing, 2001

Guarnaccia PJ: Ataque de nervios in Puerto Rico: culture-bound syndrome or popular illness? Med Anthropol 15:157–179, 1993

Paniagua FA: Diagnosis in a Multicultural Context. New York, Sage, 2001

Smart D, Smart JF: DSM-IV and culturally sensitive diagnosis: some observations for counselors. J Couns Dev 75:392–398, 1997

Questions

24.1   Who is the original Lady Marmalade?

    A. Patti LaBelle.
    B. Christina Aguilera.
    C. Yo Mama.
    D. Yo Yo Ma.

The correct answer is A.

Patti LaBelle is the lead singer of the 1974 hit song "Lady Marmalade."

24.2 The ideal, adaptive state of acculturation is

A. Segregation.
B. Assimilation.
C. Integration.
D. Marginalization.

The correct answer is C.

Integration occurs when an individual from a different culture is able to maintain a connection with their primary/native culture while successfully socially interacting within their adopted/local culture.

Phase of Life Problem

"It's Just a Phase": Phase of Life Problems and LGBT Development

JOHN K. BURTON, M.D.
LORRAINE LOTHWELL, M.D.

A PHASE OF LIFE PROBLEM is described in DSM-IV-TR as a problem that is linked to a particular developmental phase or life circumstance and either not due to a mental disorder or severe enough "to warrant independent clinical attention" (V62.89; Table 25–1) (American Psychiatric Association 2000). Lesbian, gay, bisexual, and transgender (LGBT) individuals, like all people, face life transitions that can stir up conflict; beginning school, leaving home, starting a new job, and retiring are just some examples. However, LGBT people have specific challenges when going through a phase of life problem. The physician or therapist who is aware of the needs of LGBT patients is in a position to be uniquely helpful to those who present without a primary mental disorder but are suffering nonetheless.

Although the DSM-IV-TR description of phase of life problems refers to development explicitly, development is relevant to all clinical presentations. The case that we present is of an adolescent who met DSM criteria for gender identity disorder (GID). The focus for treatment was not the GID, however, but the obstacles to her development that were created by conflicts in her community, her school, her family, and her own identity.

TABLE 25–1.   Phase of life problem (DSM-IV-TR, V62.89)

This category can be used when the focus of clinical attention is a problem associated with a particular developmental phase or some other life circumstance that is not due to a mental disorder or, if it is due to a mental disorder, is sufficiently severe to warrant independent clinical attention. Examples include problems associated with entering school, leaving parental control, starting a new career, and changes involved in marriage, divorce, and retirement.

Source.   Reprinted from *Diagnostic and Statistical Manual of Mental Disorders,* 4th Edition, Text Revision. Washington, DC, American Psychiatric Association, 2000. Used with permission. Copyright © 2000 American Psychiatric Association.

The Developmental Lens

We focus here on adolescent development in order to discuss the crucial importance this period has for LGBT individuals, but also as a model for applying a developmental perspective to all patients. Erik Erikson's "Eight Phases of Self-Development" provides a useful theoretical framework to consider clinical presentations across the life span (Table 25–2) (Sadock et al. 2009). Adults as well as children go through distinct developmental phases, each with a unique task that the individual must accomplish in order to grow as a person. For example, an LGBT 30-year-old might be conflicted about her wish to find a life partner in a society that does not recognize gay marriage; a retired LGBT activist might be struggling to feel relevant, as the homophobia he fought in the past no longer has significance to a younger generation.

The phase-specific task of adolescence is the consolidation of a stable identity. As such, this phase is of particular importance for LGBT people. It is the time when sexuality becomes realized and conflicts involving the physical self are brought to the fore. The challenges to completing the task of identity consolidation are many. There can be great variation in an adolescent's timelines for developing physical, cognitive, emotional, and social maturity. The adolescent brain is still in the process of myelination and pruning and is thus limited in its ability to control and regulate impulses. This can result in more risk-taking behaviors. Accidents, homicide, and suicide are the three most common causes of death among adolescents in the United States. As for LGBT adolescents specifically, several studies have shown that youths who are questioning their sexual or gender identity are at increased risk for suicide, nonsuicidal self-injury, and other high-risk behaviors, such as substance abuse and unprotected sex (Toomey et al. 2010). It is vital when treating an LGBT adolescent that the clinician formulate a treatment plan that will facilitate the task of developing a positive and secure adult identity.

TABLE 25–2.   Erikson: eight phases of self-development

Psychosocial conflict	Phase	Outcome
Trust versus mistrust	Infant	The infant depends on the primary caregiver for feeding/protection and develops an ability to trust others and trust in oneself (i.e., "basic trust)."
Autonomy versus shame and self-doubt	Toddler	The child becomes aware of herself as a separate and independent individual, laying the foundation for self-assertion and self-expression.
Initiative versus guilt	Preschool age	The child begins to use her improving motor skills and curiosity about the world to "test limits," learning about parental limits and developing her sense of responsibility, self-discipline, and conscience.
Industry versus inferiority	School age	The child's world expands to include schoolmates and adults outside of her family, learning the skills to love, work, and play with the rest of society.
Identity versus identity confusion	Adolescence	This stage is marked by the onset of puberty and intense growth, with the adolescent developing a sense of self-awareness in relation to herself and others.
Intimacy versus isolation	Early adult	In this stage the adult becomes psychosexually mature and begins to establish significant intimate interpersonal relationships.
Generativity versus stagnation	Middle adult	The adult creates and (re)produces in various ways during this phase, enriching the lives of others.
Integrity versus despair	Late adult	At this point, the adult reflects on her life and ideally, is able to find satisfaction and acceptance in the life she has lived.

Source.   Adapted from Erikson 1950 and Sadock and Sadock 2009.

Case Example: Jess

Evaluation

Chief complaint: Jess was the eldest of three girls born in the United States to Mexican immigrant parents. The family lived in a two-bedroom apartment in a working-class urban neighborhood, and Jess shared one room with her sisters. She was about to begin high school when her mother first took her to the child and adolescent psychiatry clinic. According to her mother, the previous 6 months had been "horrific." According to Jess, the problem was, "I can't be my true identity."

History of the presenting problem: Jess's mother reported that the problem began when Jess told her that she thought she was "born in the wrong body" and felt she "should have been a boy." This was followed by increasing conflicts at home with her parents, oppositional behavior toward her teachers, and a drop in her grades from B's to C's. Over the summer, the family visited Mexico. Jess said she initially was happy to be with her grandparents and cousins, but after a few days felt sad and angry at their refusal to accept her decision to transition to a male gender identity. Back in the United States, she told her parents that she would not return to school in September, and she refused to do any of the required summer readings. In view of Jess's increasing anger and school refusal, her mother brought her to the psychiatry clinic for further evaluation.

The initial evaluation consisted of a joint meeting with Jess and her parents, individual sessions with Jess, individual sessions with her parents, and a follow-up joint meeting to discuss treatment planning. When evaluating an adolescent, the clinician should always meet with the parents or guardian and obtain information from school and any other systems with which the youth is involved. This allows for the fullest understanding of the dynamics of the systems in which the person is functioning and provides collateral information to complement the adolescent's self-report. Most importantly, a therapeutic alliance with the parents must be established if the treatment is to have any success. This process need not conflict with the adolescent's need for autonomy and confidentiality if the goals of these sessions are made clear to both the patient and the parents (Novick and Novick 2005).

In the initial joint session, Jess was adamant that she would not be attending school in September. "I am not going back there. They're idiots." She said she felt angry most of the time when she was in school or with extended family, as if she was "about to explode." She angrily recounted the time her guidance counselor told her "You don't know what you want" when she revealed her conflict about her gender identity to him at the end of the school year. She was angry too at her parents, who were similarly dismissive; as they explained to the evaluating psychiatrist in her presence, "She's too young to understand what this all means. It's just a phase."

When speaking to the evaluating psychiatrist alone, Jess was less angry and defensive and opened up about her inner conflict. Jess revealed that she has "always felt like a boy," since age 3 or 4. She remembered other children asking if she was a boy or girl and "sometimes I'd say boy, because it felt right." Jess searched for information about sexuality and gender online at age 11, and finding a description of transgender, felt the definition applied to her. Jess said that she did not often feel sad, but when she was, it was always related to her gender variance and her desire to express her gender identity "honestly" to her family and at school. She denied active suicidal thoughts but said she sometimes thought she would kill herself if she could not pass as a boy.

In meetings with her parents, Jess's father explained that they came to see a psychiatrist because her previous therapist had not helped Jess, as she continued to have an "unnatural" desire to be a boy. However, he reported that he did not care what Jess did, "as long as she stops with the computer and gets better grades." Her mother went on to ask if there was anything that could be done, "like electric shock treatment."

Past history: Jess had no history of psychotic symptoms, panic attacks, substance abuse, trauma, obsessions, compulsions, or eating-disordered behavior. She had not been on medications or had any other psychotherapy, other than the 6 months of weekly psychotherapy in eighth grade. Her parents denied a family history of psychiatric illness, including suicide attempts or substance abuse.

Developmental history: Jess's parents immigrated to the United States 2 years before she was born. Pregnancy was uneventful and without complications, according to her mother. Jess met all developmental milestones on time and was described as a "calm" baby by her parents. She had attended the same school since kindergarten and had been an honors student in sixth and seventh grades. She had no medical problems other than mild asthma. Jess began puberty at age 9. Her mother reports she was embarrassed to talk about her menses, but the mother did take her to see her pediatrician. She had no gynecological or endocrine abnormalities. Despite being a social child prepubertally, she had become increasingly isolated and by eighth grade had no friends at all.

Appearance: Jess presented as a petite girl with shoulder-length straight black hair and an olive complexion. She wore dark jeans, sneakers, and a black oversized hooded sweatshirt. In joint sessions, she appeared sullen, played with her cell phone, and would grip the arms of her chair tightly when she became frustrated. She refused to make eye contact with either the interviewer or her parents.

Impression: Jess presented with school refusal, academic difficulties, and increased oppositionality, all linked closely to her dysphoria about her female gender. Her parents were limited in their understanding of Jess's gender identity conflict and its connection to her behavioral and academic problems. While a diagnosis of GID was warranted, the problems of school refusal, academic decline, and conflict with her parents, all linked to Jess's emerging identity, took precedence over making decisions about her gender identity.

Treatment

The primary goal of treatment was to improve Jess's ability to function in school and at home. These goals had to be achieved within the constant back-and-forth that is adolescent development, with Jess's growing autonomy on one side, and her continued need for her parents on the other. Thus, the involvement of Jess's parents was a central part of her treatment. Concomitantly, individual psycho-therapy gave Jess a private and nonjudgmental place to explore the challenge of developing a social identity congruent with her inner sense of self. Below, we discuss in turn each area of functioning that was addressed in treatment.

Behavior and academic function: At the outset of treatment, the therapist helped Jess and her parents collaboratively set up a behavior plan. The plan outlined house rules and consequences for Jess's school and homework refusal, treating school and homework as things that had to be done regardless of Jess's gender conflicts. Regular family sessions continued, alternating with individual psycho-therapy, until school attendance and academics improved. Jess made the honor roll by the spring semester.

Self-identity and internal system: Jess discussed her sexual and gender identity can-didly in her individual psychotherapy. She had done a lot of research online about what it meant to be transgender, and she felt the term applied to her. A neutral stance on the part of the therapist was essential for Jess to explore her feelings about gender fully. In this case, neutrality meant neither convincing Jess that she should become comfortable as a female nor agreeing that she should identify as male. In-stead, the therapist listened respectfully and asked questions aimed at deeper ex-plorations of her identity. Jess talked about the "difference between the sex you're born as and your gender," and "how sometimes the two don't match." The therapist asked Jess whether she preferred male or female pronouns when referring to her-self, and Jess acknowledged she was unsure. She acknowledged that this was a source of tension with her parents when they referred to her as "she" or went out of their way to introduce her as "our daughter." Now that Jess had an outlet to explore her feelings, she became less argumentative and oppositional at home and began attending school regularly and completing her homework on time.

Family system: The therapist met with Jess's parents several times to provide psy-choeducation about gender and GID. Jess's gender conflict was reframed within the larger context of adolescent identity development, thus making it something with which her parents could more easily empathize. Prognosis was understand-ably of great concern to her parents, and it was essential to maintain neutrality with them, as it had been with Jess. The therapist refocused her parents' wish to help Jess by improving their ability to be open to Jess's thoughts about gender as it came up in daily life, for example, in choosing her clothes for a family event or deciding which pronouns she preferred. These sessions helped her parents find a way to be supportive of Jess without relinquishing their parental authority. As tension at home and school decreased, family meetings became less frequent, but the therapist remained available to the parents' questions or concerns.

Physical self and bodily control: Nowhere is the adolescent conflict between au-tonomy and dependence more intensely experienced than in the bodily changes of puberty. Jess expressed a great deal of shame about her body, particularly her menses and her breasts. Jess had learned about "hormone blockers" from talking online with other transgender teenagers. In parent sessions, her mother revealed how devastated and angry Jess became each month during her menses, with fits of crying, yelling, locking herself in her room, refusing to acknowledge the need for feminine hygiene products, and repeatedly soiling her underwear and bed-sheets. Her mother had tried to talk with Jess, but Jess only responded with anger. Jess and her parents were in intense conflict around this issue, but discussions over the course of several family meetings led to improvement. Psycho-education about transgender transitioning was helpful, especially the recommendation that the individual live for at least a year as the opposite gender before undergoing any medical or surgical treatment (World Professional Association for Transgender Health Standards of Care for Gender Identity Disorder [2011]). Jess agreed to disagree with her parents about hormone therapy. Jess also wanted a chest binder to give her torso a male appearance but had no idea how to broach the subject with her parents. The therapist helped Jess plan how to bring up the topic. When Jess explained to them what she wanted, their first concern was that it would exacerbate Jess's asthma. After a series of family sessions, her parents agreed to buy the binder in time for Jess to try it out at home during winter break. These family discussions illustrate the evolving oscillation between the adolescent's growing control over her body and the need for parents to remain involved in important decisions about physical health.

School and social system: Jess's school refusal catalyzed her initial presentation to the clinic, and she soon opened up about the hostile climate at her school. She reported having things thrown at her during class and being subjected to slurs on a daily basis. She felt that most teachers ignored this behavior (Rivers 2011). As a result, Jess was dreading high school, especially gym class. She talked about her anger and shame every time she had to walk beneath the "Girls" sign that hung above the locker room door, "because it doesn't apply to me." The therapist offered to consult with school personnel to address the bullying and the possibility of gender-neutral accommodations, for example, with regard to the school uniform. Jess declined the offer for her therapist to speak with the school about the bullying, and the therapist respected Jess's need for autonomy. Jess later revealed more mixed feelings about her school, indicating that she did have positive relationships with a few teachers and her guidance counselor. Again, neutrality was central; the therapist did not push to speak with the school even though the reports of bullying were extremely concerning. Supporting Jess's autonomy allowed her to find her own ways to deal with the problem.

Romantic life: As her exploratory work in therapy continued, more typically adolescent themes came up, including the topic of dating. Jess had explained that she was sexually attracted to girls, "but as a boy, in a heterosexual way." Jess revealed that she had a crush on a girl, Ali, who knew Jess was transitioning, thought of her as a boy, and most importantly, liked her back. Jess began "officially" dating Ali when she returned from winter break. Individual psychotherapy became an important place for Jess to discuss their relationship, and it provided an opportunity to explore Jess's sexuality in more depth. Jess said she felt as if she liked Ali "like how a guy likes a girl, in a heterosexual way, not like a lesbian or anything gay like that." The hint of homophobia in Jess's comment signaled that Jess's transgender identity might be a coping mechanism for conflicts about homoerotic feelings. This possible function of Jess's GID is something that she and her therapist would explore as they went forward in their work together, always with a neutral and nonjudgmental stance.

Conclusion

Jess's case illustrates the importance of considering both development and systems when treating phase of life problems in LGBT people. The decisions about Jess's gender made during the course of her treatment were specific to her and came out of a careful exploration of her conflicts and a solid working relationship with both Jess and her family. Very different decisions about gender could reasonably be made in a different case. Our emphasis here has been on framing Jess's gender dysphoria as a phase of life problem, that is, a developmental problem, which helped her return to the path of normal development. As well, Jess's case illustrates the crucial developmental tasks that face LGBT people in adolescence, especially the integration of one's adult body and adult sexuality into a stable adult identity. Whether an LGBT person presents as an adolescent or later in life, it is crucial to explore the experience of adolescence in treatment.

Key Points

- Considering developmental context can be immensely beneficial for treatment. LGBT patients have the same developmental tasks as all patients, but the unique LGBT experience of these tasks must be recognized.

- Like all adolescents, LGBT adolescents are faced with the immense challenge of consolidating a genuine, stable, and individual identity while maintaining a healthy connection to their parents and other important figures. LGBT adolescents must deal with the additional challenge of integrating a differing gender or sexual orientation into their developing identity.

- Because identity is so central to LGBT development, an LGBT patient's experience of adolescence should be explicitly explored in treatment, even when that individual presents later in life.

References

American Psychiatric Association: Diagnostic and Statistical Manual of Mental Disorders, 4th Edition, Text Revision. Washington, DC, American Psychiatric Association, 2000

Erikson EH: Childhood and Society. New York, WW Norton, 1950

Novick K, Novick J: Working With Parents Makes Therapy Work. New York, Jason Aronson, 2005

Rivers I: Homophobic Bullying: Research and Theoretical Perspectives. New York, Oxford University Press, 2011

Sadock BJ, Sadock VA, Ruiz P (eds): Kaplan and Sadock's Comprehensive Textbook of Psychiatry, 9th Edition. Baltimore, MD, Lippincott Williams &Wilkins, 2009

Toomey RB, Ryan C, Diaz RM, et al: Gender-nonconforming lesbian, gay, bisexual, and transgender youth: school victimization and young adult psychosocial adjustment. Dev Psychol 46:1580–1589, 2010

World Professional Association for Transgender Health: Standards of Care for Gender Identity Disorders, 7th Edition, 2011. Available at: http://www.wpath.org/documents/Standards%20of%20Care%20V7%20-%202011%20WPATH.pdfocv6.pdf. Accessed March 1, 2012.

Questions

25.1 When an LGBT adolescent presents for treatment, the decision to involve parents should adhere to the following principle:

   A. Issues of confidentiality are paramount with an LGBT adolescent, especially when there is conflict with the parents; strict boundaries should be set that limit the parents' access to the therapist.

   B. LGBT adolescents are at high risk for dangerous behaviors, and therefore parents should be apprised of every issue the patient brings up; otherwise, parents will not trust the therapist.

   C. A therapeutic alliance should be established with the parents, just as it must be established and consistently evaluated and maintained with the patient. The therapeutic alliance will determine the extent to which the therapist should meet with the family.

The correct answer is C.

The therapeutic alliance with a young person's parents or guardians is essential to maintaining an effective treatment. Each case differs in terms of how much contact the therapist should have with parents, and this will also change over the course of an individual treatment. For example, usually contact with parents will be more frequent in the beginning of treatment. The therapist must rely on his or her judgment and knowledge of the importance of the patient's developing autonomy on the one hand and continued reliance on the parents on the other.

25.2 According to Erikson's model of self-development, adolescence is the period of life when the individual is faced with accomplishing the following task:

A. Consolidating a stable adult identity.
B. Finding a sense of purpose in life and work.
C. Developing the capacity for intimate relationships.
D. Strengthening the ability to function autonomously from parents.
E. All of the above.

The correct answer is A.

Although each of the tasks listed is central to healthy psychological development, it is in adolescence that consolidating a stable identity takes priority. According to Erikson, the development of intimacy takes precedence in early adulthood, after which, in middle adulthood, finding a sense of purpose in one's life is central. Autonomous functioning is important throughout the life span but is achieved first during toddlerhood, when the child develops the capacity for physical independence.

Glossary

bisexual   Erotically attracted to both males and females; a sexual identity.

cisgender   A term used in the transgender community to describe nontransgender individuals. Sometimes called *cissexual*.

the closet   A state in which a lesbian, gay, bisexual, or transgender (LGBT) person conceals his or her sexual or gender identity from self and/or others ("in the closet" or "closeted").

coming out   A process in which an LGBT person accepts his or her sexual or gender identity ("coming out to oneself") and/or discloses that identity to others ("coming out to others").

gay   Colloquial and affirmative term for *homosexual*. May refer to men or women, although some women may identify more with the term *lesbian*.

gay-friendly   Fostering an environment accepting of and open to LGBT people. Can refer to institutions or individuals.

gaydar   A colloquialism referring to the presumption of a capacity to sense someone else's sexual identity by relying on outward appearance, behaviors, and other cues such as omitted mentions of dating or home life.

gender   A cultural concept including the combination of social, psychological, and emotional traits associated with masculinity or femininity.

gender expression   Refers to how people demonstrate their gender to the outside world via manner of dress, behaviors, and appearance.

gender identity   A person's self-identification as male or female or other gender (e.g., genderqueer). Compare with *gender role*.

gender minority   Another term for transgender, intersex, and genderqueer people.

genderqueer   A colloquial term that conveys a person's internal sense of being between two genders.

gender role   Refers to the behaviors and dress that distinguish a person as male or female. Compare with *gender identity.*

heterosexism   A belief system that naturalizes and idealizes heterosexuality and either dismisses or ignores an LGB subjectivity.

heterosexual   Erotically attracted to people of the other sex; for some, a sexual identity.

homo-ignorance   Lacking information and having misinformation about homosexuality and LGB people.

homonegativity   A negative attitude toward homosexuality or LGB people. As typically used, the term has fewer political connotations than *homophobia.*

homophobia, external   The irrational fear and hatred that heterosexual people may feel toward LGB people.

homophobia, internal (internalized, interiorized)   The self-loathing that LGB people may feel for themselves.

homosexual   Erotically attracted to people of the same sex. Historical usage of the noun *homosexual* as a psychopathological term in medicine and psychiatry makes contemporary usage of the noun offensive to some LGB people.

intersex   Historically known as *hermaphroditism,* in more recent usage refers to diverse presentations of ambiguous or atypical genitals; sometimes confused by laypeople with transsexualism.

lesbian   A woman erotically attracted to women; a sexual identity.

queer   Historically a derogatory term for LGBT people, but adopted in the 1990s as a sexual identity by younger gays and lesbians and as a descriptive term for scholarship by academics who favored radical politics or a fluid conception of sexual identity (*queer theory*).

sex   The biological and anatomical attributes of male and female. Compare with *gender.*

sexual identity (sexual orientation identity)   One's subjective experience of one's sexual orientation. Although sexual orientation is usually immutable, sexual identity develops over time and in a cultural context. For example, calling oneself "gay" or "lesbian" is a subjective affirmation of one's homosexual orientation.

sexual minority   Another term for lesbian, gay, and bisexual people; some people may consider transgender people as sexual minorities, but trans people themselves may identify more with the term *gender minority.*

sexual orientation   Whether someone is attracted to same-sex partners, other-sex partners, both, or neither.

straight   Colloquial term for *heterosexual.*

transgender   Refers to someone whose gender identity (or gender expression) and sex are discordant with each other relative to social norms. Note that gender identity and sexual orientation are independent variables insofar as one's gender identity does not automatically reveal one's sexual attractions.

trans man (female-to-male [FTM])   Someone born anatomically as a woman (natal female) but identifying as a man.

transphobia   A range of negative attitudes and feelings towards transsexual or transgender people.

transsexual   An older and less inclusive term than *transgender;* refers to someone who chooses to make a physical transition by using hormonal and/or surgical sex interventions.

trans woman (male-to-female [MTF])   Someone born anatomically as a man (natal male) but identifying as a woman.

Index

*Page numbers printed in **boldface** type refer to tables or figures. Page numbers followed by an n refer to note numbers.*